THE KIDNEY
Morphology, Biochemistry, Physiology

VOLUME III

CONTRIBUTORS

Sulamita Balagura-Baruch

Gerhard Giebisch

D. Z. Levine

Donald J. Marsh

Floyd C. Rector, Jr.

K. Thurau

Mackenzie Walser

THE KIDNEY
Morphology, Biochemistry, Physiology

Edited by CHARLES ROUILLER

INSTITUT D'HISTOLOGIE
ET D'EMBRYOLOGIE
ECOLE DE MÉDECINE
GENEVA, SWITZERLAND

AND

ALEX F. MULLER

CLINIQUE MÉDICALE
HÔPITAL CANTONAL
GENEVA, SWITZERLAND

VOLUME III

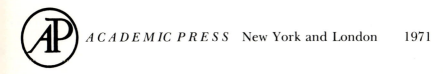

ACADEMIC PRESS   New York and London   1971

ACADEMIC PRESS, INC.
111 Fifth Avenue, New York, New York 10003

United Kingdom Edition published by
ACADEMIC PRESS, INC. (LONDON) LTD.
Berkeley Square House, London W1X 6BA

LIBRARY OF CONGRESS CATALOG CARD NUMBER: 68-28895

PRINTED IN THE UNITED STATES OF AMERICA

LIST OF CONTRIBUTORS

Numbers in parentheses indicate the pages on which the authors' contributions begin.

SULAMITA BALAGURA-BARUCH (253), Department of Physiology, Cornell University Medical College, New York, New York

GERHARD GIEBISCH (329), Yale University School of Medicine, New Haven, Connecticut

D. Z. LEVINE (1), Department of Physiology, University of Munich, Munich, Germany

DONALD J. MARSH (71), Department of Biomedical Engineering, Graduate School of Southern California, Los Angeles, California

FLOYD C. RECTOR, JR. (209), Department of Internal Medicine, University of Texas Southern Medical School, Dallas, Texas

K. THURAU (1), Department of Physiology, University of Munich, Munich, Germany

MACKENZIE WALSER (127), Department of Pharmacology and Experimental Therapeutics, Johns Hopkins University School of Medicine, Baltimore, Maryland

CONTENTS

PREFACE

This treatise, which is written for morphologists, biochemists, physiologists, pathologists, pharmacologists, and clinicians, is an attempt to present in comprehensive form present knowledge of the kidney under normal and pathological conditions, as revealed by morphological, biochemical, and physiological studies. Emphasis is placed on recent developments in the study of renal structure and function, particularly on the subcellular and molecular level. Thus, this work tries to fill the gap between the many valuable textbooks that are unavoidably limited to human pathology and the numerous excellent reviews and monographs that are concerned with special aspects of the kidney.

The first volume stresses the embryology, macroscopic, microscopic, and ultramicroscopic morphology, and histochemistry of the kidney. Volume II is devoted to explants of embryonic kidney, experimental renal diseases, tumors and intoxications, and the function of erythropoietin. Volumes III and IV discuss experimental renal transplantation, structure and function of the juxtaglomerular apparatus, and the macula densa, the gaseous and substrate metabolism of the kidney, the role of this organ in the osmotic concentration and dilution of the urine, hydrogen secretion, potassium and sodium excretion, the correlation of the kidney with vitamins and parathyroid gland, and many other aspects.

The authors of the individual chapters emphasize the results obtained by animal experimentation supported by evidence based on modern techniques. The correlation of structure with function is stressed in all instances; the participation of the kidney in metabolic systems and its relation to other organs are pointed out and discussed.

The extensive documentation by carefully compiled references should make the treatise useful for the worker active in the field. The bibliographies comprise three categories: basic publications, recent papers, and reviews containing numerous references. It is hoped that the reader interested in additional information will readily be guided to the original communications.

We are deeply grateful to the contributors who, in spite of the numerous duties and tasks with which they are burdened, nevertheless agreed to participate in the collaboration of this work. Our thanks are also due to Dr. Robert J. Schnitzer and the staff of Academic Press for their painstaking care in the production of the volumes.

CHARLES ROUILLER
ALEX F. MULLER

CONTENTS OF OTHER VOLUMES

xiii

1 THE RENAL CIRCULATION

K. Thurau and D. Z. Levine

1

I. Introduction

As knowledge of renal function becomes more complete, it is increasingly difficult to describe experimental data in the context of more conventional categories. This is particularly true when we attempt to understand the basic pattern of renal hemodynamics, the subject of this chapter. The material to be presented can best be appreciated when considered in its relation to other renal functions. Such an approach is desirable in view of recent observations that different kidney regions have distinctive blood flow and functional characteristics. For example, primary alterations of medullary blood flow may decisively influence the concentrating mechanism. Conversely, ADH may, in addition to altering collecting duct water permeability, simultaneously influence medullary blood flow and the filtration rate of juxtamedullary nephrons. This type of phenomenon is well appreciated only if a broad approach is taken. With this in mind, this chapter is intended to be selective, illustrating the interdependence of renal functions as far as possible. For example, newer micropuncture data are included which illuminate the tubular events concomitant with changes in renal artery perfusion pressure.

However, notwithstanding this stated objective, recent observations relevant to more classic situations such as hemorrhage and exercise, have been included. Indeed, we have not hesitated to reintroduce the most obscure cousin in the renal family—the lymph.

II. Total Renal Blood Flow

blood entering the kidney via the renal artery is distributed to areas which differ widely in their hemodynamic and functional characteristics. An awareness of this heterogeneity is important for the interpretation of changes in total renal blood flow.

The blood flow of the renal cortex, which comprises 75% of total kidney mass, is 400–500 ml/min per 100 gm tissue. The corresponding medullary values are approximately 120 for the outer medulla and 25 ml/min per 100 gm for the inner medulla (for details see Medullary Blood Flow, Section XIV). The predominance of cortical tissue mass and its high blood flow rate per gram are reflected in the fact that 93% of total renal blood flow perfuses the cortex alone. Therefore, total renal blood flow, as measured by different methods, is almost exclusively renal cortical blood flow. These considerations show that changes in blood flow which occur only in the renal medulla minimally influence total renal blood flow, and such changes are not discernible in measurements of whole kidney blood flow.

The analysis of phasic blood flow changes in the renal artery, as measured by electromagnetic flow meter techniques, indicates that this high tissue blood flow rate is caused not only by a high degree of vascularization but also by low resistance to flow of the arterial offshoots. This follows from the observation that under normal conditions blood flow in the renal artery is maintained throughout diastole (Gregg, 1962; Thurau, 1964a) and is on the order of 40% of the systolic flow maximum (Fig. 1). Backflow during the early phase of diastole or diastolic fluctuations in blood flow, which is a usual finding in the arteries supplying skeletal muscle, can be observed in the renal artery only when the peripheral pulse wave reflection is considerably increased by vasoconstriction. This has been shown by Okino and Spencer (1961) during the infusion of epinephrine. Increases in renal vascular resistance which occur under physiological conditions are not sufficient to create backflow during early diastole.

The kidney, because of its low vascular resistance, receives under resting conditions 1.2 liters/minute of blood, approximately 25% of the cardiac output. This important part of total blood flow is often considered with respect to the regulation of the systemic circulation. In this sense the renal vascular system has been characterized as a type of arteriovenous shunt which may participate in circulatory regulation by changes in its resistance to flow. A simple quantitative calculation raises some doubts about such a function: During exercise cardiac output

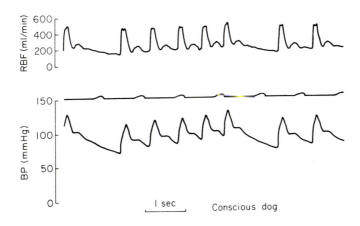

Fig. 1. Phasic characteristics of renal artery blood flow (electromagnetic flow meter) and aortic blood pressure in a conscious dog during normal respiratory arrythmia.

may increase from 5 to 15 liters/minute. If arterial blood pressure remains more or less constant, and since RBF does not increase above its normal value during exercise, a complete interruption of renal blood flow may contribute 1.2 liters/minute to the increase in cardiac output of 10 liters/minute. It is apparent that such a diversion of blood flow away from the kidney would be of little effect, especially when the increase in cardiac output is maximal.

Data about changes in renal fraction of cardiac output during hemorrhagic hypotension are contradictory (see Selkurt, 1963). This may be due to the fact that the data were obtained from anesthetized animals undergoing major, nonsterile surgery. In addition, inadequate attention has been devoted to the extracellular fluid and electrolyte status before the hemorrhagic period and the subsequent velocity of bleeding and reinfusion. Furthermore, in most instances, renal blood flow was calculated by PAH clearance without considering changes in PAH extraction. The pitfalls inherent to PAH clearance determinations during hemorrhagic hypotension have been discussed by Selkurt (1962), Bálint and Fekete (1960), and Bálint et al. (1964).

Experiments on unanesthetized dogs, in which renal blood flow was continuously recorded by means of implanted electromagnetic flow meters, show an increase in renal resistance during hemorrhagic hypotension associated with blood pressures below 70–80 mm Hg (Gregg, 1962). The increase in renal resistance concomitant with this low blood pressure is more pronounced than that of systemic circulation. This results in a decrease in the renal fraction of cardiac output.

III. Hydrostatic Pressures and Distribution of Resistance to Flow in the Renal Cortical Vascular System

Under normal nondiuretic conditions the blood pressure in the renal artery is reduced to 15–20 mm Hg by the time the blood reaches the peritubular capillaries (see Table I). This pressure range has been found in the rat and cat using the micropuncture technique of Landis (1926) as modified for the kidney by Wirz (1952). No pressure difference between peritubular capillaries and proximal convolution could be demonstrated. In the dog kidney, data on peritubular capillary pressures are not yet available. Liebau et al. (1968) found the intratubular pressure in the proximal convolution of the dog kidney to be 18.3 mm Hg. Assuming that, similar to the rat, no pressure difference exists between peritubular capillaries and proximal convolutions, these data indicate that in the dog kidney the pressure in the peritubular capillaries is only slightly higher than that in the rat.

TABLE I

COLLECTED DATA ON PRESSURES (MM HG) IN PERITUBULAR CAPILLARIES AND
PROXIMAL CONVOLUTIONS OF THE RENAL CORTEX

Authors	Arterial	Peritubular capillary	Proximal tubule	Animal
Wirz (1952)	–	17.4	14.8	Rat
Wirz (1955)	–	–	15–21	Rat
Gottschalk and Mylle (1956)	118–128	14.0	13.5–14.6[a]	Rat
Gottschalk and Mylle (1957)	–	–	12.5[a]	Rat
Thurau and Wober (1962)	80–198	–	14.3[a]	Rat
	80–140	16.6[a]	–	Rat
	108	–	17.8	Cat
Liebau et al. (1968)	95–165	–	18.3[a]	Dog
	165–215	–	19.8[a]	Dog
Koch et al. (1968)	105–130	–	12.3	Rat
	140–184	–	21.4	Rat
Schnermann et al. (1969)	–	–	15.3	Rat
Gertz et al. (1969)	–	–	12.6–16.7	Rat

[a]Independent of changes in arterial blood pressure.

Direct measurements of glomerular capillary pressure have not been performed. Such data are essential in order to determine the components of the pressure fall from the renal artery to the peritubular capillaries. This calculation allows the derivation of the segmental resistance to flow in the afferent or efferent arteriole.

Earlier calculations of glomerular capillary pressure by Winton (1953) and Pappenheimer (1955) indicated 70 mm Hg. Gertz et al. (1966) developed a micropuncture method to evaluate glomerular capillary pressure. They blocked distal flow from the first loop of a single superficial proximal tubule of rats through the microinjection of castor oil, and then observed the increase of intratubular pressure proximal to the oil. After 30 to 40 seconds, this pressure reached a plateau at a mean of 63 mm Hg. Since no visible flow could be observed in the occluded tubular segment, it was assumed that filtration ceased when the intratubular pressure reached this value. The plateau was constant with arterial pressures between 100 and 160 mm Hg. Assuming a plasma oncotic pressure of 25 mm Hg, the calculated glomerular capillary pressure would be 88 ± 4 mm Hg. The glomerular capillary pressure calculated in this way was found to be unchanged during mannitol diuresis or hydrochlorothiazide diuresis but to be increased after the administration of furosemide (Koch et al., 1967; Krause et al., 1967).

Distal to the peritubular capillaries a fall in pressure of approximately 7 mm Hg was localized in the venous segment at the intra-extrarenal border (Swann, 1952; Gottschalk and Mylle, 1956; Brun et al., 1956).

From these data it follows that in the nondiuretic state, one-third of the total resistance to flow between renal artery and peritubular capillaries derives from the afferent arteriole and the remaining two-thirds from the efferent arteriole (see Fig. 2). This pattern of resistance distribution may change considerably during certain conditions, such as osmotic diuresis, increase in pelvic pressure, or pharmacological vasodilation during which the peritubular capillary pressure may increase up to 80 mm Hg. The intrarenal venous pressure under those conditions may increase to the same extent (Brun *et al.*, 1956; Thurau and Henne, 1964). This demonstrates a compression of the renal veins at the intra–extrarenal border by the increase in intrarenal tissue pressure.

IV. Autoregulation of Renal Circulation

Central to many hemodynamic considerations of the renal circulation is the phenomenon that renal blood flow remains almost constant when arterial blood pressure is increased above 90 mm Hg (Fig. 3). This was first observed by Burton-Opitz and Lucas (1911) and later confirmed by Rein (1931) and associates and Corcoran and Page (1939). The increase in renal resistance, which correlates well with the increase in arterial blood pressure, has been observed in innervated, denervated, and isolated perfused kidneys. Accordingly, it is generally accepted that this increase in renal vascular resistance is the result of intrarenal mechanisms, which are referred to as autoregulation of renal circulation (Forster and Maes, 1947; Selkurt *et al.*, 1949; Shipley and Study, 1951; Miles *et al.*, 1954; Ochwadt, 1956; Grupp *et al.*, 1959; Thurau *et al.*, 1959b; Waugh and Shanks, 1960; Belleau and Earley, 1967).

In 1947, Forster and Maes showed that not only blood flow, but also glomerular filtration rate, is kept constant, a result which has been verified by many investigators (Selkurt *et al.*, 1949; Selkurt, 1951; Shipley and Study, 1951; Thompson *et al.*, 1957; Thurau and Kramer, 1959). The constancy of glomerular filtration rate points to a preglomerular location of autoregulatory resistance changes. This localization is further supported by the results of measurements of postglomerular pressures, which were found to be practically constant when arterial blood pressure was varied in the autoregulatory range (Thurau and Wober, 1962; Miles and de Wardener, 1954; Thurau and Henne, 1964; Gottschalk, 1952; Haddy and Scott, 1965; Gertz *et al.*, 1966; Liebau *et al.*, 1968). Furthermore, total kidney volume as well as renal interstitial and blood volume were also found to remain essentially unchanged when

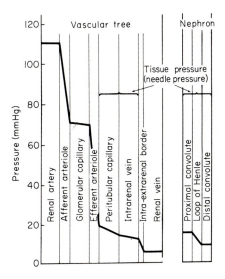

FIG. 2. Hydrostatic pressure gradients in the renal vascular and tubular system during antidiuresis.

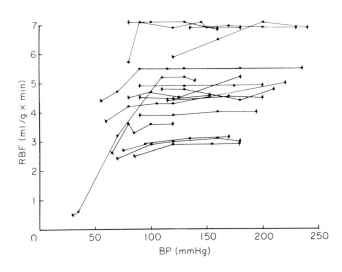

FIG. 3. Correlation between renal blood flow and renal arterial blood pressure in the nondiuretic dog. From Thurau and Henne (1964).

blood pressure was increased above 100 mm Hg (Folkow and Langston, 1964; Swann, 1964; Gärtner, 1966). Hence, the existence of a constant glomerular filtration pressure as derived from the autoregulation of GFR, can be maintained only if glomerular capillaries are buffered from variable arterial pressures by compensatory alterations of preglomerular resistance.

The first results to indicate the contribution of vascular musculature to renal autoregulation were reported by Lochner and Ochwadt (1954), who found that autoregulation can be abolished by high doses of procaine (10^{-3} gm/ml) and potassium cyanide.

Some confusion exists about the term "abolished autoregulation," because often pressure flow curves which are convex to the pressure axis (see Fig. 4) were taken *a priori* to indicate abolished autoregulation. This term, however, should be restricted only to those instances in which the increase in renal resistance, which normally occurs at a blood pressure above 90 mm Hg, is abolished. This abolition, as can be induced by papaverine, leads to a further increase in blood flow above the autoregulatory value when blood pressure is increased. This is very different from those situations during which the high renal resistance is manifest at low BP levels, as may occur during the infusion of epinephrine. Under these circumstances the pressure flow curves are at a lower level and a further increase in renal resistance does not occur when blood pressure is elevated.

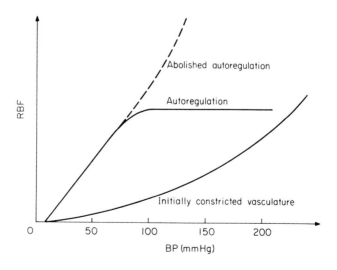

Fig. 4. Pressure flow relationship in the renal artery under normal conditions (autoregulation), in the presence of abolished autoregulation (e.g., papaverine), and associated with initially constricted vasculature (e.g., adrenaline or hemorrhage).

Following Lochner's and Ochwadt's observations, several laboratories reported data demonstrating that the preglomerular autoregulatory reactivity of the arterioles depends on the functional integrity of vascular smooth muscles, since autoregulation is abolished by smooth muscle paralyzing agents, such as papaverine (Thurau and Kramer, 1959; Gilmore, 1964a,b; Waugh, 1964; Takeuchi et al., 1965; Basar et al., 1968), procaine and chloral hydrate (Waugh and Shanks, 1960), and acetylcholine (Nahmod and Lanari, 1964).

Of the theories which were proposed in order to explain the autoregulatory mechanisms, two incorporate the myogenic response of the vasculature into the regulatory mechanisms. They differ, however, in regard to the stimulus for the vascular smooth muscle. The theories are the transmural pressure theory and the juxtaglomerular apparatus theory.

A. Transmural Pressure Theory

In this theory, the stimulus for the contraction of preglomerular smooth muscle is thought to be the increase in tangential tension of the vascular wall (T_{wall}) (Semple and de Wardener, 1959; Gilmore, 1964a,b; Nash and Selkurt, 1964; Waugh, 1964; Thurau, 1964c; Basar et al., 1968), which can be represented according to the LaPlace equation:

$$T_{wall} = r \, (P_{in} - P_{out}) \tag{1}$$

where r is the inner vascular radius; P_{in}, the intravascular hydrostatic pressure; and P_{out}, the extravascular hydrostatic pressure.

There are certain limitations in the applicability of this equation to the vascular musculature:

(1) From hemodynamic data, r of the individual arteriole cannot be derived. A radius can be calculated only for an analog vessel which simulates, as a single vessel, the same resistance to flow, which in the kidney is developed by the many vessels in parallel:

$$r_{\text{analog vessel}} = \sqrt[4]{\frac{I \, \eta \, l \, 8}{p \cdot \pi}} \tag{2}$$

where I is the blood flow rate; η, the viscosity; l, the length of arterioles; p, arterial-venous pressure difference.

(2) The vascular length l varies from arteriole to arteriole, although it is inserted in Eq. (2) as a constant.

(3) If the intravascular pressure falls linearly from the beginning to

the end of the arteriole and if the extravascular pressure is the same along the entire length of the arteriole, the transmural pressure difference would decrease from the beginning to the end of the arteriole.

At the end of the arteriole the transmural pressure difference would be practically zero. Hence, the use of the arterial blood pressure as P_{in} in Eq. (1) may approximate wall tension in the beginning of the arteriole but not along its length. Furthermore, it is not known whether the intravascular pressure declines linearly along the length of the arteriole or in an exponential fashion. Therefore, even a mean transmural wall tension for the entire arteriole cannot be calculated.

It is evident that these arguments preclude a quantitative calculation of the tangential wall tension of the preglomerular resistance vessels by means of the LaPlace equation. However, a qualitative use of this equation might be useful for the description of directional changes in tangential wall tension which accompany an increase in arterial blood pressure. The rationale behind this transmural pressure theory is that the higher the intravascular pressure, the higher the tangential wall tension and, thereby, the greater the stretch stimulus for the smooth muscle fibers.

This theory is supported by experiments in which vasodilation occurred when the tangential wall tension was reduced by increasing the extravascular pressure and by keeping the arterial pressure constant. The extravascular pressure (tissue pressure) was elevated by osmotic diuresis, increased venous pressure, and ureteral occlusion. Under those conditions, renal blood flow increases (Enger et al., 1937; Blake et al., 1949; Shave, 1952; Schirmeister et al., 1962; Kiil and Aukland, 1961; Selkurt et al., 1963; Gilmore, 1964a; Waugh, 1964; Thurau and Henne, 1964; Haddy and Scott, 1965).

The decrease in precapillary resistance, however, cannot be quantitatively calculated from the increase in blood flow since the elevated tissue pressure initiated a compression of venous vessels at the intra-extrarenal border (Brun et al., 1956; Waugh, 1964; Thurau and Henne, 1964). Thus, the actual precapillary dilation is more pronounced than calculated from the increase in blood flow. For example, even an unchanged renal blood flow at elevated ureteral and, hence, intrarenal tissue pressure implies precapillary dilation in order to compensate for the increase in intrarenal venous resistance. These considerations apply also to the quantitative evaluation of resistance changes occurring after the injection of dilating drugs which also lead to an increase in tissue pressure.

The above theory implies that the smooth muscles are capable of adjusting their lengths to changes in arterial pressure in order to keep renal blood flow and glomerular filtration rate constant. Certain limitations in this theory are apparent. No data are, in fact, available which suggest mechanisms by which changes in blood flow can be recognized at the local arteriolar level and then be translated into appropriate changes in vascular wall tension for the servoregulation of blood flow. Indeed, theoretical considerations suggest that it is most unlikely that wall tension per se is the stimulus. For example, let us assume arterial blood pressure is doubled and the autoregulatory reduction in vascular radius keeps blood flow constant. A simple calculation reveals that wall tension in the new steady state would almost double (Thurau, 1967a). If wall tension were an adequate stimulus, the smooth muscles should respond with further contraction till the initial wall tension is again attained. According to the equations of Poiseuille and LaPlace [see Eqs. (1) and (2)], the wall tension would regain its original value only if the radius is reduced to 50%, resulting in a 16-fold increase in vascular resistance. In other words, renal blood flow would decrease to 1/16th its original value when blood pressure is doubled. It is obvious, then, that a constancy of tangential wall tension does not seem to be the primary goal of renal autoregulation or that this parameter is an adequate stimulus for the autoregulatory mechanism. From an analysis of the effect of sinusoidal pressure changes upon phasic flow pattern in the isolated artificially perfused rat kidney, Basar et al. (1968) concluded that two different myogenic mechanisms may underlie autoregulatory resistance changes: (a) a fast component in vascular reaction which is stimulated by $\Delta P/t$ and (b) a long-lasting mechanism in which angiotensin might play the role of a transmitter substance.

In this context it is worth noting that complete autoregulation has been demonstrated in kidneys perfused without pulsatile changes in pressure (Goodyer and Glenn, 1951; Ritter, 1952). Accordingly, pulsatile alteration in renal artery pressure is not a necessary condition for autoregulation.

Another observation remains that is not readily explained by the transmural pressure theory. Below a blood pressure of 70 mm Hg, where glomerular filtration ceases, the smooth muscle in the renal vasculature is maximally relaxed and does not respond to changes in blood pressure that are nevertheless sufficient to alter total wall tension (Ochwadt, 1956; Thurau et al., 1959b). It is striking that this lower limit of the autoregulatory range coincides with the blood pressure just necessary to maintain the formation of a glomerular filtrate and the flow of tubular fluid. Rather than dismiss this as a simple coincidence, theories have been suggested by Thurau (1963, 1967a) and Guyton et al. (1964) which incorporate the tubular function as an essential part in the autoregulatory phenomenon and which are outlined in the following section.

B. Juxtaglomerular Feedback Theory

Recently, there has been reason to believe that renal autoregulation may not be a primary vasomotor phenomenon, but rather a consequence of an intrarenal regulating mechanism by which glomerular filtration rate, and hence the tubular sodium load, is kept constant. In terms of energy cost, the major work of the kidney is to actively reabsorb the sodium which is delivered to the tubules via GFR (Section VI). Autoregulation has an important role in the control of this work because, as first shown in 1947 by Forster and Maes, constancy of the glomerular filtration rate is a concomitant of blood flow regulation. Since plasma sodium concentration is usually invariant, it may be justified to speak of autoregulation of tubular sodium load. This theory incorporates the anatomical arrangement and the function of the juxtaglomerular apparatus.

Figure 5 shows a schematic diagram of a single nephron. Tubular cells at the end of the thick ascending limb of Henle's loop make contact with the vascular pole of the glomerulus belonging to the same nephron (Peter, 1909/1927; Michailowitsch, 1918). The point of contact is shown in detail on the left of Fig. 5 and in Fig. 6. In 1933 Zimmermann first referred to a group of tubular cells which are in contact with the vascular pole as macula densa cells. These cells, which are morphologically distinct from the adjacent tubular epithelium, are attached at their basal side to the renin-secreting granular cells in the wall of the afferent arteriole. Together with interposed lacis cells, the macula densa cells and granular cells compose the juxtaglomerular apparatus (Ruyter, 1925; Goormaghtigh, 1937, 1945; Dunihue, 1941; Bohle, 1954; Bucher and Reale, 1961, 1962; Hartroft, 1963; Barajas and Latta, 1963; Faarup, 1965; Riedel and Bucher, 1967; Hatt, 1966).

Goormaghtigh (1945) originated the concept of an endocrine function of the juxtaglomerular apparatus and there is much evidence now that the granular cells in the wall of the afferent arteriole are indeed the site of renin formation (Edelman and Hartroft, 1961; Cook, 1968; Thurau et al., 1969). Goormaghtigh also suggested the macula densa cells to be a sensing device by which changes in volume or concentration of the tubular fluid could influence the function of the granular cells, thereby regulating the blood flow rate through the glomerulus. When Schloss (1945–1946) reviewed the juxtaglomerular apparatus he wrote: "Of course the ingenious hypothesis of Goormaghtigh, concerning the function of the granular cells, is difficult to prove. However, it would be tempting to assume an autonomy of the individual nephron . . ." (translation). The juxtaglomerular feedback theory of

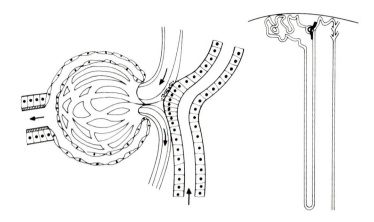

FIG. 5. Schematic representation of the anatomical relationship of the juxtaglomerular apparatus within the single nephron unit. On the left is shown in enlarged form the point of contact between the ascending limb of the loop of Henle and the vascular pole of the glomerulus of the same nephron.

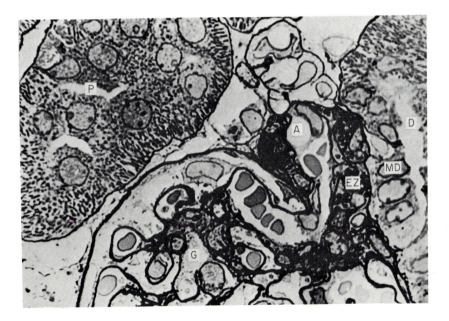

FIG. 6. Juxtaglomerular apparatus. Macula densa cells (MD) located between the distal tubular lumen (D) and the epithelial cells (EZ) of the afferent arteriolar wall in the mouse kidney. The afferent arteriole (A) in the section is cut at the point of entrance into the glomerulus (G). A proximal tubule (P) is in the upper left. Movat silver stain, microphotograph, enlarged × 1400, tissue thickness ½ μ. Courtesy of A. Bohle.

autoregulation incorporates the function of the juxtaglomerular apparatus as an essential component of the autoregulatory mechanism.

A central requirement of this theory is the ability of the juxtaglomerular apparatus to form vasoactive angiotensin II locally in the wall of the glomerular arterioles. Therefore, renin substrate, renin, and converting enzyme activity must all be present in the area of the JGA if a formation of angiotensin II at this site takes place. There is experimental evidence that all three factors are available at the juxtaglomerular site.

Lever and Peart (1962) showed the presence of renin substrate in the renal lymph, indicating that the substrate for angiotensin formation is not only distributed in plasma but also in the interstitial space of the kidney. Therefore, it is assumed that substrate is also available in the interstitial space of the juxtaglomerular apparatus.

It is now generally agreed that renin is formed in the granular cells of the juxtaglomerular apparatus, which are located in the wall of the afferent arteriole (Hartroft, 1963; Cook, 1968). An important question is the route by which renin is discharged from the granules. Renin first enters the cytoplasm of the granular cells, and from the cytoplasm it enters the extracellular or interstitial space. Since renin is 50 times more concentrated in renal lymph than in renal venous blood (Lever and Peart, 1962), it seems unlikely that renin is released directly into the lumen of the afferent arteriole. If, as seems more likely, renin is discharged into the interstitial space of the JGA, it follows that renin activity in the region of the JGA is considerably higher than might be estimated from measurements of its activity in renal venous blood or even in renal lymph.

The availability of both renin and its substrate means that angiotensin II's precursor, i.e., the decapeptide angiotensin I, can be formed locally.

Converting enzyme activity in single juxtaglomerular apparatuses has been demonstrated recently by Thurau et al. (1969). When single dissected juxtaglomerular apparatuses of rat kidneys were incubated with highly purified rat renin substrate, the pressor material formed in the incubate was identified to be angiotensin II. These authors, therefore, concluded that the converting enzyme activity in the juxtaglomerular apparatus was sufficient to convert all angiotensin I, which was formed by the renin in the juxtaglomerular apparatus, into angiotensin II. The demonstration of converting enzyme activity in the juxtaglomerular apparatus seems to contradict results obtained by Ng and Vane (1967), who showed that angiotensin I, when injected into renal arterial blood, was not converted into angiotensin II during its passage through the kidney. If, however, converting activity is located primarily in the juxta-glomerular apparatus, conversion of infused angiotensin I to angiotensin II may not be expected to occur in detectable amounts, insofar as endogenous angiotensin I is more completely exposed to the interstitially located converting enzyme. In contrast, infused (exogenous) angiotensin I in all likelihood bypasses the site of maximal converting enzyme concentration.

Following the above arguments, the prerequisites seem to exist for the intrarenal formation of vasoactive angiotensin II which may affect the preglomerular resistance.

Such a mechanism, as the cause for renal autoregulation, was proposed by Thurau (1963, 1967a), Thurau et al. (1967), and Guyton et al. (1964). Several attempts were made to characterize the nature of the stimulus for the intrarenal formation of angiotensin.

The luminal membranes of the macula densa cells are in contact with the tubular fluid leaving the ascending limb of Henle's loop. The composition of the tubular fluid in this segment is noteworthy in that its sodium concentration and osmolality are less than in peripheral plasma, because the ascending limb of the loop reabsorbs sodium actively and has restricted permeabilities to salt and water. Regardless of the diuretic state, the sodium concentration is approximately only 25–50 mEq/liter (Malnic et al., 1966; Schnermann et al., 1966; Cortney et al., 1966).

Using micropuncture techniques, Thurau and Schnermann (1965) varied sodium concentration and osmolality in single macula densa segments of the rat kidney. They observed that an increase of sodium concentration toward isotonic levels produced a decrease in proximal tubular diameter in the same nephron, indicating a reduction in single nephron filtration rate and hence tubular sodium load, and that this effect was less prevalent in renin-depleted kidneys. Because the response of the glomerular filtration rate to an increase in sodium concentration was restricted to the individual nephron unit receiving the injection, it was suggested that this reaction is mediated by the local control of angiotensin formation in the juxtaglomerular apparatus, thereby regulating the preglomerular resistance to blood flow.

Recently, Gottschalk and Leyssac (1968) have offered data to suggest that the effect on proximal tubular diameter may have been the result of a technical artifact. However, the observations of Thurau and Schnermann (1965) that proximal tubular collapse was regularly observed in high-renin but rarely in low-renin kidneys, and that the collapse was not observed during mannitol or choline chloride perfusions, may argue against this criticism.

The incorporation of a tubulovascular feedback mechanism for the autoregulation of glomerular filtrate would imply that some tubular fluid characteristics at the macula densa vary with filtration rate, thereby acting as a controller of glomerular filtration rate. Also, of course, the existence of a tubular flow rate would be a prerequisite for this type of regulation, as already discussed on p. 11.

Using an analog computer simulation of hypothetical feedback mechanisms, Guyton *et al.* (1964) concluded that the afferent arteriolar resistance might be controlled by the tubular fluid osmolality at the macula densa site. Several lines of evidence, however, suggest that the feedback mechanism is sensitive to sodium.

Tobian's (1967) critical review of the literature on this subject makes it appear likely that the juxtaglomerular apparatus plays an important role in the Na balance of the organism. Vander (1967) reported evidence against the concept that the granular cells in the afferent arterioles may be stretch receptors. The rise in the renal venous concentration of renin, which can be induced in dogs by infusing catecholamines or by stimulating the renal nerves, could be prevented by simultaneous osmotic diuresis, even though renal arterial pressure was kept constant. The increase in renal venous renin concentration, which normally accompanies a reduction in arterial pressure, can also be inhibited by mercurial diuretics. He therefore suggests that some change in the composition of tubular fluid, possibly at the macula densa site, may regulate renin secretion.

From their microinjection experiments, Thurau and Schnermann (1965) suggested that the intratubular sodium concentration in the macula densa segment could be the adequate stimulus for the reduction in filtration rate. Consistent with this concept were data of Cortney *et al.* (1966), who microperfused single loops of Henle and found a positive correlation between loop of Henle flow rate and sodium concentration at the end of the perfused loop. These data were later confirmed by Morgan and Berliner (1969) and Schnermann *et al.* (1970), although both groups reported that at the lowest perfusion rates such a positive correlation between loop flow rate and early distal sodium concentration could not be demonstrated. This might be due to the fact that the puncture site is several hundred microns away from the macula densa segment. The modifying influence of the reabsorptive epithelium between macula densa segment and distal puncture site upon intratubular fluid composition will be exaggerated at the lowest perfusion rates when the contact time between fluid and epithelium is longest.

Theoretically, such a functional characteristic of the loop which translates flow rate alterations into changes of sodium concentration, would result in autoregulation. It is apparent that this type of filtrate regulation reflects nothing else than the adjustment of tubular sodium load to tubular sodium reabsorptive activity. Autoregulation of blood flow would then only be a byproduct of this sodium load-adjusting mechanism. Consistent with the assumption of sodium at the macula densa as a controller for preglomerular resistance is the renal vasodilatory effect of mannitol. During mannitol diuresis, early distal sodium concentration declines below control values to 7 mEq/liter, because of the inclusion of a poorly reabsorbable substance into the tubular fluid.

It is clear that such observations can only furnish indirect evidence for this hypothesis. An inherent difficulty in the quantitative analysis of this sodium feedback mechanism is caused by the inaccessibility of the macula densa segment for direct micropuncture evaluation. The closest approach is the analysis of tubular fluid in the first distal segment seen at the renal surface. Hence, the changes observed in tubular fluid composition at this site may only approximate the conditions at the macula densa cells.

Any attempt to further characterize and quantify the functional pattern of the feedback mechanism implies simultaneous measurements of fluid composition at the macula densa segment and of the glomerular filtration rate of the same nephron. This type of analysis was recently carried out in micropuncture experiments by Schnermann et al. (1970). They perfused single loops of Henle with various test solutions, measured flow rate at the end of the loop simultaneously with filtration rate of the glomerulum belonging to this nephron unit, and analyzed the collected perfusion fluid. They found that when the loop perfusion rate was high, the corresponding filtration rate was low, and vice versa (Fig. 7). This inverse correlation, which clearly demonstrates the existence of a feedback mechanism, appeared not to be triggered by the tubular flow rate in the macula densa segment per se or by the intratubular pressure at this site, but rather by changes in the chemical composition of the intratubular fluid induced by changes in flow rate. From their data, Schnermann et al. (1970) concluded that the most probable stimulus for the reduction in filtration rate is the concentration of sodium ions, which are free to permeate the tubular cell membranes. This conclusion followed from the observation that an increase in intratubular sodium concentration at the macula densa, when associated with an increase in poorly permeable SO_4^{2-} anions, did not reduce single glomerular filtration rate. These results are the first indications that either the electrical potential difference of the luminal membrane of the macula densa, the transmembrane sodium flux, or some other cellular parameters are important factors in the feedback mechanism. In any event, the data indicate that the intratubular sodium at the

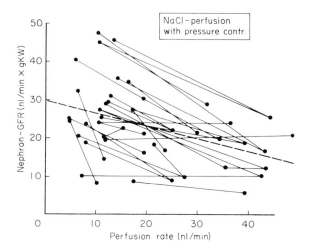

Fig. 7. Correlation between perfusion rate of loop of Henle and nephron filtration rate of the perfused nephron. The perfusion fluid is isotonic Ringer's solution; the lines connect data from identical nephrons. "Pressure control" refers to fluid collection in the early proximal convolution with continuously adjusting the applied negative pressure to a constant proximal hydrostatic pressure of 15 mm Hg. From Schnermann *et al.* (1970).

macula densa is a parameter which initiates changes in these cellular functions, rather than one which directly regulates the filtration rate.

V. The Influence of Renal Artery Perfusion Pressure on Renal Tubular Function

While the autoregulation of renal blood flow and whole kidney glomerular filtration rate is the major subject of this chapter, in view of new techniques of investigation it is appropriate to consider the extent to which other renal parameters are influenced by changes in arterial pressure. Recent studies involving acute and chronic changes in arterial perfusion pressure have, by means of micropuncture techniques, provided data on tubular function, such as fractional reabsorption of salt and water, flow velocity, and intratubular pressure. Liebau *et al.* (1968) have shown that acute changes of systemic blood pressure within the autoregulatory range were not associated with changes in fractional reabsorption, intratubular pressure, single nephron GFR, or flow velocity in superficial proximal tubules of the dog kidney. In these studies autoregulation of renal blood flow and whole kidney glomerular filtration rate were demonstrated during the time that the micropuncture maneuvers were carried out.

Previous data from studies on the rat kidney are inconsistent with respect to proximal tubular function in the presence of acute changes in arterial perfusion pressure. Gertz et al. (1965) showed that within the range of blood pressure of 100–150 mm Hg fractional reabsorption and tubular transit time in the proximal convolution varied; at lower blood pressures fractional reabsorption was increased and transit time was prolonged. Koch et al. (1968) showed that at higher blood pressures the transit time was slightly prolonged and fractional reabsorption was reduced. The reasons for these discrepancies are not clear. There is also lack of agreement on the response of proximal intratubular pressure when perfusion pressure is changed. Thurau and Wober (1962) showed that free-flow proximal intratubular pressure in the rat kidney was not dependent on blood pressure, whereas Gertz et al. (personal communication) found different results: proximal intratubular pressure was dependent on systemic blood pressure.

In a later study Koch et at. (1968) also found a dependency of proximal intratubular pressure on renal artery perfusion pressure but noted that when the renal capsule was removed, the intratubular pressure remained constant. Relevant to this controversy is the fact that the data of Koch et al. (1968) were obtained in kidneys in which autoregulation was demonstrated. No other demonstration of autoregulation of renal blood flow and glomerular filtration rate in the rat kidney is known to us. Another interesting aspect of the data of Koch et al. (1968) is their demonstration that acute elevations in perfusion pressure were associated with prolongation of the reabsorptive half-time using the Gertz split-droplet technique, suggesting an impairment of reabsorptive function of the proximal convolution. However, in decapsulated kidneys this change during acute hypertension could not be demonstrated; reabsorptive half-time was normal. The Goldblatt model of chronic elevations in renal artery perfusion pressure has recently been studied by Lowitz et al. (1968) in the rat kidney, and detailed information on tubular function was obtained in the clamped and unclamped kidney. It was shown that the unclamped kidney excreted salt and water at a higher rate than either normal controls or the clamped kidney. The clamped kidney did not show excretion rates that were different from normal. This change in the unclamped kidney was primarily due to a reduction in salt and water reabsorption along the short loops of Henle. Proximal tubular function in both kidneys was normal. These data suggest that the allegedly higher inulin concentration and lower sodium concentration seen in clinical renal artery stenosis may, in fact, be normal, while the nonstenotic kidney may be excreting a higher rate of salt and water. The same authors also demonstrated an enhanced capacity for distal tubular sodium reabsorption in the unclamped kidney and decreased sodium retrieval in the distal tubule of the clamped kidney. They suggested that this difference may be a reflection of the renin contents of the two kidneys.

VI. Renal Oxygen Consumption

The unique nature of renal oxygen uptake in relation to renal blood supply can be readily appreciated if the characteristics of oxygen consumption in striated muscle are kept in mind. It has been shown (Pappenheimer, 1941) that oxygen consumption of muscle remains constant over a wide range of decreasing blood flow so that the arterial venous oxygen difference increases. Accordingly, the arteriovenous (a.v.) oxygen difference varies inversely with blood flow, as shown in Fig. 8. In contrast, when blood flow in the kidney decreases, the renal a.v. oxygen difference remains constant (van Slyke et al., 1934; Kramer and Winton, 1939; Kramer and Deetjen, 1960; Lassen et al., 1961). This suggests that renal oxygen consumption may be a function of blood flow over a wide range and that muscle oxygen consumption is for the most part independent of it.

Another important characteristic of the kidney is that renal blood flow is higher (400 ml/minute per 100 gm kidney weight) and a.v. oxygen difference (1–2 vol %) is smaller than in almost all other organs. It is also worth noting that in muscle a high rate of oxygen consumption, manifested in a high a.v. oxygen difference, is often the stimulus for a higher blood flow mediated through various metabolites. The high renal blood flow is almost certainly not to be explained on this basis since in relation to the oxygen supplied, the oxygen consumption is not large in the sense that the resulting a.v. oxygen difference is very low, as noted above. Indeed, the kidney is the only organ that shows minimal reactive hyperemia (Grupp and Heimpel, 1958). This observation is not surprising in view of the fact that—as outlined below—the tubular transport of sodium is the determinant of about 75% of renal oxygen consumption (Fig. 9), while only the remaining 25% represent the basal oxygen consumption of renal tissue itself. Insofar as a reduction in blood flow to the kidney is associated with a reduction in sodium load, and, hence, a diminution in transported sodium, it is not surprising that the oxygen debt that develops, accrues only from basal oxygen needs. Hence, the extent of renal reactive hyperemia is very modest at best, never approaching the 10–20-fold increase in blood flow rate in peripheral musculature after a period of ischemia. It is also relevant to note that under a normal perfusion pressure (about 100

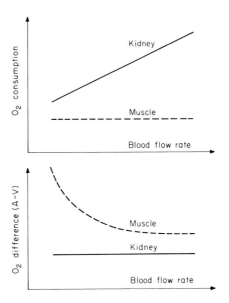

FIG. 8. Schematic representation of oxygen consumption and a.v. oxygen difference in muscle and kidney as a function of varying blood flow rates. (For details see text.)

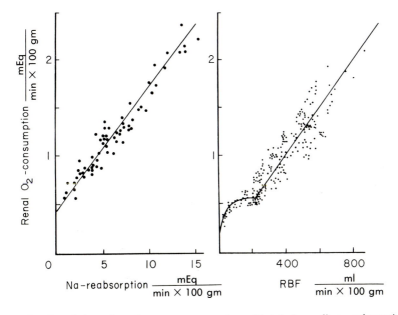

FIG. 9. Correlation of renal oxygen consumption with tubular sodium reabsorption (left graph) and renal blood flow (right graph). From Kramer and Deetjen (1963).

mm Hg), renal vasculature is almost maximally dilated, thereby leaving little possibility of further dilatation and higher blood flow (Ochwadt, 1956; Thurau et al., 1959b).

For many years it was unclear what function was served by the kidney's high rate of oxygen consumption. Attempts to correlate the extent of urinary osmotic concentration with renal oxygen uptake failed (Eggleton et al., 1940). The observations of Zerahn (1956), showing that the oxygen uptake of an isolated frog skin above the resting level is proportional to active sodium transport, paved the way for an explanation of the direct relation between renal blood flow and oxygen consumption. It is well established that renal sodium reabsorption is an active process and represents the overwhelming fraction of all tubular processes. Several laboratories have described a positive correlation between tubular sodium reabsorption and renal oxygen consumption (Lassen et al., 1961; Deetjen and Kramer, 1961; Thurau, 1961; Kiil et al., 1961; Bálint and Forgács, 1966; Eisner et al., 1964). As already noted, the portion of the oxygen uptake of the kidney, which is the result of tubular sodium reabsorption, accounts for approximately 75% of renal oxygen consumption under normal conditions (see Fig. 9). The remaining 25% of renal oxygen uptake, which is not correlated to sodium reabsorption, is considered to be the basal renal oxygen consumption. This fraction is in the order of 0.06–0.1 mmole O_2/minute per 100 gm kidney (Lassen et al., 1961; Deetjen and Kramer, 1961; Thurau, 1961).

From the correlation between suprabasal oxygen consumption and amount of reabsorbed sodium, a ratio of Na^+ (eq)/O_2 (mole) ranging from 28 to 31 has been derived (Lassen et al., 1961; Deetjen and Kramer, 1961; Thurau, 1961; Kiil et al., 1961; Bálint and Forgács, 1966; Eisner et al., 1964). This ratio is considerably higher than the ratio of 16–20, which was found on the isolated frog skin by Zerahn (1956). A reduction of this sodium/oxygen ratio in the kidney to values of 20–24 was observed during mannitol diuresis by Kiil et al. (1961) and by Deetjen and Kramer (1961). These authors explained the reduction in the sodium/oxygen ratio by the fact that during mannitol diuresis the intratubular sodium concentration in the proximal tubule may be lowered below plasma values, thereby establishing a sodium concentration gradient between tubular fluid and peritubular plasma. Presumably, the transport of sodium against a sodium concentration gradient is more "expensive" in terms of oxygen needed. There is experimental evidence that the correlation between renal O_2 consumption and glomerular filtration rate, and thereby the amount of sodium to be reabsorbed, is also maintained in renal disease, as shown by Cargill and

Hickam (1949) and Crosley *et al.* (1961). The data of Crosley *et al.* (1961) may be taken to indicate that the slope of the correlation between glomerular filtration rate and renal O_2 consumption in man is less steep than that observed in the dog kidney. The significance of this finding, however, remains obscure, since Eisner *et al.* (1964) reported data obtained on man which agree with the correlation found in the dog kidney.

Since under normal conditions about 99% of the filtered sodium is reabsorbed actively by the tubular cells, it is obvious that the amounts of sodium filtered and reabsorbed are almost identical. From this it follows that an increase in renal blood flow which is accompanied by an increase in glomerular filtration rate and thereby in tubular sodium load results in an increase in renal O_2 consumption (see Fig. 9). This correlation, however, is valid only for renal blood flow rates associated with glomerular filtrate formation. At low blood flow rates (less than $\frac{1}{3}$ of normal), during which glomerular filtration ceases, O_2 consumption in the kidney can no longer be correlated to renal blood flow. Under those conditions, a reciprocal correlation between renal a.v. oxygen difference and blood flow exists (Kramer and Deetjen, 1960; Lassen *et al.*, 1961). Thus, in this low range of blood flow, the kidney resembles muscle tissue in several respects (see above).

In contrast to other organs, the correlation between blood flow and energy-consuming sodium reabsorption in the kidney results in the peculiar situation that the work done by the kidney is a function of blood flow rate. This leads to the following consequences:

(a) At a constant filtration fraction and normal tubular sodium reabsorption, the a.v. oxygen difference remains constant and the suprabasal O_2 consumption varies directly with renal blood flow rate.

(b) The renal a.v. oxygen difference falls when (1) the filtration fraction is decreased (Table II), or (2) if at a constant filtration fraction the tubular sodium reabsorption is reduced, for example, either by diuretic agents or in osmotic diuresis.

The afore-mentioned conditions are valid only insofar as circulatory changes occur homogeneously in the entire kidney. If these variations are restricted to only parts of the kidney, the situation is more complicated. For example, Fig. 10 depicts a situation in which 50% of a 100-gm kidney is perfused with only one-tenth of normal blood flow rate, so that in this ischemic half of the kidney there is no filtration and no sodium reabsorption. The a.v. oxygen difference is high (5 vol %) in this ischemic part as a result of continuing basal O_2 consumption. This partial renal ischemia, however, is not reflected in the a.v. oxygen dif-

TABLE II

BLOOD FLOW, ARTERIOVENOUS OXYGEN DIFFERENCE AND OXYGEN CONSUMPTION IN
THE DOG KIDNEY DURING REDUCTION OF FILTRATION FRACTION BY MEANS OF
URETERAL OCCLUSION IN MANNITOL DIURESIS[a]

	RBF (ml/min)	a.v. O_2 Difference (Vol%)	O_2 Consumption (cc/min)
Control	402	2.52	10.10
Stop flow (2 min)	498	1.92	9.60
(4 min)	498	1.43	7.14
(6 min)	454	0.93	4.22
(10 min)	412	0.93	3.86
Release (1 min)	320	2.60	8.30
(4 min)	320	2.86	8.60

[a]Courtesy of K. Kramer and P. Deetjen.

ference of the entire kidney since the low blood flow rate through the
ischemic part, associated with the large a.v. oxygen difference, is mixed
in the renal vein with the 200 ml of blood which perfuses the normal
half of the kidney and which has a normal a.v. oxygen difference of 1.8
vol %. Therefore, the whole kidney a.v. oxygen difference is increased
only to 2.1 vol %. This example may demonstrate the difficulties involved in detecting renal hypoxia by measuring a.v. oxygen differences.

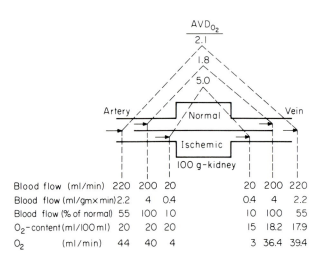

FIG. 10. The influence of partial renal ischemia on renal a.v. oxygen difference
(AVD_{O_2}). (For details see text.)

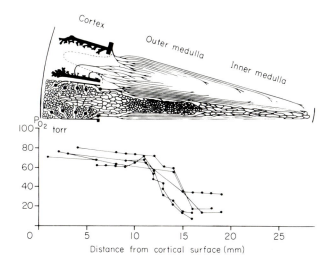

FIG. 11. Renal tissue oxygen tension in different parts of the kidney. The upper part illustrates schematically the renal vascular pattern. Adapted from Deetjen (1968).

VII. Partial Pressure of Oxygen in Kidney

When a platinum oxygen electrode is pushed into the cortex of the kidney and then progressively deeper into the medullary structures, a clear profile of decreasing oxygen tension is apparent (Aukland and Krogh, 1960) (see Fig. 11). When the P_{O_2} in the kidney is quantitatively measured, it becomes obvious that papillary tissue P_{O_2} and urine P_{O_2} are remarkably lower than that of renal venous blood (Aukland and Krogh, 1960; Ulfendahl, 1962a; Kramer and Deetjen, 1963; Strauss et al., 1968). The existence of this gradient of oxygen tension in the kidney, and the absolute low level of P_{O_2} in the papilla are intimately concerned with the countercurrent arrangement of medullary structures and the characteristics of cortical and medullary blood supply.

The possibility of renal O_2 shunting in cortical and medullary structures was investigated by Levy and Sauceda (1959) and Levy and Imperial (1961). By selectively cooling the cortical or inner layers of the isolated kidney and then injecting blood of high O_2 tension and containing methemoglobinemic erythrocytes into the renal artery, densometric tracings of renal venous blood revealed a shorter transit time for oxygen than for erythrocytes. A contribution of oxygen shunting to the medullary P_{O_2} gradient must be predicated upon oxygen consumption of the medullary tissue. It is this oxygen utilization which maintains the P_{O_2} difference between descending and ascending vasa recta in steady-state conditions and, hence, makes shunting possible. This view would, then, relegate medullary oxygen consumption to a role of a multiplication factor ("Einzeleffekt") for the countercurrent handling of oxygen.

Of course, it is conceivable that a high inner medullary oxygen consumption in the presence of a low blood supply can alone explain the low papillary P_{O_2}, i.e., the papillary P_{O_2} would surely reflect the medullary a.v. oxygen difference. However, data obtained on medullary blood flow and on *in vivo* estimations of inner medullary O_2 consumption (Kramer *et al.*, 1960) (calculated from the rate of hemoglobin desaturation) bear critically upon this; it is clear that the rate of medullary oxygen consumption is not sufficient to account for the low P_{O_2}. The plasma skimming theory would also provide a mechanism for the low papillary P_{O_2} insofar as this theory holds that deeper renal structures are perfused with an erythrocyte-poor and, hence, low O_2-containing blood (Pappenheimer and Kinter, 1956). Although most of the basis for this theory has been weakened by more experimental evidence (for a literature review, see Thurau, 1964b), it is still possible that an element of skimming in the medullary region does exist. Indeed, the low hematocrit of vasa recta blood is an established fact (see Thurau, 1964b). Accordingly, we would expect some depression of medullary tissue oxygen tension on this basis.

The P_{O_2} of urine, which is below renal venous P_{O_2}, is thought to be in equilibrium with papillary P_{O_2} and is, of course, determined by the mechanisms mentioned above. These and other considerations in this section are treated in a recent review by Deetjen (1968).

VIII. Intrarenal Blood Volume and Intrarenal Hematocrit

Table III contains available data on intrarenal blood volume. The studies are grouped according to the methods by which they were obtained. Using the passage time method (Lilienfield *et al.*, 1957; Ochwadt, 1957), the intrarenal blood volume (Vol$_{intrarenal}$) may be calculated according to the following equation:

$$\text{Vol}_{\text{intrarenal}} = \text{RFB} \left(1 - \text{Hct}\right) \cdot \bar{t}_{\text{plasma}} + \text{Hct} \cdot \bar{t}_{\text{ery}} \qquad (3)$$

in which RBF is the renal blood flow rate; Hct the hematocrit in the arterial blood; $\bar{t}_{\text{plasma}}$ the mean renal passage time for plasma; and $\bar{t}_{\text{ery}}$, the mean renal passage time for erythrocytes.

TABLE III
COLLECTED DATA ON INTRARENAL BLOOD VOLUME AND HEMATOCRIT

Reference	Intrarenal blood volume (% of kidney)	System Hct / Intraren. Hct	Animal
	Passage time method		
Lilienfield *et al.* (1958)	24.0	0.89	Dog
Ochwadt (1957)	20.0	0.90	Dog
Chinard *et al.* (1964)	19.8	0.88	Dog
	Tissue analysis method		
Emery *et al.* (1959)	34.0	0.45	Dog
Lilienfield *et al.* (1958)	32.8	0.49	Dog
Pappenheimer and Kinter (1956)	24.8	0.48	Cat
Ulfendahl (1962b)	20.0	0.53	Rabbit

Other methods are (a) the *in vivo* or *in vitro* analyses of tissue in order to determine plasma content and erythrocyte content in the tissue (Lilienfield *et al.*, 1958; Emery *et al.*, 1959; Wolgast, 1968) and (b) washout techniques of labeled erythrocytes and plasma (Polosa and Hamilton, 1962; Ochwadt, 1964).

The intrarenal hematocrit has been measured either from the mean circulation time for erythrocytes and plasma or from the relationship between plasma content and erythrocyte content in the tissue. For details in intrarenal distribution of blood volume, see Table IV. Table III shows that the values for intrarenal blood volume obtained from tissue analysis are higher than those obtained by the passage time method. Most likely, this difference is due to the fact that the apparent plasma volume measured by tissue analysis contains part of the extravascular volume. This may also explain the low hematocrit values and the observation that the values for blood volumes are higher when more time is allowed to elapse between the injection of the indicator and the moment at which the tissue was analyzed. Therefore, the data obtained by the passage time methods seem to be more credible (Ochwadt, 1957; Lilienfield and Rose, 1958; Chinard *et al.*, 1964). Nevertheless, the following reservations should be made:

(a) The arteriovenous passage time for erythrocytes and plasma includes the passage through the main arterial and venous vessels of the kidney in which the hematocrit is identical with the hematocrit of peripheral blood. A correction, therefore, would lead to a lower hematocrit in the small intrarenal vessels compared to the data listed in Table III.

TABLE IV

Collected Data on Intrarenal Hemodynamics

Localization and object		Weight (% of total kidney)	Intrarenal circulation times (min)	Vascular volume			Blood flow rates			Investigators
				ml/100 gm tissue	ml/100 gm kidney	% of total intra-renal vascular volume	ml/100 gm tissue/min	ml/100 gm kidney/min	% of total renal blood flow	
Cortex	Dog	70	0.021	19.2	13.5	69.0	458	321.0	92.5	Kramer et al. (1960)
	Dog	75	—	—	—	—	472	354.0	94.1	Thorburn et al. (1963)
	Dog	—	—	—	—	—	476	—	—	Harsing and Pessey (1965)
	Dog	—	—	—	—	—	481	—	85.0	Carrière et al. (1966)
	Dog	—	0.022–0.035[a]	—	—	—	—	—	—	Wolgast (1968)
	Rat	—	—	—	—	—	347–499	—	—	Haining and Turner (1966)
	Rat	—	—	—	—	—	564	—	—	Girndt and Ochwadt (1969)
	Man	—	0.13	—	—	69.4	—	—	87.0	Reubi et al. (1966)
Outer medulla	Dog	20	0.086	19.2	3.9	20.0	112	22.4	6.5	Deetjen et al. (1964)
	Dog	—	—	—	—	—	135	—	—	Harsing and Pessey (1965)
	Dog	15	—	—	—	—	132	20.0	5.3	Thorburn et al. (1963)

Region	Species									Reference
	Dog	—	—	—	—	—	111	—	12.0	Carrière et al. (1966)
	Dog	—	0.065–0.087[a]	—	—	—	190–380	—	—	Wolgast (1968)
	Rat	—	—	—	—	—	190	—	—	Girndt and Ochwadt (1969)
Outer and inner medulla	Man	—	0.358	—	—	30.6	—	—	13.0	Reubi et al. (1966)
Inner medulla	Dog	10	0.75	22.0	2.2	11.0	29	2.9	1.0	Kramer et al. (1960)
	Dog	—	—	—	—	—	66	—	—	Harsing and Pessey (1965)
	Dog	10	—	—	—	—	17	2.0	0.6	Thorburn et al. (1963)
	Dog	—	—	—	—	—	22	—	—	Lilienfield et al. (1961)
	Dog	—	—	—	—	—	18	—	3.0	Carrière et al. (1966)
	Dog	—	0.18–0.5[a]	—	—	—	40–120	—	—	Wolgast (1968)
	Rat	—	—	—	—	—	104	—	—	Girndt and Ochwadt (1969)
Papilla	Rat	—	—	—	—	—	72	—	—	Girndt and Ochwadt (1969)
Compartment I + II (Cortex and parts of the outer medulla)	Dog	—	0.095 0.073[a]	—	17.3	74.0	—	209.5	96.9	Ochwadt (1964)

TABLE IV (*Continued*)

Localization and object	Weight (% of total kidney)	Intrarenal circulation times (min)	Vascular volume			Blood flow rates			Investigators
			ml/100 gm tissue	ml/100 gm kidney	% of total intra-renal vascular volume	ml/100 gm tissue/min	ml/100 gm kidney/min	% of total renal blood flow	
Compartment III (parts of outer medulla and inner medulla) Dog	—	1.4 1.1[a]	—	5.1	26.0	—	6.5	3.1	Ochwadt (1964)

[a] Erythrocytes.

(b) As indicated by the results of Chinard *et al.* (1964), labeled plasma, even during a single passage through the kidney, leaves the intravascular space and distributes in the extravascular compartment. Therefore, the prolonged passage time for plasma when compared to that for erythrocytes may not only be a result of the greater intravascular plasma volume but also of the permeability of the capillary membranes for plasma.

Von Kügelgen and Braunger (1962) published an extensive study on the capillary system of the dog kidney. For detailed data about the density of capillaries, spatial arrangement of capillaries, surface area of capillaries and capillary volumes, the reader is referred to this publication.

IX. Nervous Control of Renal Blood Flow

It is widely accepted that under normal conditions there is little or no neurogenic sympathetic constrictor tone in the kidney, since acute surgical or pharmacological denervation, as well as chronic denervation of the kidney, does not change RBF and GFR (Smith, 1951). It has often been recorded in the literature that renal blood flow may increase after denervation. However, this is true only in anesthetized animals in which the sympathetic vasoconstrictor tonus is elevated by the anesthesia. This has been demonstrated in the dog by Berne (1952), who denervated one kidney 6–40 days prior to the experiment. After introduction of anesthesia (Nembutal or Chloralose) renal blood flow was found to be as much as 13% higher in the denervated kidney when compared with the control. In the absence of anesthesia these differences between denervated and innervated kidney could not be demonstrated. Similar results were obtained for glomerular filtration rate. The most convincing demonstration comes from data on transplanted kidneys on human subjects with renal blood flow and glomerular filtration rate values in the normal range (Bricker *et al.*, 1956). Of course, some species differences may exist. In unanesthetized rabbits, Korner (1963a) observed a higher blood flow rate in denervated kidneys.

A neurogenic increase in vascular tonus leading to a decrease in GFR and RBF can also be observed during arterial hypoxemia (Fig. 12). When inspired O_2 tension is acutely lowered to 50–70 mm Hg, renal vasoconstriction occurs (Kramer, 1952; Korner, 1963b). The vasoconstriction does not occur in denervated kidneys, nor does it occur after bilateral dissection of chemoreceptors and pressoreceptors (Korner, 1963b). This points to the importance of the chemoreceptors in this

Endexpiratory
O_2 concentration

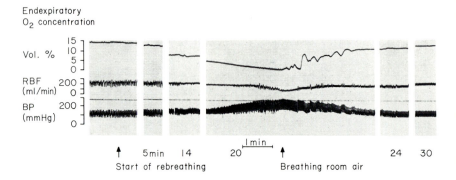

FIG. 12. Renal blood flow (electromagnetic flow meter) and blood pressure measurements in a conscious dog subjected to progressive hypoxemia. Hypoxemia was induced by rebreathing and simultaneous CO_2 absorption.

chain of events. The neurogenic origin of the renal vasoconstriction during hypoxemia is also consistent with the data of Kramer (1959), who showed a return of renal blood flow to normal values during hypoxemia when the pressoreceptors in the carotid sinus and aortic arch are stimulated.

There is some controversy as to whether or not neurogenic renal vasoconstriction occurs when the inhibitory effect of pressoreceptor activity upon the sympathetic system is diminished. These differences may arise from the observation that the arterial blood pressure increases simultaneously and that constancy of renal blood flow under those conditions may be interpreted as exhibiting autoregulation of renal blood flow instead of a neurogenic mechanism. By the use of phenoxybenzamine, Gilmore (1964b) was able to abolish in some experiments the increase in renal vascular resistance induced by a diminished pressoreceptor activity. Although this indicates some contribution of the nervous system for the adjustment of vascular resistance under these conditions, it is well established that denervated kidneys also exhibit the same response (Thurau and Henne, 1964). After clamping both carotid arteries in conscious hydrated dogs, PAH clearance remained unchanged (Somlay et al., 1962). Similar results were obtained by Perlmutt (1963) on hydrated anesthetized dogs. Although there is no doubt that a direct stimulation of renal nerves leads to a depression in renal blood flow rate (Study and Shipley, 1950; Houck, 1951; Block et al., 1952; Celander, 1954), it is obvious that there is little or no nervous control of renal blood flow under normal conditions.

The renal vascular response to exercise remains a matter of controversy, possibly because PAH clearance has usually been determined immediately after the end of exercise with the subject in a recumbent position. It is interesting to note that Freeman *et al.* (1955) found a decrease in PAH clearance in man exercising in the upright position but a constant PAH clearance when exercising in the recumbent position. These results suggest that a major part of the vasoconstriction found during exercise may be due to an orthostatic effect. Recently, however, Castenfors (1967) reported that even during supine exercise C_{PAH} decreases in man. E_{PAH} simultaneously measured remained unchanged. Consistent with the interpretation that the major factor responsible for the fall in renal blood flow during erect exercise is orthostasis *per se*, are data obtained in conscious dogs. In these experiments renal blood flow was recorded continuously by means of an implanted electromagnetic flow meter. A decrease in RBF was invariably noted when the animal was made to stand on its hind legs, but renal blood flow remained constant when the dog exercised in its normal horizontal posture (Fig. 13).

In isolated kidney preparations and by experiments involving con-

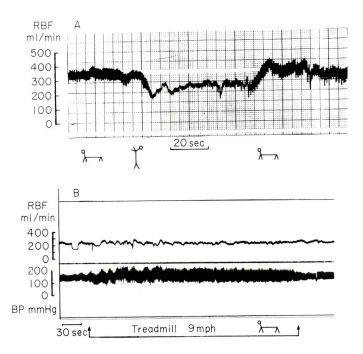

FIG. 13. (A) Renal blood flow in a conscious dog in normal standing and in head-up position. (B) Renal blood flow and arterial blood pressure in a conscious dog during rest and exercise. Renal blood flow measured by electromagnetic flow meter, implanted on the left renal artery. Blood pressure recorded via Teflon tube implanted into the aorta above the origin of the renal arteries. Implantations 3 weeks prior to the experiment. From Thurau (1964b).

stant infusion into the renal artery *in situ*, it has been demonstrated that drugs that paralyze smooth muscle increase renal blood flow (Ochwadt, 1956; Thurau and Kramer, 1959; Waugh and Shanks, 1960). The action of these drugs on renal blood flow after a single injection, however, may be very different in the intact organism, since changes in systemic hemodynamics occur simultaneously, thus initiating powerful nervous constriction in the kidney. For instance, when papaverine is injected in a single dose into the aorta above the renal artery of a conscious dog, vasodilation occurs only initially. This is followed by a marked vasoconstriction, probably induced by the decrease in systemic blood pressure (Fig. 14), since the constrictive phase is prevented after pretreatment with ganglionic blocking drugs, which is in accordance with a reflexly induced increase in resistance.

The efferent innervation of the mammalian kidney has been investigated by electrophysiological methods (Engelhorn, 1957). These analyses confirm data obtained from measurements of blood flow rate: the frequency of efferent discharges increased during hypoxemia, clamping of the carotid artery, and hemorrhage. An increase in frequency was also observed when blood pressure was reduced by means of acetylcholine or histamine. The efferent discharges were inhibited after blood pressure was increased by infusion of epinephrine, norepinephrine, and high doses of ADH.

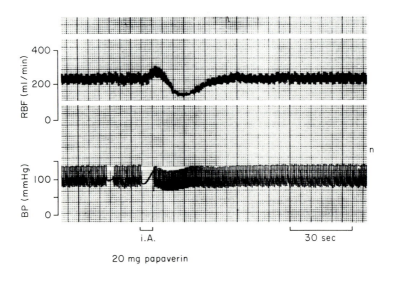

Fig. 14.   The effect on renal blood flow of injecting papaverine into the aorta above the origin of the renal arteries. Techniques for measurement as for Fig. 13, conscious dog. From Thurau (1964b).

X. Renal Blood Flow following Renal Ischemia

Numerous experiments have been carried out to investigate the recovery of renal function after interruption of renal blood flow (Sarre and Ansorge, 1939; Selkurt, 1946; Phillips and Hamilton, 1948; Roof *et al.*, 1951; Dutz and Kretzschmar, 1954; Birkeland *et al.*, 1959; Neely and Turner, 1959). In this section only the changes of renal blood flow and filtration rate following an ischemic period will be discussed.

Renal blood flow and filtration rate are only slightly affected by interruption of renal blood flow up to 20 minutes (Dutz and Kretzschmar, 1954; Sarre and Ansorge, 1939; Fajers, 1955). After a 30-minute period of ischemia, control values are again obtained when measured 30 minutes later. After 45 minutes of ischemia, PAH clearance and inulin clearance remain below control values, even 2 hours after cessation of clamping. Following an ischemic period the PAH clearance can no longer be taken as a valid measure for renal blood flow rate since PAH extraction (E_{PAH}) may change in an unpredictable manner (Bálint *et al.*, 1965). E_{PAH} is only slightly affected by ischemic periods up to 50 minutes (Dutz and Kretzschmar, 1954) but changes considerably after longer periods. Phillips and Hamilton (1948) found E_{PAH} reduced from a normal of 0.87 to 0.74 after 20 minutes ischemia, to 0.53 after 60 minutes, and to 0.22 after 120 minutes. These values for E_{PAH} were measured 2 hours following restoration of the renal circulation. Similar results were obtained by Selkurt (1946) and Friedman *et al.* (1954). Little is known about the cause of the reduction in PAH extraction. Both tubular secretory processes for PAH may be inhibited or an increased permeability of the tubular cells for PAH may facilitate the back-diffusion of PAH from the tubular fluid into the peritubular capillary blood.

The data of Selkurt (1946) allow a comparison of postischemic blood flow rates as determined either directly or by the ratio of C_{PAH}/E_{PAH}. The data clearly indicate that the values obtained by direct methods are always higher than those obtained by clearance methods. These data indicate that PAH is either stored in the renal parenchyma or destroyed by the kidney. If one considers the latter possibility unlikely, it appears likely that PAH may either be stored in the cells or secreted into tubular fluid of those nephrons which in the postischemic period contribute only little to the final urine.

A large body of information is available demonstrating renal vasoconstriction after periods of renal ischemia (Friedman *et al.*, 1954; Selkurt, 1946; Phillips and Hamilton, 1948; Roof *et al.*, 1951; Dutz and Kretzschmar, 1954). By direct measurement of renal blood flow, Selkurt (1946) found renal blood flow to be reduced to 55%, 1 hour following a 20-minute period of renal ischemia. A similar reduction was observed for glomerular filtration rate. Indeed, about 25 years ago Selkurt made the observation that mannitol infused prior to interruption of renal blood flow exhibits some protecting effect against postischemic renal vasoconstriction. Similar results were obtained when the kidney was cooled to 5–17°C during the period of ischemia (Birkeland et al., 1959). Under those conditions renal function was observed to recover completely even after an ischemic period up to 7–12 hours. A reduction in renal temperature to 31–33°C is not sufficient to protect the kidney against ischemia.

There is not much evidence that the sustained renal vasoconstriction following renal ischemia is of neurogenic origin. Franklin et al. (1951) suggested the existence of an intrarenal nervous reflex. This hypothesis may be discarded since it has been found that blockade of the intrarenal ganglia does not affect renal resistance to flow (Ochwadt, 1956; Waugh and Shanks, 1960). There is much evidence that the renal vasoconstriction is maintained by a humoral mechanism, particularly by the intrarenal formation of angiotensin. The participation of the intrarenal renin-angiotensin system on regulation of renal resistance to flow has been described in detail on p. 14. According to this view, the sodium concentration in the tubular fluid at the end of the loop of Henle is an important factor for the activation of this system. The sodium concentration at the macula densa is normally 25–50 mEq/liter and can only be maintained at these low levels if the transfer functions of the ascending limb are intact. Any damage to renal cells should not only decrease sodium reabsorption along the entire nephron but should also increase the sodium concentration at the macula densa toward plasma values. Such an increase in sodium concentration following renal ischemia has been observed in micropuncture studies by Schnermann et al. (1966). The increase in early distal sodium concentration under those conditions again was inversely related to the glomerular filtration rate. In this context it is interesting to note that Phillips and Hamilton in 1948 made the observation in unilaterally nephrectomized dogs, that 2 hours following ischemia of the remaining kidney, renal blood flow was restored to 81–85% of control independent of whether the period of renal ischemia was 20, 60, or 120 minutes. Gross et al. (1963) have shown that renin content in the remaining kidney is considerably decreased. The reduced vasoconstrictory response following unilateral nephrectomy, therefore, is consistent with the assumption that the renin-angiotensin system participates in the maintenance of renal vasoconstriction. Similar results were obtained in kidneys depleted of renin by high salt intake prior to the experiment (Wolff et al., 1964).

The importance of an adjustment of glomerular filtration rate in a damaged kidney to the reduction in tubular reabsorptive capacity is stressed by a consideration of what would result if tubular sodium load (GFR) remained normal with tubular reabsorption reduced by 50%. Under these circumstances urinary sodium excretion would be half of the filtered sodium load and urine volume would likewise be half of GFR. It is obvious from this that the reduced GFR and the vasoconstriction which usually occur in a damaged kidney are vital compensatory reactions which prevent this fatal course of sodium and water loss. The restoration of GFR and consequently of RBF then depends upon the restoration of the tubular competency to reabsorb salt and thereby to lower sodium concentration at the macula densa.

XI. Renal Lymphatic Function

A consideration of renal hemodynamics should properly concern itself with renal lymph formation, since this represents one of the routes by which the large renal plasma flow leaves the kidney. Reviews on the renal lymphatics (Goodwin and Kaufman, 1956; Mayerson, 1963; Rusznyak et al., 1967) have emphasized the many difficulties involved in the determination of the anatomy of the renal lymphatic system and the chemical nature of its lymph fluid. In this section no attempt will be made to review again these many difficulties, but rather, a few points will be discussed, in the hope of both illustrating the problems of the past and, at the same time, suggesting a way in which the role of the renal lymphatic system may be tied in with current problems of renal tubular transport.

At present, there is no agreement as to the anatomical distribution of the lymphatics within the kidney. Recently, Bell et al. (1968) were unable to demonstrate medullary lymphatics in the dog kidney. This anatomical observation was further strengthened by studies of the same group (Bell et al., 1969) suggesting that renal lymph composition bears no direct relationship to the countercurrent system of the renal medulla. However, other investigators (Cockett et al., 1969) appear to be satisfied that two intrarenal lymphatic networks exist. Differences in potassium and glucose concentration of hilar and capsular lymph samples led these investigators to believe that the hilar lymphatics drain, at least in part, the outer medulla. LeBrie (1968) showed a large increase in capsular lymph flow during osmotic diuresis and believed this to be due to lymph drainage of the medulla.

The view that lymph is composed in part of a protein-free reabsorbate is supported by the observation that the renal lymph protein concentration is half that of plasma (LeBrie and Mayerson, 1959). One of the earliest studies concerning the origin of renal lymph (Kaplan *et al.*, 1943) demonstrated that renal lymph inulin concentration was 32% lower than that of arterial plasma. This observation was accepted as evidence that renal lymph is composed in part of an inulin-free tubular reabsorbate. This rationale, however, neglects the fact that the renal venous inulin concentration which is supposed to be identical with that in renal lymph is lower than that of renal arterial plasma as a result of the addition of an inulin-free reabsorbate to renal venous blood. This concentration difference in the nondiuretic state practically equals the filtration fraction, and is about 25% ($E_{Inulin} = 0.25$). Accordingly, the lowered inulin concentration in renal lymph when compared to arterial blood reported by Kaplan *et al.* (1943) cannot be taken as indication of a tubular fluid component of lymph.

Relatively little information is available which permits conclusions concerning the influence of lymphatic function on renal blood flow, GFR and other renal transport parameters. Ligation of the renal lymphatics in one study (Rusznyak *et al.*, 1967) was reported to be without significant influence on RBF and GFR. However, these conclusions were based on endogenous creatinine clearances and C_{PAH} was not accompanied by PAH extraction ratios. Kaiserling and Soostmeyer (1939) and Rusznyak *et al.* (1967) have observed that impaired lymphatic drainage is associated with a salt and water diuresis. Insofar as GFR and RBF in this association are constant (see above), this would indicate impaired reabsorptive function. In the context of current hypotheses of tubular transport the following possibilities exist whereby the lymphatic system may modulate reabsorptive function:

(a) A large part of transtubular fluid reabsorption is isosmotic, and has been postulated to be critically dependent upon the geometry of the tubular intercellular channels (Diamond, 1969). The intercellular reabsorptive pathways are held to be in free communication with the extracellular space. The transporting membranes are thought to deliver solutes into the intercellular and basal labyrinthine spaces, and at this point, because of local osmotic gradients, water flows from the tubular lumen into these channels. Hydrostatic forces may then direct the isotonic fluid into the extracellular space. With this in mind, it is reasonable to assume that impairment of extracellular lymphatic drainage may well alter the oncotic and hydrostatic pressures of the fluid in the intercellular spaces or the geometry of the spaces itself.

(b) The above considerations are also relevant to Windhager's *et al.*

proposal (1969) which assigns peritubular protein concentration to the role of a determinant of proximal tubular fluid reabsorption. They suggested that the oncotic pressure of peritubular capillary blood may influence the volume of a hypothetical compartment interposed between the transporting cell membranes and the capillary endothelium. In their model, a decrease in peritubular protein concentration will impede reabsorbate entry into the capillaries at a time when the basal labyrinthine extrusion of reabsorbate proceeds. This situation would cause expansion of the hypothetical space which subsequently may inhibit net reabsorption. This sequence of events may be equally well triggered by impairment of lymphatic flow, which would also lead to an enlargement of the hypothetical compartment and, hence, reduction in reabsorption.

(c) The more conventional belief is that the importance of renal lymph lies in the conjecture that the oncotic pressure of the medullary interstitium must be kept low in order for the vasa recta to act as a countercurrent exchanger (e.g., Mayerson, 1963). This theory has serious limitations in that it has been shown by Wilde and Vorburger (1967), Bethge et al. (1962), Lassen et al. (1958), Ulfendahl (1962b), Young and Wissing (1964) that the medullary interstitium has a high albumin concentration. Furthermore, since the existence of medullary lymphatic vessels in the mammalian kidney has been doubted, the data of several authors (Kaiserling and Soostmeyer, 1939; Rusznyak et al., 1967) which have been interpreted as evidence for a lymphatic role in medullary function, may represent a cortical effect only. It is attractive to speculate that lymphatic ligation primarily impedes proximal tubular fluid reabsorption, perhaps in the sense of the models described above. Such a view would be consistent with current anatomical and functional data but must await direct experimental confirmaton.

XII. Pharmacology of Renal Blood Flow

Many investigators have evaluated the pharmacological activity of the various substances by infusing them into the renal artery and subsequently observing changes in renal function. This approach, however, has a basic limitation in that there is no complete mixing of the substance with the renal arterial blood. Accordingly, the test material can only exert its influence on a portion of the kidney. This phenomenon can be readily demonstrated if a dye is infused into the renal artery. Observation of the renal surface shows that staining is irregular. It follows then, that a quantitative correlation between the doses of the test substance used and its effect on total renal blood flow is probably erroneous. The following example illustrates this point:

Epinephrine in doses of 1 μg/minute is infused into the renal artery of the dog. Renal blood flow rate is reduced to almost 0 after 60 seconds. This time course cannot be taken as indicating a reaction time of 60 seconds for the individual vessel. This is true because in the beginning of the infusion epinephrine reaches only few areas in the kidney and leads to a maximal vasoconstriction in these segments. Because of the continuing infusion of epinephrine, the remaining blood flow rate distributes the epinephrine to other areas of the kidney, which again are constricted. These considerations preclude the temporal description of the effect of substances infused into the renal artery.

Both epinephrine and norepinephrine constrict renal vessels (Corcoran and Page, 1947; Burn and Hutcheon, 1949; Kramer, 1952; Spencer et al., 1954; Ahlquist et al., 1954; Marson, 1956; Mehrizi and Hamilton, 1959; Nahmod and Lanari, 1964). In man the reduction in PAH clearance following 20.4 μg/minute norepinephrine is more pronounced than following the same doses of epinephrine (Werkö et al., 1951). Glomerular filtration rate is only little affected by these doses. In dogs 4–8 μg/kg i.v. or 10 μg injected into the renal artery is sufficient to interrupt renal blood flow temporarily. After a single injection of epinephrine, renal blood flow is restored after 40–50 seconds have elapsed. During the recovery phase Spencer et al. (1954) observed an increase in renal blood flow above control levels. There seems to be little doubt that the afferent arterioles are constricted by epinephrine, since glomerular filtration rate is simultaneously reduced. However, the increase in filtration fraction (Barclay et al., 1947) also indicates that there is an increase in resistance to flow in the postglomerular vessels (Mehrizi and Hamilton, 1959; Zimmermann et al., 1964).

Attempts to differentiate renal vascular reactions into α- and β-receptor-type responses have been unsuccessful until now. In conscious dogs, Corcoran and Page (1947) found a slight decrease in renal resistance to flow following the infusion of isoproterenole. Using the same compound, Spencer (1956) observed a slight increase in renal resistance. PAH clearance in man remains unchanged during infusion of β-stimulating agents (Schirmeister et al., 1966).

Angiotensin II reduces renal blood flow by 45% in man when intravenously infused at a rate of 7.5 μg/minute from 605 to 330 ml/min (Bock and Krecke, 1958). Simultaneously, glomerular filtration rate is reduced from 111 to 78 ml/minute (-29%) together with an increase in filtration fraction from 0.18 to 0.24. When angiotensin infusion is continued, PAH clearance and inulin clearance both return to control values. Similar results were obtained by Schröder (1963), who observed control values for RBF and GFR after 20 minutes of continuous infusion of 0.01 μg/kg per minute of angiotensin II.

5-Hydroxytryptamine (Serotonin) exerts a different effect upon PAH clearance and inulin clearance. During intravenous infusion of 15 μg/kg per minute, inulin clearance is reduced by 11% and at 25 μg/kg per minute by 26%. Simultaneously, PAH clearance is maximally increased by 22% (Spinazzola and Sherrod, 1957; Blackmore, 1958). In these experiments, arterial blood pressure was constant or only little changed. At higher doses (up to 100 μg/minute) Serotonin leads to vasoconstriction in the dog kidney. Similar observations were made in the isolated perfused rat kidney, where serotonin in the perfusate in the concentration ranging from 0.034 to 10.0 μg/ml led to a reversible vasoconstriction (Passow et al., 1960).

Acetylcholine in low doses dilates renal vessels. Similar to the action of other dilating substances, such as papaverine, aminophyline, and Apresoline, glomerular filtration rate does not increase parallel to the increase in RBF (Pinter et al., 1964; Vander, 1964). This divergent behavior may be explained by the dilation of the efferent arterioles and by the increase in the intratubular hydrostatic pressure which occurs during renal vasodilation (Thurau and Kramer, 1959; Schirmeister et al., 1962). Acetylcholine abolishes renal autoregulation completely (Nahmod and Lanari, 1964), indicating that afferent arteriole smooth muscles are paralyzed. The action of acetylcholine may be abolished by atropine (Vander, 1964). Atropine per se has no effect upon renal hemodynamics or the excretory functions of the kidney. This observation led Vander (1964) to conclude that there is no endogenous formation of acetylcholine in the kidney.

Åström et al. (1964) have reported that injection of 0.2–200 μg acetylcholine into the renal artery of cats and dogs is followed by a vasocontrictory effect. Lower doses (0.002–0.02 μg) led to vasodilation. The constrictory effect of acetylcholine could be potentiated by the use of neostigmine (30 mg/kg i.v.) and abolished by atropine (0.02 mg/kg i.v.). A vasoconstrictory effect of acetylcholine was demonstrated even after pretreatment of the animals with dihydroergotamine (0.5 mg/kg i.v.) and reserpine (5 mg/kg i. p.) 24 hours prior to the experiment. On the basis of these experiments, the authors concluded that acetylcholine exerts a direct constrictory effect upon renal vasculature. These data, however, do not exclude the possibility of intrarenal formation of angiotensin in the presence of high doses of acetylcholine.

Bradykinin. Little is known about the action of the polypeptides Bradykinin, Kallidine and Eledoisine upon renal hemodynamics (Barer, 1963, Mertz, 1963, Heidenreich *et al.*, 1964). In contrast to the significance of Bradykinin for blood flow rate in secretory glands, this polypeptide seems to be of little importance to the kidney. In man, inulin clearance and PAH clearance were found to be increased slightly by the injection of 0.15–0.3 μg/kg/min i.v. (Mertz, 1963). Similar results were obtained by Barer (1963) in cats. In contrast to these findings, Heidenreich *et al.*, 1964, did not find any change in PAH clearance in the dog following i.v. infusion of 0.5–1.0 μg/kg/min of Bradykinin.

XIII. The Intrarenal Distribution of Glomerular Filtrate

The heterogeneity of intrarenal blood flow distribution has recently been shown to have a parallel in the partitioning of the total filtrate within the kidney. The first indication of the fact that total filtrate is unequally partitioned among glomeruli in different cortical layers were Hanssen's (1961) early observations using ferrocyanide as an indicator of the single nephron filtrate. Recently, this has been supported by more direct investigations using micropuncture techniques. Horster and Thurau (1968) found superficial single nephron GFR in salt-depleted antidiuretic rats to be approximately 50% of that found in juxtamedullary nephrons (Fig. 15). This heterogeneity of single nephron filtrate is consistent with anatomical data indicating that in the rat

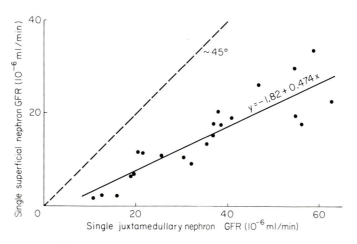

Fig. 15. Correlation between simultaneously determined single superficial and single juxtamedullary nephron filtration rate in salt-depleted rats. The slope of the regression line indicates a ratio between juxtamedullary and superficial filtration rate of 2.47. From Horster and Thurau (1968).

kidney 80% of glomeruli belong to the superficial layers, the remainder being juxtamedullary in location and having long loops of Henle. The possibility of a specific role of antidiuretic hormone in this phenomenon of filtrate redistribution has been further investigated by Horster *et al.* (1969). In rats with hereditary diabetes insipidus it was found that administration of ADH was associated with a large increase in filtrate of juxtamedullary nephrons. As noted elsewhere in this review, blood flow studies have shown a decrease in medullary blood flow (Thurau *et al.*, 1960a) concomitant with antidiuresis. Aukland (1968), however, using hydrogen gas clearance techniques, did not show this. The increase in juxtamedullary filtrate following ADH administration is consistent with all of these data in that it can be postulated that antidiuretic hormone causes efferent arteriolar constriction of juxtamedullary glomeruli and thereby increases the effect of filtration pressure. It is quite possible that in Aukland's studies an increased hydrogen gas clearance, associated with higher urine flow rates through juxtamedullary nephrons, masked the decrease in gas clearance that resulted from lower medullary blood flows. Finally, another factor which may influence the intrarenal distribution of glomerular filtrate is acute saline infusion. Although direct evidence is not yet available, micropuncture data obtained from superficial nephrons during saline infusion lead to the inference that deeper nephrons must be filtering at a very low rate, since the increase in filtrate in superficial nephrons proportionally far exceeds the increase in total kidney filtrate (Seldin, personal communication).

XIV. Medullary Blood Flow

The countercurrent theory of Kuhn, Wirz, and Hargitay has greatly advanced our understanding of renal concentrating mechanisms. It has become apparent, however, that a complete understanding of this process requires a quantitative consideration of medullary hemodynamics (Berliner *et al.*, 1958). In a mathematical treatment of this problem Günzler (in Thurau and Deetjen, 1962) showed that the osmolar concentration at the tip of the medulla is inversely proportional to a value of blood flow between F and F^2, *ceteris paribus*

$$C_1 = C_o + \frac{\Phi m_a}{F} \left(1 + 2 \frac{Pm_i}{F} L\right)x - \frac{\Phi m_a \cdot Pm_i}{F^2} x^2 \qquad (4)$$

where

C_1 is the osmolar concentration at the tip of the medulla; C_o, the osmolar concentration of plasma; Φm_a, the influx of osmotically active substances into vasa recta blood per unit length; Pm_i, countercurrent diffusion of osmotically active substances per unit length; L, total length of loop; x, distance from beginning of the loop; and F, flow rate. This influence of medullary blood flow upon the concentration ability of the kidney is particularly relevant to experimental work on medullary hemodynamics.

A. Anatomy of Medullary Vessels

Following the classical work of von Möllendorff (1930) and of Trueta *et al.* (1948), recent more detailed descriptions of the medullary vascular system have been published by several groups who questioned the existence of true vascular loops in the medulla (Moffat and Fourman, 1963; Plakke and Pfeiffer, 1964; Rollhäuser *et al.*, 1964; Kriz, 1967; Moffat, 1967).

Medullary vasa recta are derived from efferent arterioles of juxta-medullary glomeruli which also supply the outer medullary capillary network. Juxtamedullary glomeruli may have two efferent arterioles, one breaking into an adjacent capillary network and the other passing into the medulla as vasa recta.

The widely accepted assumption that all blood perfusing medullary vessels is of postglomerular origin probably needs revision. Ljungqvist (1964) studied the anatomical arrangement of vascular poles in different zones of the human kidney by combining stereo-microangiographic and histological techniques. In most of the vascular poles of juxtamedullary glomeruli, the afferent and efferent arterioles were connected directly by a vessel bypassing the glomerular capillaries. Such bypasses were not found in the more superficial glomeruli.

Rollhäuser *et al.* (1964) showed that the capillary network adjacent to the bundles in the outer medulla is the densest capillary system of the entire kidney. The vasa recta, located in the center of the bundles, pass into the inner medulla and branch into capillary networks at different levels along the axis of the medulla (see Fig. 16). The capillary system in the inner medulla is less dense than that in the outer medulla and forms elongated meshes between the straight limbs of the vasa recta in the inner medulla. Thus, there is an abrupt transition between outer and inner medulla, as demonstrated in Fig. 17. No descending vasa recta were found looping back to form ascending (venous) vasa recta without first breaking into a capillary network. The venous vasa recta enter the bundles at different levels of the medulla, similar to the various branching points of the arterial vasa recta.

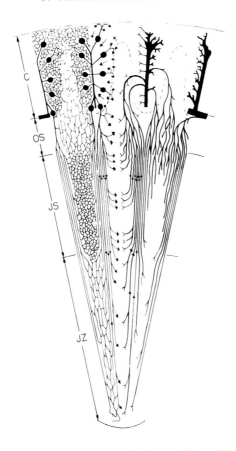

Fig. 16.   Diagram of the vascular pattern in the rat kidney. The arterial vessels and capillaries are shown on the left half of the figure and venous vessels on the right. The arrows along the center line indicate the direction of flow. The picture should be imagined folded vertically along the center line at which time the interrelationship between arterial and venous vasa recta will be projected. C, Cortex; OS, outer stripe of the medulla; IS, inner stripe of the medulla; IZ, inner zone of the medulla (papilla). From Rollhäuser *et al.* (1964).

In the rat kidney each vascular bundle in the inner stripe of the outer medulla is composed of 40–170 (mean 84) vessels (Kriz, 1967). At the transition from outer to inner medulla, the average number of vasa recta in a single bundle is reduced to a mean of 33, which decreases further along the axis of the papilla. Descending and ascending vasa recta lie closely mingled, so that the bundles form *rete mirabile* (Fig. 18). The outer ring of the bundles is primarily composed of ascending (venous) vasa recta, which are in close association with the thin de-

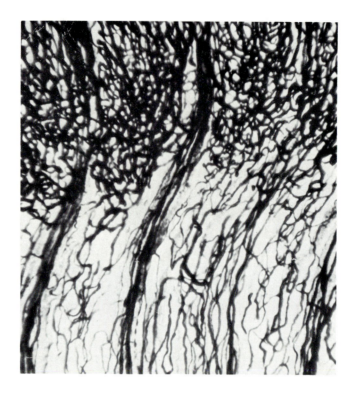

Fig. 17. Section to show the abrupt transition between the outer and inner zones of the medulla in the rat kidney. Above is the outer medullary plexus with vascular bundles surrounded by a capillary plexus. Below lies the elongated capillary plexus of the inner medullary zone. From Moffat and Fourman (1963).

scending limbs of loops of Henle, surrounding the vascular bundles. The endothelium of descending vasa recta is relatively thick, while that of the ascending vessels appears to be thin and fenestrated (see Fig. 19).

Recent studies of the ultrastructure of the vasa recta in the rat kidney by Moffat (1967) clearly indicate that the efferent arterioles of juxta-medullary glomeruli and the proximal parts of vasa recta (i.e., in the outer stripe of the outer medulla) are surrounded by smooth muscle cells (Fig. 20). This is in contrast to the efferent arterioles of superficial glomeruli. In the deeper zones of the medulla smooth muscle cells are gradually replaced by perivascular cells (Longley et al., 1960; Dietrich, 1968). Hence, there is sufficient anatomical evidence to support the

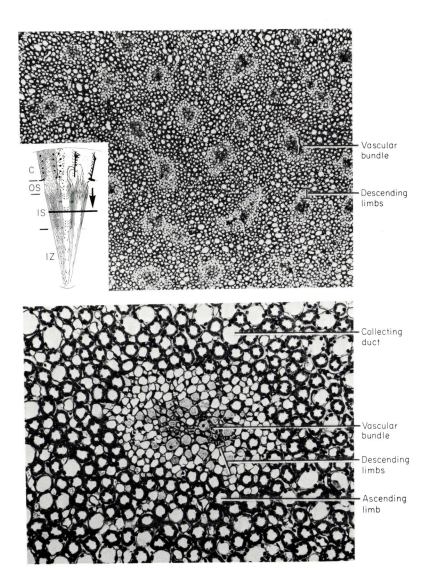

FIG. 18.   Transverse section through the inner stripe of the rat medulla. The insert
shows the level of the section. The vascular bundles form the center of concentric systems
of descending limbs, ascending limbs and collecting ducts. Magnification: above approx.
×80, below approx. ×200. From Kriz (1967).

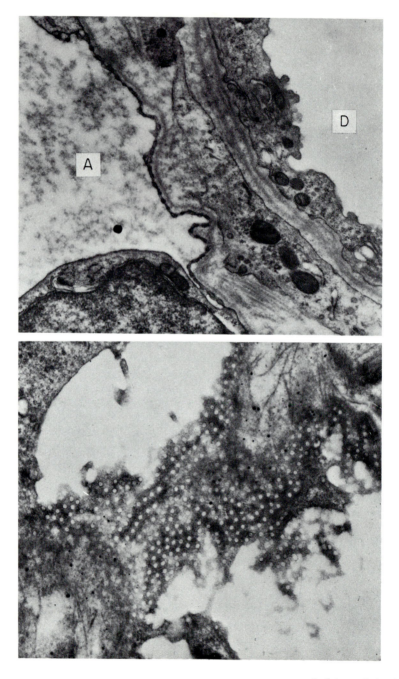

See facing page for legend →

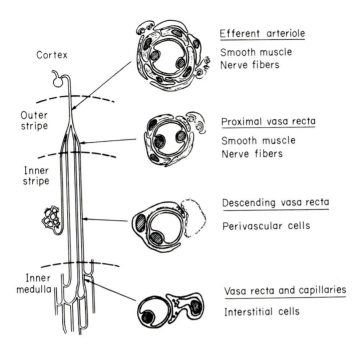

Cortex

Outer stripe

Inner stripe

Inner medulla

Efferent arteriole

Smooth muscle
Nerve fibers

Proximal vasa recta

Smooth muscle
Nerve fibers

Descending vasa recta

Perivascular cells

Vasa recta and capillaries

Interstitial cells

FIG. 20.   Diagram of the blood supply of the renal medulla to indicate the cell types that are found in relation to the vessels at different levels. From Moffat (1967).

assumption that the resistance to blood flow in the efferent arterioles of juxtamedullary glomeruli can be regulated actively. This would permit a simultaneous, but reciprocal change in juxtamedullary nephron filtrate and medullary blood flow (see below).

B. Medullary Hemodynamics

In recent years methods have been developed to determine the intrarenal distribution of blood flow and blood flow rates per unit tissue in the various parts of the kidney. Based on the assumption that PAH is not extracted from the blood perfusing the medulla, but completely extracted from blood perfusing the cortex, it was suggested that med-

FIG. 19.   *Upper*: Section through adjacent walls of descending (D) and ascending (A) vasa recta in the outer medulla of the rat. The endothelium of the ascending vasa recta is thin and fenestrated. *Lower*: Tangential section of the endothelium of the ascending vas rectum showing the fenestrations of the wall. This section was obtained from an animal which was kept on drinking water with silver nitrate. The dark dots are silver granules. Courtesy of D. B. Moffat. ×36,000.

ullary blood flow could be calculated from the PAH extraction ratio (Reubi, 1960; Pilkington *et al.*, 1965):

$$\text{Medullary blood flow} = \text{RBF} \, (1 - E_{\text{PAH}}) \qquad (5)$$

For example, if 90% of the PAH is extracted from blood flowing through the kidney ($E_{PAH} = 0.9$), cortical blood flow would then be 90%, and the blood perfusing the medulla, 10% of total renal blood flow. Although this value is consistent with that obtained by other methods (see Table IV, pp 28–30), several reservations concerning the general applicability of this approach have been raised (Slotkoff *et al.*, 1968). For example, Harvey (1966), using Eq. (5), has calculated medullary blood flow rates of 14 ml/gm minute during acetylcholine infusion, an implausibly high value, which led him to question the applicability of this method.

Using small photocells and dye dilution techniques, Kramer and associates (1960) measured plasma passage times in the cortex and medulla of the dog (Fig. 21). Table IV contains these data together with those for regional blood volumes from which regional blood flow rates were calculated. Thorburn *et al.* (1963) calculated regional blood flow rates from the nonexponential slope of disappearance curves of γ-emission after a single injection of [85]Kr into the renal artery (Table IV). The advantage of this method is its applicability in conscious animals. However, this method yields correct values for blood flow rate only when the removal of the test substance from renal tissue is solely affected by blood flow. This is apparently true for the renal cortex. There is evi-

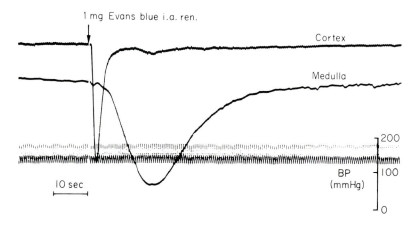

FIG. 21.   Dye dilution curves in the renal cortex and medulla of the dog after rapid injection of Evans blue into the renal artery. The passage of Evans blue was measured by small photo cells, which separately picked up reflected light from the cortex (upper curve) and transmitted light from the medulla (lower curve). From Kramer *et al.* (1960).

dence, however, that in the inner and to a lesser extent in the outer medulla, the removal of highly diffusible substances such as krypton and hydrogen is also affected by tubular and vascular countercurrent exchange diffusion and by urine flow. Accordingly, the derived values tend to be smaller than the true medullary flow rates.

Local hydrogen gas clearance measured polarographically with small platinum electrodes was used by Aukland and Berliner (1964) and Haining and Turner (1966) to calculate local blood flow rates. Again, this method seems to be quantitatively inapplicable to the inner medulla since hydrogen clearance in this region has been demonstrated to be influenced by urine flow. For the rat renal cortex Haining and Turner calculated a blood flow rate of 3.8–4.9 ml/gm kidney per minute, a value similar to that found in dogs and man.

In a recent extensive study, Wolgast (1968) used ^{32}P-labeled erythrocytes as an indicator for red cell passage time through cortex and medulla, a method originally applied to the kidney by Thurau et al. (1959a). Local indicator dilution curves are recorded by β-sensitive needle-shaped detectors plunged into the kidney at different layers after labeled erythrocytes are injected as a single slug into the renal artery. Local blood flow rate, however, can be calculated only if intravascular dynamic hematocrit and local blood volume are known.

Table IV contains data available in the literature on medullary blood flow rate. Blood flow rates in the outer and inner medulla per unit tissue weight are considerably lower than in the cortex and together account only for 6 or 7% of total renal blood flow. The inner medulla is perfused by approximately 1% of total renal blood flow and has the lowest perfusion rate per unit tissue of these areas. However, the term "low" medullary blood flow is relative only, in comparison to the renal cortex. After all, inner medullary blood flow per unit tissue weight is about 15 times that in resting muscle and approximately 50% that in the brain and 30% that in the heart under basal conditions.

The low blood flow rate through the medulla, when compared to that through the cortex, does not seem to be caused by a low vascular volume per unit tissue. Similar to the cortex, the vascular volume in the medulla accounts for approximately 1/5 of tissue mass (see Table IV). It is more likely that the extraordinary length of the vasa recta (in the dog up to 40 mm) accounts primarily for the medullary resistance to flow. Therefore, it is expected that blood flow rate per unit tissue decreases towards the tip of the papilla. Consistent with the idea of a reduction in flow rate along the longitudinal axis of the medulla are measurements of transit times of erythrocytes in different levels of the medulla by Wolgast (1968), as shown in Fig. 22.

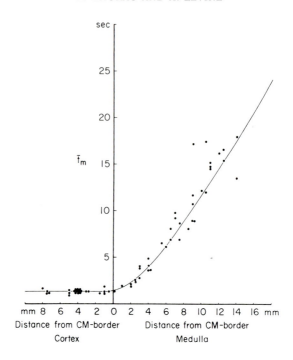

Fɪɢ. 22. Mean transit time (t_m) of ^{32}P-labeled red cells in different layers of the dog kidney. From Wolgast (1968).

Hydrostatic pressure measurements in vasa recta of the golden hamster papilla show that the resistance to blood flow is not uniformly distributed over the entire length of these vessels, but occurs primarily in the descending limb. The pressure drop was 6.5 mm Hg/mm vessel length along the descending limbs, but none was measurable along the ascending limbs (Thurau, 1963). From this pressure drop and a total length of the descending limb of 6–8 mm, a hydrostatic pressure at the beginning of the vasa recta of 60–70 mm Hg was calculated. Consistent with these data are recent measurements of vasa recta pressure in the rat papilla by Wunderlich and Schnermann (1969). Using a micropressure transducer attached to the micropuncture capillary, they recorded a pressure in the vasa recta close to the papillary tip of 8.3 ± 2.3 mm Hg.

The lower vascular resistance of the ascending limbs could be due either to a greater vessel diameter or to a greater number of vessels, or both. One should be cautious in applying Poiseuille's equation to these measurements for two reasons. First, Poiseuille's equation is applicable only when volume flow is constant along the vessel, but water ex-

changes between vasa recta and interstitial fluid, so that flow is not uniformly isovolumetric. Second, Poiseuille's equation assumes constant
viscosity, but changes of plasma protein and osmolar concentration as
well as of erythrocyte volume in the vasa recta make it most unlikely
that this condition is fulfilled. Therefore, Poiseuille's equation does not
permit a precise determination of vasa recta radius, and, hence, of vascular capacity.

However, it does seem justified in a qualitative sense to conclude that
the vascular volume of the descending limbs is smaller than that of the
ascending limbs. Blood flow velocity should then be higher in the descending vasa recta than in the ascending, and this relationship can
easily be verified by observing vessels in the exposed papilla.

More precise measurements of vascular volume distribution in the
vasa recta were made by Meier *et al.* (1964) by means of a modification
of the transillumination transit time technique designed to study local
plasma flow velocity. According to their data, the descending limbs of
vasa recta contain only 37% of the medullary vascular volume and the
ascending limbs 63%. This estimate divides the vascular volume of the
true capillaries equally between the two limbs, rather than retaining it
as a separate entity. These values were obtained from antidiuretic
dog kidneys; no data are available to indicate whether this pattern is
retained when the concentrating ability of the kidney changes.

The high resistance to flow of the vasa recta when compared to the
cortical vessels might in part also be due to an increase in blood viscosity, since, as demonstrated by micropuncture techniques (Thurau *et al.*,
1960b; Ullrich *et al.*, 1961; Gottschalk *et al.*, 1962; Wilde *et al.*, 1963,
microspectrophotometry (Wilde and Vorburger, 1967), and tissue analysis (Lassen *et al.*, 1958; Bethge *et al.*, 1962; Ulfendahl, 1962b; Young
and Wissig, 1964), the protein concentration in vasa recta blood during
antidiuresis is approximately 2 times that in systemic blood. A quantitative evaluation of the increased protein concentration upon blood viscosity in the medulla is not feasible, since the hematocrit of vasa recta
blood simultaneously is lowered and crenation of red cells occurs in the
hypertonic environment of the medulla. In *in vitro* experiments
Schmid-Schönbein *et al.* (1969) has demonstrated that the plasticity of
red cells is markedly reduced when osmolarity is increased above 300
mosm/kg, which in turn increases the apparent viscosity of the blood.
The lowered hematocrit might in part compensate for this effect of an
increased osmolarity. Wells *et al.* (1965) tried to assess the influence of
osmolality on medullary blood flow by using mesenteric vessels of dogs
covered with bathing media of varying osmolarity. With increasing
osmolality blood flow velocity was reduced, indicating that the medul-

lary osmolality per se may in part contribute to the decrease in medullary blood flow in the concentrating kidney.

C. Correlation between Medullary Blood Flow and Concentrating Ability

Little is known about the precise relation between rate of medullary blood flow and efficiency of the concentrating mechanism. From theoretical considerations [see Eq. (4)] it is apparent that an increase in medullary blood flow rate per se reduces the osmotic gradient in the medulla. Up to the present time, however, there is no experimental proof for this hypothesis. The difficulties arise from the fact that any experimental design developed in order to change medullary blood flow also affects the juxtamedullary glomerular function and, hence, tubular flow rate in the long loops of Henle. Thus, a quantitative examination of the influence of medullary flow rate on the concentrating mechanism cannot be made.

It is now generally agreed (Berliner and Bennett, 1967; Thurau, 1967b; Wilde and Vorburger, 1967) that the hydrostatic pressure difference between adjacent descending and ascending vasa recta is not sufficient to act as an osmotic multiplier. Such a possibility, originally rejected by Kuhn and Ramel (1959), was reconsidered by Lever (1965).

In contrast to the cortical blood flow, inner medullary blood flow in dogs, measured as dye passage time, is only poorly autoregulated and therefore increases with increasing blood pressure (Thurau et al., 1960; Thurau and Deetjen, 1962). These authors explained the loss of renal concentrating ability which accompanies an increase in arterial blood pressure on the basis of an increase in medullary blood flow (Fig. 23). Glomerular filtration rate and total renal blood flow were little or not at all affected by changes in blood pressure, indicating autoregulation of cortical circulation. The decline in U/P_{osm} below 1.0 indicated that medullary osmolarity was reduced to or close to plasma isotonicity. The osmotic disequilibrium between final urine and medullary tissue water may in part be due to a high flow velocity in the collecting ducts. This would prevent the urine from attaining full osmotic equilibrium with medullary interstitium. Additional support for the existence of a reduced medullary osmolality at an increased arterial blood pressure is presented by analysis of medullary tissue sodium concentration at two levels of arterial pressure (Selkurt et al., 1965). At a high blood pressure range, tissue sodium concentration was significantly reduced in the papillary region of the medulla. Such a loss in concentrating ability by increased medullary blood flow is consistent with mathematical treatments of the correlation between osmolar concentration at the tip

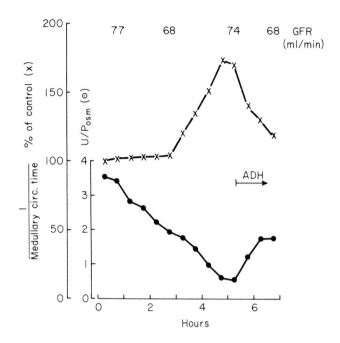

FIG. 23. Medullary blood flow, estimated as the reciprocal of medullary circulation time, in a dog during the development of a water diuresis, and its inhibition by ADH. Modified from Thurau *et al.* (1960a).

of a countercurrent system and flow rate in the system, as noted on p. 43 [Eq. (4)].

For the outer medulla, Aukland (1966) and Wolgast (1968) interpreted their data as indicating the existence of autoregulation in the renal medulla. As outlined above, the difficulties inherent in the interpretation of the experimental data might be the reason for the discrepancies. It is unlikely that the regulation of blood flow in the outer medulla differs qualitatively from that in the inner medulla because the vascular systems in both areas are derived from efferent arterioles of juxtamedullary glomeruli.

Consistent with the absence of autoregulation in the renal medulla are recent measurements by Girndt and Ochwadt (1969) of medullary blood flow in rats with renal hypertension. In unclamped kidneys, which were exposed to an arterial blood pressure of 200 mm Hg, cortical blood flow remained unchanged while blood flow in the outer medulla increased by 40%, in the inner medulla by 50%, and in the papilla by 70%.

D. Medullary Blood Flow during Water and Osmotic Diuresis

When renal function changes from antidiuresis to water or osmotic diuresis, a decrease in medullary circulation time was measured (Thurau *et al.*, 1960a). Figure 24 shows dye dilution curves in the inner medulla of a dog kidney during antidiuresis, water diuresis, and following inhibition of the water diuresis by ADH. Assuming no change in vascular volume, 1/circulation time is a relative measure of medullary blood flow. The assumption that medullary blood volume is not decreased during water diuresis is supported by measurements of red cell and albumin distribution spaces in frozen medullary tissue slices, which may in fact be increased during water diuresis (Ulfendahl, 1962b). Figure 25 summarizes such an experiment and indicates that, during water diuresis, medullary blood flow may increase by approximately 70%.

Recent observations have shed further light on the mechanisms associated with the increase of medullary blood flow during change from antidiuresis to water diuresis. The increase in medullary blood flow was recently confirmed by Fourman and Kennedy (1966). Using the injection of a fluorescent dye, they demonstrated an extensive staining of vasa recta in water-loaded normal rats and in diabetes insipidus rats whether hydrated or dehydrated, whereas dehydration or the injection of ADH, independent of water load, in normal rats prevented or reduced considerably the staining of the vasa recta. These results together with the finding of extensive distribution of smooth muscles in the efferent arteriole of juxtamedullary glomeruli by Moffat (see Fig. 20) strengthen the concept that ADH exhibits a vasoconstrictory effect upon the efferent arterioles of juxtamedullary glomeruli. Consistent with a vasoconstrictory effect of ADH upon postglomerular vasa recta are the results of Horster *et al.* (1969), who showed an increase in filtration rate of juxtamedullary glomeruli when ADH was given to rats with hereditary hypothalamic diabetes insipidus. Further support comes from measurements of vasa recta pressure in the rat papilla during water diuresis and ADH-induced (subpressor doses) antidiuresis. Vasa recta pressure fell from 13.0 ± 4.2 mm Hg during water diuresis to 8.3 ± 2.3 when ADH was given (Wunderlich and Schnermann, 1969). Similar conclusions were drawn by Moffat, who found evidence for a reduced perfusion rate of juxtamedullary glomeruli in dehydrated rats in which, presumably, ADH activity was elevated, when compared to normally hydrated rats.

Aukland (1968), using the hydrogen gas clearance method in dogs, reported that outer medullary hydrogen clearance was not changed when antidiuresis was induced in hydrated dogs by ADH. He, there-

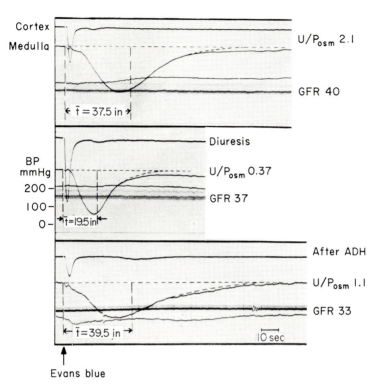

FIG. 24. Dye dilution curves in the cortex and inner medulla of a dog kidney during antidiuresis, water diuresis and during inhibition of the water diuresis by ADH. $\bar{t}$ = medullary circulation time. (From Thurau *et al.* 1960a).

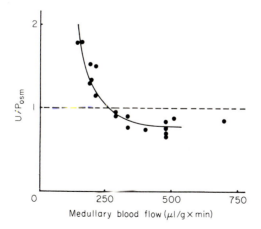

FIG. 25. Urine to plasma osmolal ratio as a function of medullary blood flow. From Thurau and Deetjen (1962).

fore, concluded that ADH does not selectively reduce medullary blood flow. However, hydrogen clearance from the medullary tissue is equally affected by flow in both vasa recta *and* loops of Henle. If, as shown by Horster *et al.* (1969), ADH increases juxtamedullary GFR's and hence loop flow rates, hydrogen clearance can only be kept constant when vasa recta flow rate is decreased simultaneously. Therefore, Aukland's finding of an unchanged hydrogen clearance when diuresis is changed to antidiuresis is consistent with a reduced medullary blood flow rate.

E. Medullary Blood Flow during Hemorrhagic Hypotension

Recently, there has been some controversy concerning the influence of hemorrhagic hypotension on medullary blood flow. It is likely that the nature of the methods used for these studies underlie the discrepant results (see Medullary Blood Flow, section XIV). Carrière *et al.* (1966), using [85]Kr washout curves and radioautographs in dogs (see Thorburn *et al.*, 1963), offer results to indicate that severe hemorrhage is not associated with a fall in medullary blood flow (BP = 50 mm Hg, 35–60% loss of blood volume) despite the marked decrease in cortical perfusion. Such a constancy of medullary blood flow implies a decrease of approximately 50% of medullary vascular resistance. Aukland and Wolgast (1968), on the other hand, using local hydrogen gas clearance for the outer medulla and local [85]K clearance for the inner medulla, showed that hemorrhagic hypotension of the same degree is associated with a fall in medullary blood flow to 25% of control, indicating a doubling of vascular resistance similar to the changes calculated for cortical resistance. These data support the earlier work of Kramer (1962) who showed, by means of Evans blue transit times, a proportional decrease in cortical and medullary blood flow during hemorrhagic hypotension.

Aukland and Wolgast (1968) believe that the demonstration of a constant medullary blood flow by Carrière *et al.* (1966) is predicated on an erroneous interpretation of the [85]K washout curves.

REFERENCES

Ahlquist, R. P., Taylor, J. P., Rawson, C. W., and Sydow, V. L. (1954). Comparative effects of epinephrine and levarterenol in intact anaesthetized dogs. *J. Pharmacol. Exp. Therap.* **110**, 352.

Åström, A., Crafoord, J., and Samelius-Broberg, U. (1964). Vasoconstrictor action of acetylcholine on kidney blood vessels. *Acta Physiol. Scand.* **61**, 159.

Aukland, K. (1966). Study of renal circulation with inert gas, measurements in tissue. *Proc. 3rd Intern. Congr. Nephrol. Washington, D.C.* **1**, 188.

Aukland, K. (1968). Vasopressin and intrarenal blood flow distribution. *Acta Physiol. Scand.* **74**, 173.

Aukland, K., and Berliner, R. W. (1964). Renal medullary countercurrent system studied with hydrogen gas. *Circulation Res.* **15**, 430.

Aukland, K., and Krogh, J. (1960). Renal oxygen tension. *Nature (London)* **188**, 671.

Aukland, K., and Wolgast, M. (1968). Effect of hemorrhage and retransfusion on intrarenal distribution of blood flow in dogs. *J. Clin. Invest.* **47**, 488.

Bálint, P., and Fekete, A. (1960). Das Verhalten des Minutenvolumens und der Nierendurchblutung bei stagnierender Hypoxie. *Arch. Ges. Physiol.* **270**, 575.

Bálint, P., and Forgács, I. (1966). Natriumreabsorption und Sauerstoffverbrauch der Niere bei osmotischer Belastung. *Arch. Ges. Physiol.* **288**, 332.

Bálint, P., Fekete, A., and Forgács, I. (1964). Quantitative considerations on the storage of clearance substances in the kidney. *Clin. Sci.* **26**, 345.

Bálint, P., Forgács, I., and Palásti, E. (1965). Renal responses to different forms of arterial hypotension. *Acta Physiol. Acad. Sci. Hung.* **27**, 33.

Barajas, L., and Latta, H. (1963). A three-dimensional study of the juxtaglomerular apparatus in the rat. *Lab Invest.* **12**, 257.

Barclay, J. A., Cooke, W. T., and Kenney, R. A. (1947). Observations on the effects of adrenaline on renal function and circulation in man. *Am. J. Physiol.* **151**, 621.

Barer, G. R. (1963). The action of vasopressin, a vasopressin analogue (PLV₂) oxytocin, angiotensin, bradykinin and theophylline ethylene diamine on renal blood flow in unaesthetized cat. *J. Physiol. (London)* **169**, 62.

Basar, E., Tischner, H., and Weiss, C. (1968). Untersuchungen zur Dynamik druckinduzierter Änderungen des Strömungswiderstandes der autoregulierenden, isolierten Rattenniere. *Pfluegers Arch. Ges. Physiol.* **299**, 191.

Bell, R. D., Keyl, M. J., Shrader, F. R., Jones, E. W., and Henry, L. P. (1968). Renal lymphatics: the internal distribution. *Nephron* **5**, 454.

Bell, R. D., Keyl, M. J., and Shrader, F. R. (1969). Effects of renal medullary concentrating ability on canine renal lymph composition. *Am. J. Physiol.* **216**, 4.

Belleau, L. J., and Earley, L. E. (1967). Autoregulation of renal blood flow in the presence of angiotensin infusion. *Am. J. Physiol.* **213**, 1590.

Berliner, R. W., and Bennett, C. M. (1967). Concentration of urine in the mammalian kidney. *Am. J. Med.* **42**, 777.

Berliner, R. W., Levinsky, N. G., Davidson, D. G., and Eden, M. (1958). Dilution and concentration of the urine and the action of antidiuretic hormone. *Am. J. Med.* **24**, 730.

Berne, R. M. (1952). Hemodynamics and sodium excretion of denervated kidney in anaesthetized and unanaesthetized dogs. *Am. J. Physiol.* **171**, 148.

Bethge, H. B., Ochwadt, B., and Weber, R. (1962). Der scheinbare Verteilungsraum von 131-J Albumin in verschiedenen Schichten der Niere bei Diurese und Antidiurese. *Arch. Ges. Physiol.* **276**, 236.

Birkeland, S., Vogt, A., Krog, J., and Semb, C. (1959). Renal circulatory occlusion and local cooling. *J. Appl. Physiol.* **14**, 227.

Blackmore, W. P. (1958). Effect of serotonin on renal hemodynamics and sodium excretion in the dog. *Am. J. Physiol.* **193**, 639.

Blake, W. D., Wégria, R., Keating, R. P., and Ward, H. P. (1949). Effect of increased renal venous pressure on renal function. *Am. J. Physiol.* **157**, 1.

Block, M. A., Wakim, K. G., and Mann, F. C. (1952). Circulation through the kidney during stimulation of the renal nerves. *Am. J. Physiol.* **169**, 659.

Bock, K. D., and Krecke, H. J. (1958). Die Wirkung von synthetischem Hypertensin II auf die PAH- und Inulin-Clearance, die renale Hämodynamik und die Diurese beim Menschen. *Klin. Wochschr.* **36**, 69.

Bohle, A. (1954). Kritischer Beitrag zur Morphologie einer endokrinen Nierenfunktion und deren Bedeutung für den Hochdruck. *Arch. Kreislaufforsch.* **20**, 193.

Bricker, N. S., Guild, W. R., Reardan, J. B., and Merrill, J. P. (1956). Studies of the functional capacity of a denervated homotransplanted kidney in an identical twin with parallel observation in the donor. *J. Clin. Invest.* **35**, 1364.

Brun, C., Crone, C., Davidsen, H. G., Fabricius, J., Hansen, A. T., Lassen, N. A., and Munck, O. (1956). Renal interstitial pressure in normal and anuric man: based on wedged renal vein pressure. *Proc. Soc. Exptl. Biol. Med.* **91**, 199.

Bucher, O., and Reale, E. (1961). Zur elektronenmikroskopischen Untersuchung der juxtaglomerulären Spezialeinrichtungen der Niere. II. Über die Macula densa des Mittelstücks. *Z. Mikroskop.-Anat. Forsch.* **67**, 514.

Bucher, O., and Reale, E. (1962). Zur elektronenmikroskopischen Untersuchung der juxtaglomerulären Spezialeinrichtungen der Niere. III. Mitteilung: Die epitheloiden Zellen der arteriola afferens. *Z. Zellforsch. Mikroskop. Anat.* **56**, 344.

Burn, J. H., and Hutcheon, D. E. (1949). Action of noradrenaline. *Brit. J. Pharmacol.* **4**, 373.

Burton-Opitz, R., and Lucas, D. R. (1911). *J. Exptl. Med.* **13**, 308.

Cargill, W. H., and Hickam, J. B. (1949). The oxygen consumption of the normal and the diseased human kidney. *J. Clin. Invest.* **28**, 526.

Carrière, S., Thorburn, G. D., O'Morchoe, C. C. C., and Barger, C. A. (1966). Intrarenal distribution of blood flow in dogs during hemorrhagic hypotension. *Circulation Res.* **19**, 167.

Castenfors, J. (1967). Renal function during exercise. *Acta Physiol. Scand.* **70**, Suppl. 293.

Celander, O. (1954). Range of control exercised by the sympathoco-adrenal system. *Acta Physiol. Scand.* **32**, 116.

Chinard, F. P., Enns, T., and Nolan, M. F. (1964). Arterial hematocrit and separation of cells and plasma in the dog kidney. *Am. J. Physiol.* **207**, 128.

Cockett, A. T. K., Roberts, A. P., and Moore, R. S. (1969). Renal lymphatic transport of fluid and solutes. *Invest. Urol.* **7**, 10.

Cook, W. F. (1968). The detection of renin in juxtaglomerular cells. *J. Physiol. (London)* **194**, 73.

Corcoran, A. C., and Page, I. H. (1939). The effect of renin, pitressin, and pitressin and atropine on renal blood flow and clearance. *Am. J. Physiol.* **126**, 354.

Corcoran, A. C., and Page, I. H. (1947). Renal hemodynamic effects of adrenaline and isuprel. *Proc. Soc. Exptl. Biol. Med.* **66**, 148.

Cortney, M. A., Nagel, W., and Thurau, K. (1966). A micropuncture study of the relationship between flow-rate through the loop of Henle and sodium concentration in the distal tubule. *Arch. Ges. Physiol.* **287**, 286.

Crosley, A. P., Castillo, C., and Rowe, G. G. (1961). The relationship of renal oxygen consumption to renal function and weight in individuals with normal and diseased kidneys. *J. Clin. Invest.* **40**, 836.

Deetjen, P. (1968). Normal and critical oxygen supply of the kidney. In: "Oxygen Transport in Blood and Tissue." p. 212. (H. Lübbers, ed.) Thieme, Stuttgart.

Deetjen, P., and Kramer, K. (1961). Die Abhängigkeit des O_2-Verbrauchs der Niere von der Na-Rückresorption. *Arch. Ges. Physiol.* **273**, 636.

Deetjen, P., Brechtelsbauer, H., and Kramer, K. (1964). Hämodynamik des Nierenmarks. III. Mitteilung: Farbstoffpassagezeiten in äußerer Markzone und V. renalis. Die Durchblutungsverteilung in der Niere. *Arch. Ges. Physiol.* **279**, 281.

Diamond, J. M. (1969). The coupling of solute and water transport in epithelia. *In* "Renal Transport and Diuretics" (K. Thurau and H. Jahrmärker, eds.). Springer, Berlin.

Dietrich, H. J. (1968). Die Ultrastruktur der Gefäßbündel im Mark der Rattenniere. *Z. Zellforsch. Mikroskop. Anat.* **84**, 350.

Dunihue, F. W. (1941). Effect of cellophane perinephritis on the granular cells of the juxtaglomerular apparatus. *Arch. Pathol.* **32**, 211.

Dutz, H., and Kretzschmar, G. (1954). Die Veränderungen in der Funktion beider Nieren nach einseitiger vollständiger Ischämie. *Z. Ges. Exptl. Med.* **123**, 497.

Edelman, R., and Hartroft, P. M. (1961). Localization of renin in juxtaglomerular cells of rabbit and dog through the use of the fluorescent antibody techniques. *Circulation Res.* **9**, 1069.

Eggleton, M. G., Pappenheimer, J. R., and Winton, F. R. (1940). The influence of diuretics on the osmotic work done and on the efficiency of the isolated kidney of the dog. *J. Physiol. (London)* **97**, 363.

Eisner, G. M., Slotkoff, L. M., and Lilienfield, L. S. (1964). Sodium reabsorption and oxygen consumption in the human kidney. *Proc. 2nd Intern. Congr. Nephrol., Prague* p. 118. Excerpta Med. Found., Amsterdam.

Emery, E. W., Gowenlock, A. M., Riddel, A. G., and Black, D. A. K. (1959). Intrarenal variations in haematocrit. *Clin. Sci.* **18**, 205.

Engelhorn, R. (1957). Aktionspotentiale der Nierennerven. *Arch. Exptl. Pathol. Pharmakol.* **231**, 219.

Enger, R., Gerstner, H., and Sarre, H. (1937). Die Abhängigkeit der Nierendurchblutung vom Ureterendruck. *Zentr. Inn. Med.* **58**, 865.

Faarup, P. (1965). On the morphology of the juxtaglomerular apparatus. *Acta Anat.* **60**, 20.

Fajers, C. M. (1955). On the effect of brief unilateral renal ischemia. *Acta Pathol. Microbiol. Scand. Suppl.* **106**.

Folkow, B., and Langston, J. (1964). The interrelationship of some factors influencing renal blood flow autoregulation. *Acta Physiol. Scand.* **61**, 165.

Forster, R. P., and Maes, J. P. (1947). Effects of experimental neurogenic hypertension on renal blood flow and glomerular filtration rates in intact denervated kidneys of unanesthetized rabbits with adrenal glands demedullated. *Am. J. Physiol.* **150**, 534.

Fourman, J., and Kennedy, G. C. (1966). An effect of antidiuretic hormone on the flow of blood through the vasa recta of the rat kidney. *J. Endocrinol.* **35**, 173.

Franklin, K. J., McGee, L. E., and Ullmann, E. A. (1951). Effects of severe asphyxia on the kidney and urine flow. *J. Physiol. (London)* **112**, 43.

Freeman, O. W., Mitchell, G. W., Wilson, J. S., Fitzhugh, F. W., and Merrill, A. J. (1955). Renal hemodynamics, sodium and water excretion in supine exercising normal and cardiac patients. *J. Clin. Invest.* **34**, 1109.

Friedman, M., Johnson, R. L., and Friedman, C. L. (1954). The pattern of recovery of renal function following renal artery occlusion in the dog. *Circulation Res.* **2**, 231.

Gärtner, K. (1966). Das Volumen der interstitiellen Flüssigkeit der Niere bei Änderungen ihres hämodynamischen Widerstandes; Untersuchungen am Kaninchen. *Arch. Ges. Physiol.* **292**, 1.

Gertz, K. H., Mangos, J. A., Braun, G., and Pagel, H. D. (1965). On the glomerular tubular balance in the rat kidney. *Arch. Ges. Physiol.* **285**, 360.

Gertz, K. H., Mangos, J. A., Braun, G., and Pagel, H. D. (1966). Pressure in the glomerular capillaries of the rat kidney and its relation to arterial blood pressure. *Arch. Ges. Physiol.* **288**, 369.

Gertz, K. H., Brandis, M., Braun-Schubert, G., and Boylan, J. W. (1969). The effect of saline infusion and hemorrhage on glomerular filtration pressure and single nephron filtration rate. *Arch. Ges. Physiol.* **310**, 193.

Gilmore, J. P. (1964a). Influence of tissue pressure on renal blood flow autoregulation. *Am. J. Physiol.* **206**, 707.

Gilmore, J. P. (1964b). Renal vascular resistance during elevated ureteral pressure. *Circulation Res. Suppl.* **1**, 148.

Gilmore, J. P. (1964c). Contribution of baroreceptors to the control of renal function. *Circulation Res.* **14**, 301.

Girndt, J., and Ochwadt, B. (1969). Durchblutung des Nierenmarks, Gesamtnierendurchblutung und cortico-medulläre Gradienten beim experimentellen renalen Hochdruck der Ratte. *Arch. Ges. Physiol.* **313**, 30.

Goodwin, W. E., and Kaufman, J. J. (1956). The renal lymphatics. I. Review of some of the pertinent literature. *Urol. Surv.* **6**, 305.

Goodyer, A. V. N., and Glenn, W. W. L. (1951). Relation of arterial pulse pressure to renal function. *Am. J. Physiol.* **167**, 689.

Goormaghtigh, N. (1937). L'appareil neuromyoartériel juxtaglomérulaire du rein: ses reactions en pathologie et ses rapports avec le tube urinifère. *Compt. Rend. Soc. Biol.* **124**, 293.

Goormaghtigh, N. (1945). Facts in favour of an endocrine function of the renal arterioles. *J. Pathol. Bacteriol.* **57**, 392.

Gottschalk, C. W. (1952). A comparative study of renal interstitial pressure. *Am. J. Physiol.* **169**, 180.

Gottschalk, C. W., and Leyssac, P. P. (1968). Proximal tubular function in rats with low inulin clearance. *Acta Physiol. Scand.* **74**, 453.

Gottschalk, C. W., and Mylle, M. (1956). Micropuncture study of pressures in proximal tubules and peritubular capillaries of the rat kidney and their relation to ureteral and venous pressures. *Am. J. Physiol.* **185**, 430.

Gottschalk, C. W., and Mylle, M. (1957). Micropuncture study of pressures in proximal and distal tubules and peritubular capillaries of the rat kidney during osmotic diuresis. *Am. J. Physiol.* **189**, 323.

Gottschalk, C. W., Lassiter, W. E., and Mylle, M. (1962). Studies of the composition of vasa recta plasma in the hamster kidney. *Excerpta Med. Found. Intern. Congr. Ser.* **47**, 375.

Gregg, D. E. (1962). Hemodynamic factors in shock. *In* "Shock-Pathogenesis and Therapy" (K. D. Bock, ed.). Springer, Berlin.

Gross, F., Schaechtelin, G., Brunner, H., and Peters, G. (1963). The role of the renin-angiotensin system in blood pressure regulation and kidney function. *Can. Med. Assoc. J.* **90**, 258.

Grupp, G., and Heimpel, H. (1958). Zum Problem der "reaktiven Hyperämie" der Niere. *Arch. Ges. Physiol.* **267**, 426.

Grupp, G., Heimpel, H., and Hierholzer, K. (1959). Über die Autoregulation der Nierendurchblutung. *Arch. Ges. Physiol.* **269**, 149.

Guyton, A. C., Langston, J. B., and Navar, G. (1964). Theory for renal autoregulation by feedback of the juxtaglomerular apparatus. *Circulation Res.* **14/15**, Suppl. 1, 187.

Haddy, F. J., and Scott, J. B. (1965). Role of transmural pressure in local regulation of blood flow through kidney. *Am. J. Physiol.* **208**, 825.

Haining, J. L., and Turner, M. D. (1966). Tissue blood flow in rat kidneys by hydrogen desaturation. *J. Appl. Physiol.* **21**, 1705.

Hanssen, O. E. (1961). The relationship between glomerular filtration and length of proximal convoluted tubules in mice. *Acta Pathol. Microbiol. Scand.* **53**, 265.

Harsing, L., and Pessey, K. (1965). Die Bestimmung der Nierenmarkdurchblutung auf Grund der Ablagerung und Verteilung von ^{86}Rb. *Arch. Ges. Physiol.* **285**, 302.

Hartroft, P. M. (1963). Juxtaglomerular cells. *Circulation Res.* **12**, 525.

Harvey, R. B. (1966). Effects of acetylcholine infused into renal artery of dogs. *Am. J. Physiol.* **211**, 487.

Hatt, P. Y. (1966). L'appareil juxtaglomérulaire. *Presse Med.* **74**, 2269.

Heidenreich, O., Keller, P., and Kook, Y. (1964). Wie Wirkungen von Bradykinin und Kallidin auf die Nierenfunktion des Hundes. *Arch. Exp. Pathol. Pharmakol.* **247**, 243.

Horster, M., and Thurau, K. (1968). Micropuncture studies on the filtration rate of single superficial and juxtamedullary glomeruli in the rat kidney. *Arch. Ges. Physiol.* **301**, 162.

Horster, M., Schnermann, J., and Thurau, K. (1969). Die Funktion der juxtamedullären Nephrone in Wasserdiurese und ADH-induzierter Antidiurese. *Symp. Ges. Nephrol.*, *4th, Vienna, 1968* Verlag Wien. Med. Akad., Vienna.

Houck, C. R. (1951). Alteration of renal hemodynamics and function in separate kidneys during stimulation of the renal artery nerves in dogs. *Am. J. Physiol.* **167**, 523.

Kaiserling, H., and Soostmeyer, T. (1939). Die Bedeutung des Nierenlymphgefäβsystems für die Nierenfunktion. *Wien. Klin. Wochschr.* **52**, 1113.

Kaplan, A., Friedman, M., and Krieger, H. E. (1943). Observation concerning the origin of renal lymph. *Am. J. Physiol.* **138**, 553.

Kiil, F., and Aukland, K. (1961). Renal concentration mechanism and hemodynamics at increased ureteral pressure during osmotic and saline diuresis. *Scand. J. Clin. Lab. Invest.* **13**, 276.

Kiil, F., Aukland, K., and Refsum, H. E. (1961). Renal sodium transport and oxygen consumption. *Am. J. Physiol.* **201**, 511.

Koch, K. M., Dume, T., Krause, H. H., and Ochwadt, B. (1967). Intratubulärer Druck, glomerulärer Capillardruck und Glomerulumfiltrat während Mannit-Diurese. *Arch. Ges. Physiol.* **295**, 72.

Koch, K. M., Aynedjian, H. S., and Bank, N. (1968). Effect of acute hypertension on sodium reabsorption by the proximal tubule. *J. Clin. Invest.* **47**, 1696.

Korner, P. I. (1963a). Renal blood flow, glomerular filtration rate, renal PAH extraction ratio, and the role of the renal vasomotor nerves in the unanesthetized rabbit. *Circulation Res.* **12**, 353.

Korner, P. I. (1963b). Effects of low oxygen and of carbon monoxide on the renal circulation in unanesthetized rabbits. *Circulation Res.* **12**, 361.

Kramer, K. (1952). Zur Vasomotorik des intrarenalen Kreislaufs. *Sitzgsber. Ges. Befoerder. Ges. Naturw. Marburg* **75**, 26.

Kramer, K. (1959). Die Stellung der Niere im Gesamtkreislauf. *Verhandl. Deut. Ges. Inn. Med.* **65**, 225.

Kramer, K. (1962). Das akute Nierenversagen im Schock. *In* "Schock, Pathogenese und Therapie" (K. D. Bock, ed.). Springer, Berlin.

Kramer, K., and Deetjen, P. (1960). Beziehungen des O_2-Verbrauchs der Niere zu Durchblutung und Glomerulumfiltrat bei Änderung des arteriellen Druckes. *Arch. Ges. Physiol.* **271**, 782.

Kramer, K., and Deetjen, P. (1963). Oxygen Consumption and Sodium Reabsorption in the Mammalian Kidney. *In* "Symposium on Oxygen" (F. Dickens and E. Neil, eds.), p. 411. Macmillan (Pergamon), New York.

Kramer, K., and Winton, F. R. (1939). The influence of urea and of change in arterial pressure on the O_2 consumption of the isolated kidney of the dog. *J. Physiol. (London)* — 96, 87.

Kramer, K., Thurau, K., and Deetjen, P. (1960). Hämodynamik des Nierenmarks. I. Mitteilung: Capilläre Passagezeit, Durchblutung, Gewebshämatokrit und O_2-Verbrauch des Nierenmarks in situ. *Arch. Ges. Physiol.* 270, 251.

Krause, H. H., Dume, T. Koch, K. M., and Ochwadt, B. (1967). Intratubulärer Druck, glomerulärer Capillardruck und Glomerulumfiltrat nach Furosemid und Hydrochlorothiazid. *Arch. Ges. Physiol.* 295, 80.

Kriz, W. (1967). Der architektonische und funktionelle Aufbau der Rattenniere. *Z. Zellforsch. Mikroskop. Anat.* 82, 495.

Kuhn, W., and Ramel, A. (1959). Aktiver Salztransport als möglicher (und wahrscheinlicher) Einzeleffekt bei der Harnkonzentrierung in der Niere. *Helv. Chim. Acta* 42, 628.

Landis, E. M. (1926). The capillary pressure in frog mesentery as determined by microinjection methods. *Am. J. Physiol.* 75, 548.

Lassen, N. A., Longley, J. B., and Lilienfield, L. S. (1958). Concentration of albumin in renal papilla. *Science* 128, 720.

Lassen, N. A., Munck, O., and Thaysen, J. H. (1961). Oxygen consumption and sodium reabsorption in the kidney. *Acta Physiol. Scand.* 51, 371.

LeBrie, S. J. (1968). Renal lymph and osmotic diuresis. *Am. J. Physiol.* 215, 116.

LeBrie, S. J., and Mayerson, H. S. (1959). Composition of renal lymph and its significance. *Proc. Soc. Exptl. Biol. Med.* 100, 378.

Lever, A. F. (1965). The vasa recta and countercurrent multiplication. *Acta Med. Scand.* 178, Suppl. 434, 1.

Lever, A. F., and Peart, W. S. (1962). Renin and angiotensin-like activity in renal lymph. *J. Physiol. (London)* 160, 548.

Levy, M. N., and Imperial, E. S. (1961). Oxygen shunting in renal cortical and medullary capillaries. *Am. J. Physiol.* 200, 159.

Levy, M. N., and Sauceda, G. (1959). Diffusion of oxygen from arterial to venous segments of renal capillaries. *Am. J. Physiol.* 196, 1336.

Liebau, G., Levine, D. Z., and Thurau, K. (1968). Micropuncture studies on the dog kidney. I. The response of the proximal tubule to changes in systemic blood pressure within and below the autoregulatory range. *Arch. Ges. Physiol.* 304, 57.

Lilienfield, L. S., and Rose, J. C. (1958). Effect of blood pressure alterations on intrarenal red cell-plasma separation. *J. Clin. Invest.* 37, 1106.

Lilienfield, L. S., Rose, J. C., and Porfido, F. A. (1957). Evidence for a red cell shunting mechanism in the kidney. *Circulation Res.* 5, 64.

Lilienfield, L. S., Rose, J. C., and Lassen, N. A. (1958). Diverse distribution of red cells and albumin in the dog kidney. *Circulation Res.* 6, 810.

Lilienfield, L. S., Maganzini, H. C., and Bauer, M. H. (1961). Blood flow in the renal medulla. *Circulation Res.* 9, 614.

Ljungqvist, A. (1964). Structure of the arteriole-glomerular units in different zones of the kidney. Micro-angiographic and histologic evidence of an extraglomerular medullary circulation. *Nephron* 1, 329.

Lochner, W., and Ochwadt, B. (1954). Über die Beziehung zwischen arteriellem Druck, Durchblutung, Durchflußzeit und Blutfüllung an der isolierten Hundeniere. *Arch. Ges. Physiol.* 258, 275.

Longley, J. B., Banfield, W. G., and Brindley, D. C. (1960). Structure of the rete mirabile in the kidney of the rat as seen with the electron microscope. *J. Biophys. Biochem. Cytol.* **7**, 103.

Lowitz, H. D., Stumpe, K. O., and Ochwadt, B. (1968). Natrium- und Wasserresorption in den verschiedenen Abschnitten des Nephrons beim experimentellen renalen Hochdruck der Ratte. *Arch. Ges. Physiol.* **304**, 322.

Malnic, G., Klose, R. M., and Giebisch, G. (1966). Micropuncture study of distal tubular potassium and sodium transport in rat nephron. *Am. J. Physiol.* **211**, 529.

Marson, F. G. (1956). Effect of noradrenaline on urine and renal blood flow. *Brit. J. Pharmacol.* **11**, 431.

Mayerson, H. S. (1963). The physiologic importance of lymph. *In* "Handbook of Physiology Vol. II: Circulation" (W. F. Hamilton, P. Dow, eds.) p. 1055. American Physiol. Society, Washington, D.C.

Mehrizi, A., and Hamilton, W. F. (1959). Effect of levarterenol on renal blood flow and vascular volume in dogs. *Am. J. Physiol.* **197**, 1115.

Meier, M., Brechtelsbauer, H., and Kramer, K. (1964). Hämodynamik des Nierenmarks. IV. Mitteilung: Farbstoffverdünnungskurven in verschiedenen Abschnitten des Nierenmarks. *Arch. Ges. Physiol.* **279**, 294.

Mertz, D. P. (1963). Renotrope Wirkungen von synthetischem Bradykinin. *Arch. Exptl. Pathol. Pharmakol.* **244**, 405.

Michailowitsch, V. (1918). Wie verhält sich der aufsteigende Schenkel der Henle'schen Schleife zum Corpusculum renis. Unpublished dissertation, Univ. of Bern, Bern, Switzerland.

Miles, B. E., and de Wardener, H. E. (1954). Intrarenal pressure. *J. Physiol. (London)* **123**, 131.

Miles, B. E., Ventom, M. G., and de Wardener, H. E. (1954). Observations on the mechanism of circulatory autoregulation in the perfused dog's kidney. *J. Physiol. (London)* **123**, 143.

Moffat, D. B. (1967). The fine structure of the blood vessels of the renal medulla with particular reference to the control of the medullary circulation. *J. Ultrastruct. Res.* **19**, 532.

Moffat, D. B., and Fourman, J. (1963). The vascular pattern of the rat kidney. *J. Anat.* **97**, 543.

Morgan, T., and Berliner, R. W. (1969). A study by continuous microperfusion of water and electrolyte movements in the loop of Henle and distal tubule of the rat. *Nephron* **6**, 388.

Nahmod, V. E., and Lanari, A. (1964). Abolition of autoregulation of renal blood flow by acetylcholine. *Am. J. Physiol.* **207**, 123.

Nash, F. D., and Selkurt, E. E. (1964). Effects of elevated ureteral pressure on renal blood flow. *Circulation Res.* **14/15**, Suppl. 1, 142.

Neely, W. A., and Turner, M. D. (1959). The effect of arterial, venous, and arteriovenous occlusion on renal blood flow. *Surg. Gynecol. Obstet.* **108**, 669.

Ng, K. K. F., and Vane, J. R. (1967). Conversion of angiotensin I to angiotensin II. *Nature* **216**, 762.

Ochwadt, B. (1956). Zur Selbststeuerung des Nierenkreislaufes. *Arch. Ges. Physiol.* **262**, 207.

Ochwadt, B. (1957). Durchflußzeiten von Plasma und Erythrocyten, intrarenaler Hämatokrit und Widerstandsregulation der isolierten Niere. *Arch. Ges. Physiol.* **265**, 112.

Ochwadt, B. (1964). The measurement of intrarenal blood flow distribution by wash-out technique. *Proc. 2nd Intern. Congr. Nephrol., Prague* p. 62. Excerpta Med. Found., Amsterdam.

Okino, H., and Spencer, M. P. (1961). Analysis of the dynamic pressure flow relationship in renal artery. *Federation Proc.* **20**, 109.

Pappenheimer, J. R. (1941). Blood flow, arterial oxygen saturation, and oxygen consumption in the isolated perfused hindlimb of the dog. *J. Physiol. (London)* **99**, 283.

Pappenheimer, J. R. (1955). Über die Permeabilität der Glomerulummembranen in der Niere. *Klin. Wochschr.* **33**, 362.

Pappenheimer, J. R., and Kinter, W. B. (1956). Hematocrit ratio of blood within mammalian kidney and its significance for renal hemodynamics. *Am. J. Physiol.* **185**, 377.

Passow, H., Schniewind, H., and Weiss, C. (1960). Die Wirkung von 5-Hydroxytryptamin auf das Gefäβsystem der isolierten Rattennieren. *Arch. Exptl. Pathol. Pharmakol.* **240**, 179.

Perlmutt, J. H. (1963). Reflex antidiuresis after occlusion of common carotid arteries in hydrated dogs. *Am. J. Physiol.* **204**, 197.

Peter, K. (1927). "Untersuchungen über Bau und Entwicklung der Niere." Gustav Fischer Verlag, Jena.

Phillips, R. A., and Hamilton, P. B. (1948). Effect of 20, 60 and 120 minutes of renal ischemia on glomerular and tubular function. *Am. J. Physiol.* **152**, 523.

Pilkington, L. A., Binder, R., de Haas, J. C. M., and Pitts, R. F. (1965). Intrarenal distribution of blood flow. *Am. J. Physiol.* **208**, 1107.

Pinter, G. G., O'Morchoe, C. C. C., and Sikand, R. S. Effect of acetylcholine on urinary electrolyte excretion. (1964). *Am. J. Physiol.* **207**, 979.

Plakke, R. K., and Pfeiffer, E. W. (1964). Blood vessels of the mammalian renal medulla. *Science* **146**, 1683.

Polosa, C., and Hamilton, W. F. (1962). The relation between cells and plasma within the renal vasculature. *Arch. Intern. Pharmacodyn. Therap.* **140**, 294.

Rein, H. (1931). Vasomotorische Regulationen. *Ergeb. Physiol. Biol. Chem. Exptl. Pharmakol.* **32**, 28.

Reubi, F. (1960). "Nierenkrankheiten" Huber, Bern.

Reubi, F., Gossweiler, N., and Gürtler, R. (1966). Renal circulation in man studied by means of a dye-dilution method. *Circulation* **33**, 426.

Riedel, B., and Bucher, O. (1967). Die Ultrastruktur des juxtaglomerulären Apparates des Meerschweinchens. *Z. Zellforsch. Mikroskop. Anat.* **79**, 244.

Ritter, E. R. (1952). Pressure flow relations in the kidney. Alleged effects of pulse pressure. *Am. J. Physiol.* **168**, 480.

Rollhäuser, H., Kriz, W., and Heinke, W. (1964). Das Gefäβsystem der Rattenniere. *Z. Zellforsch. Mikroskop. Anat.* **64**, 381.

Roof, B. S., Lauson, H. D., Bella, S. T., and Eder, H. A. (1951). Recovering of glomerular and tubular function, including PAH-extraction, following two hours of renal artery occlusion in the dog. *Am. J. Physiol.* **166**, 666.

Rusznyak, I., Földi, M., and Szabo, G. (1967). "Lymphatics and Lymph Circulation." Macmillan (Pergamon), New York.

Ruyter, J. H. C. (1925). Über einen merkwürdigen Abschnitt der vasa afferentia der Mäuseniere. *Z. Zellforsch. Mikroskop. Anat.* **2**, 242.

Sarre, H., and Ansorge, H. (1939). Über die reaktive Hyperämie der Niere. *Arch. Ges. Physiol.* **242**, 79.

Schirmeister, J., Schmidt, L., and Söling, H. D. (1962). Über die Autoregulation des Glomerulumfiltrates bei intratubulärem Druckanstieg am Hund. *Klin. Wochschr.* **40**, 884.

Schirmeister, J., Decot, M., Hallauer, W., and Willmann, H. (1966). β-Receptoren und renale Hämodynamik des Menschen. *Arzneimittel-Forsch.* **16**, 847.

Schloss, G. (1945–1946). Der Regulationsapparat am Gefäßpol des Nierenkörperchens in der normalen menschlichen Niere. *Acta Anat.* **1**, 365.

Schmid-Schönbein, H., Wells, R. E., and Goldstone, J. (1969). Influence of deformability of human red cells upon blood viscosity. *Circulation Res.* **25**, 131.

Schnermann, J., Nagel, W., and Thurau, K. (1966). Die frühdistale Natriumkonzentration in Rattennieren nach renaler Ischämie und hömorrhagischer Hypotension. *Arch. Ges. Physiol.* **287**, 296.

Schnermann, J., Horster, M., and Levine, D. Z. (1969). The Influence of sampling technique on the micropuncture determination of GFR and reabsorptive characteristics of single rat proximal tubules. *Arch. Ges. Physiol.* **309**, 48.

Schnermann, J., Wright, F. S., Davis, J. M., von Stackelberg, W., and Grill, G. (1970). Regulation of superficial nephron filtration rate by tubulo-glomerular feedback. *Arch. Ges. Physiol.* **318**, 147.

Schröder, R. (1963). Die Beeinflussung der Angiotensinwirkung auf die renale Elektrolyt- und Wasserausscheidung durch Aldosteronvorbehandlung. *Klin. Wochschr.* **41**, 620.

Selkurt, E. E. (1946). Renal blood flow and renal clearance during hemorrhagic shock. *Am. J. Physiol.* **145**, 699.

Selkurt, E. E. (1951). Effect of pulse pressure and mean arterial pressure modification on renal hemodynamics and electrolyte and water excretion. *Circulation* **4**, 541.

Selkurt, E. E. (1962). Nierendurchblutung und renale Clearances bei Blutverlust und im hämorrhagischen Schock. *In* "Schock-Pathogenese und Therapie" (K. D. Bock, ed.) Springer, Berlin.

Selkurt, E. E. (1963). The renal circulation. *In* "Handbook of Physiology. Vol. II: Circulation" (W. F. Hamilton, P. Dow, eds.) p. 1457. Amer. Physiol. Soc., Washington, D. C.

Selkurt, E. E., Hall, P. W., and Spencer, M. P. (1949). Influence of graded arterial pressure decrement on renal clearance of creatinine, p-aminohippurate and sodium. *Am. J. Physiol.* **159**, 369.

Selkurt, E. E., Elpers, M. J., Womack, I., and Dailey, W. N. (1963). Effect of ureteral blockade on renal blood flow and urinary concentrating ability. *Am. J. Physiol.* **205**, 286.

Selkurt, E. E., Womack, I., and Dailey, W. N. (1965). Mechanism of natriuresis and diuresis during elevated renal arterial pressure. *Am. J. Physiol.* **209**, 95.

Semple, S. J. G., and de Wardener, H. E. (1959). Effect of increased renal venous pressure on circulatory autoregulation of isolated dog kidneys. *Circulation Res.* **7**, 643.

Shave, L. (1952). Effect of increased ureteral pressure on renal function. *Am. J. Physiol.* **168**, 97.

Shipley, R. E., and Study, R. S. (1951). Changes in renal blood flow, extraction of inulin, glomerular filtration rate, tissue pressure and urine flow with acute alterations of renal arterial blood pressure. *Am. J. Physiol.* **167**, 676.

Slotkoff, L. M., Eisner, G. M., and Lilienfield, L. S. (1968). Functional separation of renal cortical-medullary circulation: significance of Diodrast extraction. *Am. J. Physiol.* **214**, 935.

Smith, H. W. (1951). "The Kidney. Structure and Function in Health and Disease." Oxford Univ. Press, London and New York.

Somlay, L., Thron, H. L., Petran, K., and Carl, G. (1962). Die Nierenfunktion während doppelseitiger Carotisabklemmung am wachen Hund. *Arch. Ges. Physiol.* **276**, 117.

Spencer, M. P. (1956). The renal vascular response to vasodepressor sympathomimetics. *J. Pharmacol. Exptl. Therap.* **116**, 237.

Spencer, M. P., Denison, A. B., and Green, H. D. (1954). Direct renal vascular effects of epinephrine and norepinephrine before and after adrenergic blockade. *Circulation Res.* **2**, 537.

Spinazzola, A. J., and Sherrod, T. R. (1957). The effect of serotonin (5-hydroxytryptamine) on renal hemodynamics. *J. Pharmacol. Exptl. Therap.* **119**, 114.

Strauss, J., Beran, A. V., Brown, C. T., and Katurich, N. (1968). Renal oxygenation under normal conditions. *Am. J. Physiol.* **215**, 1482.

Study, R. S., and Shipley, R. E. (1950). Comparison of direct with indirect renal blood flow, extraction of inulin and Diodrast before and during acute renal nerve stimulation. *Am. J. Physiol.* **163**, 442.

Swann, H. G. (1964). Some aspects of renal blood flow and tissue pressure. *Circulation Res.* **14/15**, 1.

Takeuchi, J., Kubo, T., Sawada, T., Funaki, E., Sanada, M., Kitagawa, T., and Nakada, Y. (1965). Autoregulation of renal circulation. *Japan. Heart J.* **6**, 243.

Thompson, D. D., Kavaler, F., Lozano, R., and Pitts, R. F. (1957). Evaluation of the cell separation hypothesis of autoregulation of renal blood flow and filtration rate. *Am. J. Physiol.* **191**, 493.

Thorburn, G. D., Kopald, H. H., Herd, J. A., Hollenberg, M., O'Morchoe, C. C. C., and Barger, A. C. (1963). Intrarenal distribution of nutrient blood flow determined with krypton[85] in the unanesthetized dog. *Circulation Res.* **13**, 290.

Thurau, K. (1961). Renal sodium reabsorption and O_2 uptake in dogs during hypoxia and hydrochlorothiazide infusion. *Proc. Soc. Exptl. Biol. Med.* **106**, 714.

Thurau, K. (1963). Fundamentals of renal circulation. *Proc. 2nd Intern. Congr. Nephrol., Prague* 1963, p. 51. Excerpta Med. Found., Amsterdam.

Thurau, K. (1964a). Diskussion *In* "Kreislaufmessungen" (A. Fleckenstein, ed.) p. 182. Werkverlag Dr. Edmund Banaschewski, Muenchen-Graefelfing.

Thurau, K. (1964b). Renal hemodynamics. *Am. J. Med.* **36**, 698.

Thurau, K. (1964c). Autoregulation of RBF and GFR including data on tubular and peritubular capillary pressure and vessel wall tension. *Circulation Res.* **14/15**, Suppl. 1, 132.

Thurau, K. (1967a). The nature of autoregulation of renal blood flow. *Proc. 3rd Intern. Congr. Nephrol., Washington, D.C.* (J. S. Handler, ed.), Vol. 1, p. 62. Huber, Basel.

Thurau, K. (1967b). Blutkreislauf der Niere. *Verhandl. Deut. Ges. Kreislaufforsch.* **33**, 1.

Thurau, K., and Deetjen, P. (1962). Die Diurese bei arteriellen Drucksteigerungen. Bedeutung der Hämodynamik des Nierenmarkes für die Harnkonzentrierung. Mit einem theoretischen Beitrag von H. Günzler: "Gegenstromsysteme mit Stoffzufuhr durch die Außenwände." *Arch. Ges. Physiol.* **274**, 567.

Thurau, K., and Henne, G. (1964). Die transmurale Druckdifferenz der Widerstandsgefäße als Parameter der Widerstandsregulation in der Niere. *Arch. Ges. Physiol.* **279**, 156.

Thurau, K., and Kramer, K. (1959). Weitere Untersuchungen zur myogenen Natur der Autoregulation des Nierenkreislaufes. *Arch. Ges. Physiol.* **269**, 77.

Thurau, K., and Schnermann, J. (1965). Die Natriumkonzentration an den Macula densa-Zellen als regulierender Faktor für das Glomerulumfiltrat. *Klin. Wochschr.* **43**, 410.

Thurau, K., and Wober, E. (1962). Zur Lokalisation der autoregulativen Widerstandsänderungen in der Niere. *Arch. Ges. Physiol.* **274**, 553.

Thurau, K., Deetjen, P., and Kramer, K. (1959a). Farbkonzentrationskurven, Erytrocytenpassage, kapilläre O_2-Sättigung im Nierenmark. *Arch. Ges. Physiol.* **270**, 50.

Thurau, K., Kramer, K., and Brechtelsbauer, H. (1959b). Die Reaktionsweise der glatten Muskulatur der Nierengefäße auf Dehnungsreize und ihre Bedeutung für die Autoregulation des Nierenkreislaufes. *Arch. Ges. Physiol.* **268**, 188.

Thurau, K., Deetjen, P., and Kramer, K. (1960a). Hämodynamik des Nierenmarks. II. Mitteilung: Wechselbeziehung zwischen vasculärem und tubulärem Gegenstromsystem bei arteriellen Drucksteigerungen, Wasserdiurese und osmotischer Diurese. *Arch. Ges. Physiol.* **270**, 270.

Thurau, K., Sugiura, T., and Lilienfield, L. S. (1960b). Micropuncture of renal vasa recta in hydropenic hamsters. *Clin. Res.* **8**, 338.

Thurau, K., Schnermann, J., Nagel, W., Horster, M., and Wahl, M. (1967). Composition of tubular fluid in the macula densa segment as a factor regulating the function of the juxtaglomerular apparatus. *Circulation Res.* **20/21**, Suppl. 2, 79.

Thurau, K., Dahlheim, H., and Granger, P. (1969). On the local formation of angiotensin at the site of the juxtaglomerular apparatus. *Proc. 4th Intern. Congr. Nephrol., Stockholm.*

Tobian, L. (1967). Renin release and its role in renal function and control of salt balance and arterial pressure. *Federation Proc.* **26**, 48.

Trueta, J., Barclay, A. E., Daniel, P. M., Franklin, J., and Prichard, M. M. C. (1948). "Studies of the Renal Circulation." Blackwell, Oxford.

Ulfendahl, H. R. (1962a). Intrarenal oxygen tension. *Acta Soc. Med. Upsalien.* **67**, 95.

Ulfendahl, H. R. (1962b). Distribution of red cells and plasma in rabbit and cat kidneys. *Acta Physiol. Scand.* **52**, 1.

Ullrich, K. J., Pehling, G., and Espinar-Lafuente, M. (1961). Wasser- und Elektrolytfluβ im vasculären Gegenstromsystem des Nierenmarks. Mit einem theoretischen Beitrag von R. Schlögl: "Salztransport durch ungeladene Porenmembranen." *Arch. Ges. Physiol.* **273**, 562.

Vander, A. J. (1964). Effects of acetylcholine, atropine and physostigmine on renal function in the dog. *Am. J. Physiol.* **206**, 492.

Vander, A. J. (1967). Control of renin release. *Physiol. Rev.* **47**, 359.

van Slyke, D. D., Rhoads, C. P., Hiller, A., and Alving, A. S. (1934). Relationships between urea excretion, renal blood flow, renal oxygen consumption, and diuresis. *Am. J. Physiol.* **109**, 336.

von Kügelgen, A., and Braunger, B. (1962). Quantitative Untersuchungen über Kapillaren und Tubuli der Hundeniere. *Z. Zellforsch. Mikroskop. Anat.* **57**, 766.

von Möllendorff, W. (1930). Der Excretionsapparat, p. 245. *In* "Handbuch der mikroskopischen Anatomie des Menschen" (W. v. Möllendorff, ed.) Bd. 7, I. Springer, Berlin.

Waugh, W. H. (1964). Circulatory autoregulation in the fully isolated kidney and in the humorally supported, isolated kidney. *Circulation Res.* **15**, Suppl. 1, 156.

Waugh, W. H., and Shanks, R. G. (1960). Cause of genuine autoregulation of the renal circulation. *Circulation Res.* **8**, 871.

Wells, C. H., Bond, T. P., and Guest, M. M. (1965). Changes in capillary blood flow induced by the extravascular application of hypertonic solutions: a possible mechanism for the control of renal medullary blood flow. *Texas Rept. Biol. Med.* **23**, 128.

Werkö, L., Bucht, H., Josephson, B., and Ek, J. (1951). The effect of nor-adrenaline and adrenaline on renal hemodynamics and renal function in man. *Scand. J. Clin. Lab. Invest.* **3**, 255.

Wilde, W. S., and Vorburger, C. (1967). Albumin multiplier in kidney vasa recta analyzed by microspectrophotometry of T-1824. *Am. J. Physiol.* **213**, 1233.

Wilde, W. S., Thurau, K., Schnermann, J., and Prchal, K. (1963). Counter current multiplier for albumin in renal papilla. *Arch. Ges. Physiol.* **278**, 43.

Windhager, E. E., Lewy, J. E., and Spitzei, A. (1969). Intrarenal control of proximal tubular reabsorption of sodium and water. *Nephron* **6**, 247.

Winton, F. R. (1953). Hydrostatic pressures affecting the flow of the urine and blood in the kidney. *Harvey Lectures* **47**, 67.

Wirz, H. (1952). Druckmessung in Kapillaren und Tubuli der Niere durch Mikropunktion. *Helv. Physiol. Pharmacol. Acta* **13**, 42.

Wirz, H. (1955). Der Einfluß des antidiuretischen Hormones auf den intratubulären Druck der Rattenniere. *Helv. Physiol. Pharmacol. Acta* **13**, C42.

Wolff, G., Nagel, W., Weichert, G., Dräger, U., Schwager, R., and Thurau, K. (1964). Die Verminderung des Glomerulumfiltrates nach hämorrhagischer Hypotension in Abhängigkeit vom Reningehalt der Niere. *Arch. Ges. Physiol.* **281**, 95.

Wolgast, M. (1968). Studies on the regional renal blood flow with P^{32}-labelled red cells and small beta-sensitive semiconductor detectors. *Acta Physiol. Scand. Suppl.* **313**.

Wunderlich, P., and Schnermann, J. (1969). Fortlaufende Registrierung des hydrostatischen Drucks in Nierentubuli und Blutkapillaren. *Arch. Ges. Physiol.* **312**, R95.

Young, D., and Wissig, S. L. (1964). A histologic description of certain epithelial and vascular structures in the kidney of the normal rat. *Am. J. Anat.* **115**, 43.

Zerahn, K. (1956). Oxygen consumption and active sodium transport in the isolated and short circuited frog skin. *Acta Physiol. Scand.* **36**, 300.

Zimmermann, B. G., Abboud, F. M., and Eckstein, J. W. (1964). Effects of norepinephrine and angiotensin on total and venous resistance in the kidney. *Am. J. Physiol.* **206**, 701.

Zimmermann, K. W. (1933). Über den Bau des Glomerulus der Säugerniere. *Z. Mikroskop-Anat. Forsch.* **32**, 176.

2

OSMOTIC CONCENTRATION AND DILUTION OF THE URINE*

Donald J. Marsh†

I. Introduction

Modern theories of renal concentrating and diluting mechanisms date to 1951 when the late Werner Kuhn, Professor of Physical Chemistry at the University of Basel, called attention to similarities between

*The research of the author cited in this article was supported in part by NIH Grant AM 06864.

†Career Scientist of the Health Research Council of the City of New York, Contract No. I-391.

71

tubules in the renal medulla and countercurrent heat exchangers used in chemical processing industries (Hargitay and Kuhn, 1951; Kuhn and Ryffel, 1942). He noted that such counterflow systems can produce strong concentrating effects and suggested that loops of Henle provide the elements of a countercurrent system serving to concentrate tubular urine in collecting ducts passing nearby. This insight is certainly one of the more significant breakthroughs in contemporary physiology. When he advanced his idea, most workers thought the kidney concentrated urine by active transport of water, but this notion is faulty on thermodynamic (Brodsky *et al.*, 1955) and evolutionary (Smith, 1959) grounds. Kuhn's hypothesis began to dominate thinking in the latter half of the 1950s, and although some disagreement about detail persists, each of the alternative proposals is lineally descended from the organizational principles he established.

II. Anatomy of the Renal Medulla

A. Tubules

The anatomical features that led Kuhn to draw his analogy are illustrated in Fig. 1. The kidney has three main subdivisions—the cortex, outer medulla, and inner medulla. Proximal convoluted tubules lie exclusively in the cortex and lead into the pars recta of the proximal tubule in the outer stripe of the outer medulla. The pars recta joins the thin descending limb of Henle's loop at the junction of the outer and inner stripe.

Two classes of nephrons are differentiated on the basis of the length of the loop of Henle. One has a short descending limb that turns at the junction of the inner and outer medulla to lead directly into the thick ascending limb; the descending limb of the second continues into the inner medulla before turning (Sperber, 1944). Thin ascending limbs of Henle's loop are morphologically distinct from both thin descending and thick ascending limbs (Lapp and Nolte, 1962; Osvaldo and Latta, 1966a).

Thick ascending limbs begin at the junction of the inner and outer medulla and cross through the outer medulla to become the distal tubule at the macula densa. Collecting ducts form from several distal tubules in the cortex, receive no further branches in the outer medulla, but then fuse progressively during their passage through the inner medulla until there are only a few ducts of Bellini at the tip of the papilla. Each of the different tubular types runs straight through the

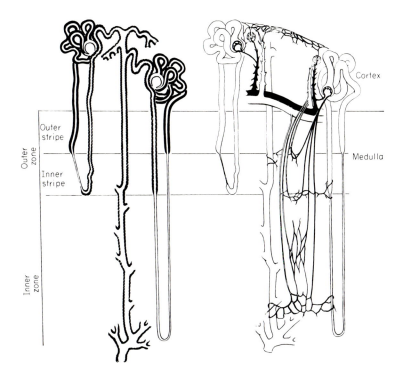

Cortex

Outer stripe

Inner stripe

Outer zone

Inner zone

Medulla

FIG. 1. Schematic diagram of the renal vascular pattern with two nephrons. For details, see text. (Reprinted, with permission, from Gottschalk, 1964.)

medulla parallel to its axis and with a minimum of convolutions. This orderly array contrasts with the random displacement of convoluted proximal and distal tubules in the cortex. The percentage of short- and long-looped nephrons is constant within a species but varies from species to species. The relative length of the medullary zone, defined as the ratio of medulla to cortex thickness, correlates well with maximum urinary osmolality; the percentage of long-looped nephrons does not (Table I).

B. Blood Vessels

The blood supply to the medulla is distributed through a vascular network as well-ordered as the tubular arrangement. Almost all the region's blood is postglomerular. Branches from vasa efferentia of juxtamedullary nephrons form long straight vessels that penetrate directly into the medulla for variable distances (Moffat and Fourman, 1963;

TABLE I

MAXIMUM URINARY OSMOLALITY AND PROPERTIES OF RENAL MEDULLA FOR SEVERAL
SPECIES[a]

Animal	% of long-looped nephrons	Relative medullary thickness[b]	Maximum urinary osmolality (mosmol/kg H_2O)
Beaver	0	1.3	515
Pig	3	1.6	1075
Man	14	3.0	1400
Dog	100	4.3	2600
Cat	100	4.8	3110
Rat	28	5.8	2600
Kangaroo rat	27	8.5	5600
Jerboa	33	9.3	6450
Psammomys	100	10.7	5000

[a]After Schmidt-Nielsen and O'Dell (1961).
[b]Defined as the ratio of medullary length to cortical thickness.

Plakke and Pfieffer, 1964; Rollhäuser *et al.*, 1964). These descending vasa recta remain unbranched until they reach their target depth in the medulla, where they break up completely into a capillary plexus. Ascending (venous) vasa recta are also straight and unbranched; they run in vascular bundles with the descending vasa recta. In the outer medulla, the vascular bundles are subdivided into a central core consisting of alternating arterial and venous vasa recta, and a peripheral ring containing venous vasa recta and most of the descending limbs of Henle's loops. The collecting ducts and thick ascending limbs lie outside the vascular bundles but are enmeshed in a capillary plexus derived from the vasa recta of the bundles (Kriz, 1967; Lever and Kriz, 1966).

A similar pattern is retained in the inner medulla, although the vascular bundles become less prominent proceeding toward the tip of the papilla as the vasa recta reach their respective capillary plexuses and disappear. The descending limbs of Henle's loop continue to penetrate the medulla with the vascular bundles, and the ascending thin limbs are set among the collecting ducts. The inner medullary collecting ducts and thin ascending limbs are also supplied with a capillary plexus derived from the vascular bundles but spatially separated from them. This subdivision of the medulla suggests that medullary tubules receive blood that has remained isolated from the tubular environment except for a brief passage through the capillaries.

Although vasa recta are unbranched and make connections with a capillary plexus, they are true capillaries because they lack smooth muscle (Longley *et al.*, 1960) and because they exchange solutes and water across their endothelia. Descending vasa recta have closed walls; their ascending counterparts are either fenestrated (Longley *et al.*, 1960) or have 200 Å pores (Lapp and Nolte, 1962). The medullary circulation receives a fraction of its supply from the pelvic plexus (von Kügelgen and Braunger, 1962), but there are no measurements of the flow from this source; it is likely to be small.

III. Principles of Countercurrent Systems

A. Countercurrent Multiplication

A clear example of how countercurrent devices can produce concentrating effects is the hydrostatic multiplier model first discussed by Kuhn (Hargitay and Kuhn, 1951; Kuhn and Ryffel, 1942), and illustrated in Fig. 2A. A tube is bent into a hairpin shape so that its ascending and descending limbs share a common wall which is a semipermeable membrane. A hydrostatic pressure difference is imposed between the inflow and outflow tubes. The major pressure drop is across the constriction at the bend; the hydrostatic pressure gradients along the two limbs are negligible. Thus, at all points along the semi-

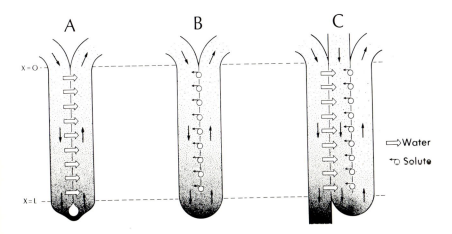

Fig. 2. Model countercurrent multipliers: (A) The single effect is filtration of water across the semipermeable membrane separating the two limbs; a gradient of hydrostatic pressure supplies the driving force. (B) The single effect is solute transport across a water-impermeable membrane. (C) Similar to B, except that a third tube (collecting duct) shares a common semipermeable membrane with the descending limb of the multiplier.

permeable membrane there is a constant gradient of hydrostatic pressure. Consider now an arbitarily small element of volume within the descending limb. The pressure gradient causes water to flow from the descending to the ascending limb, reducing the volume of fluid in the descending limb and concentrating the solutes because the membrane is impermeable to them. The element of volume, now more concentrated, moves farther down the descending limb where again the pressure gradient causes filtration of water into the ascending limb, and the solutes in the descending limb are concentrated still further. If the filtration process occurs along the entire length of the descending limb, the solute concentration in the fluid will increase with length down the tube and reach a maximum at the bend of the loop. The fluid passes the constriction and enters the ascending limb where it recollects the water filtered through the semipermeable membrane; the concentration in the ascending limb decreases progressively until the outflowing fluid has returned to the concentration of the inflowing fluid.

An alternate model, one much closer to the real operation of the kidney, is shown in Fig. 2B (Kuhn and Ramel, 1959). The membrane separating the two limbs now transports solute from the ascending to the descending limb; the membrane is water-impermeable and concentrating effects arise from solute transport rather than water transport. Solute is added to the first volume element in the descending limb, raising its concentration. The volume element moves to the next position, more solute is added, and the concentration increases still more. Repetition of this "single effect" along the length of the loop system leads to a steadily increasing concentration of the tubular fluid with a maximum at the bend. The operation of this model achieves the same result as the hydrostatic pressure model, except that one works by recirculating solute and the other by short-circuiting water.

Kuhn and Ramel (1959) assumed that the rate of solute transport is proportional to the local concentration, which leads to the result that the solute concentration in the loops is an exponential function of the length of the multiplier and of the intensity of the transport operation, as shown in Fig. 3. Alternatively, if the membrane transports solute at a constant rate, independent of local concentration, there is a linear dependence of concentration on length and transport rate.

The model of Fig. 2B performs no useful work; in a steady state both the concentration and volume flow of the effluent fluid from the ascending limb are the same as in the descending limb fluid entering the system. Work can be done by the system if a third tube is juxtaposed, as in Fig. 2C (Kuhn and Ramel, 1959). A semipermeable membrane (solute-impermeable, water-permeable) separates the descending limb

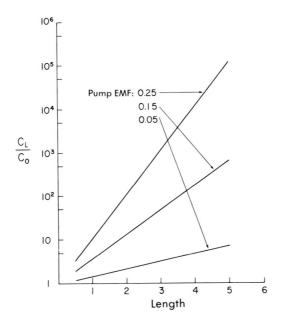

FIG. 3.   Dependency of concentrating ability on the length of the countercurrent multiplier, and on the intensity of the single effect. Curves were generated for the model shown in Fig. 2B. C_L is the concentration at $X = L$, C_0 the concentration at $X = 0$. Length and pump EMF (electromotive force) are in arbitrary units.

from the third tube (collecting duct). Suppose that the fluids entering the descending limb and collecting duct have identical concentrations. As solute transport between the two limbs concentrates descending limb fluid, osmosis removes water from the collecting ducts, leaving its solutes more concentrated. Volume flow in the loops increases to the extent that water is removed from the collecting ducts; the effluent from the ascending limb must leave at a higher flow rate than fluid enters the descending limb. The ascending limb fluid must also exit with a lower concentration than the solution entering the descending limb; this is the route taken by the water extracted from the collecting ducts as it leaves the system. The concentration difference between the two limbs at $X = 0$ represents the magnitude of the single effect. It need be only a fraction of the concentration difference developed along the length of the model, and this is really the crux of the countercurrent idea. Nowhere must the lateral differences be very great — large gradients arise from small differences repeated often enough along a longitudinal axis.

The geometry of this model is not too dissimilar from that of the kidney. Kuhn and Ramel (1959) analyzed the model's operation; their equations lead to some useful conclusions which are shown in Fig. 4. The smaller the volume flow in the loops, the greater the maximum concentration achieved at the bend. The concentration change produced in an element of volume from addition of a given amount of solute depends on the volume flow rate. The greater the volume flow rate, the less will be the effect on the concentration of the addition of a given amount of solute. The transport rate depends on local concentrations; if concentrations are reduced by increasing the volume flow, the efficacy of the concentrating effect is compromised still further. The inverse relationship between volume flow and concentrating ability is a recurrent theme in much of the discussion that follows.

Another determinant of the concentration at $X = L$ is the ratio of collecting duct to loop flows. The membrane separating collecting duct and descending limb is water-permeable; osmosis continues until osmotic equilibration occurs. As volume flow into the collecting duct is increased, more water must cross from collecting duct to descending limb to achieve equilibration and so the rise of descending limb concentration due to the solute pump is lessened. The collecting duct comes more and more to dominate the system as its flow increases in comparison to flow in the loops.

B. Countercurrent Exchange

Renal tubules do not adjoin each other directly but are separated by a common interstitial space through which the vasa recta also run. Countercurrent multiplication works in such a system by raising interstitial solute concentrations, forcing loops and vasa recta to cross twice through a zone of steadily changing concentration, and producing transmural concentration differences as they travel. Exchanges between blood or tubular fluid and interstitium caused by these differences are important for the overall function of the region.

Figure 5 shows an arbitrarily small region of interstitium containing a looped structure. The descending limb fluid enters the region less concentrated than interstitial fluid because it comes from more dilute areas; the ascending limb enters more concentrated because it has equilibrated with regions nearer the apex of the countercurrent multiplier system. If the vessel walls have relatively free permeability to both solute and water there is a tendency for the descending limb to lose water and gain solute while the ascending limb takes up water and gives off solute. The interaction between vasa recta and interstitium tends to exclude from the depths of the countercurrent region those materials

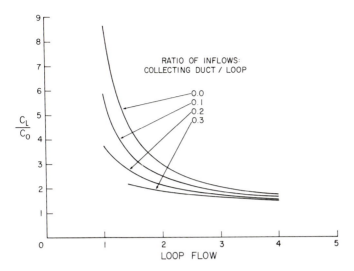

FIG. 4.   Dependence of concentrating ability on flow through the loops and collecting duct. Curves were generated for the model shown in Fig. 2C. C_L is the concentration of collecting duct fluid at $X = L$, C_0 is the concentration at $X = 0$. Flows are in arbitrary units. The topmost curve (flow ratio = 0) corresponds to the behavior of the model without a collecting duct, as in Fig. 2B.

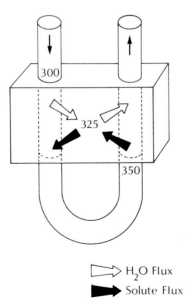

FIG. 5.   Countercurrent exchange. A looped structure penetrates a region of interstitial space. The descending limb comes from a less concentrated region, the ascending from a more concentrated one.

already there in low concentration (water) while retaining those present in higher concentration (solute). This arrangement serves to maintain gradients built up along the axis of the countercurrent system.

It should be emphasized that, by itself, a countercurrent exchanger can do no work and so it cannot contribute to the buildup of longitudinal concentration gradients. Indeed, large flows through an exchanger can dissipate much of the work done by a countercurrent multiplier on the interstitial region. As volume flow rate increases, time for equilibration decreases; the descending limbs carry water deeper into the medullary zones and the ascending vessels bring solute farther out. This relationship between flow and the dissipation of the countercurrent gradient has been emphasized by Berliner et al. (1958), by Thurau and Deetjen, (1962), and by Niesel and Röskenbleck (1963b).

IV. Application of the Countercurrent Hypothesis to the Kidney

A. The Hypothesis

Application of the countercurrent multiplier model to the kidney can be made in a straightforward way (Berliner et al., 1958; Gottschalk and Mylle, 1959; Windhager and Giebisch, 1965; Wirz, 1953, 1956) (Fig. 6). Active salt reabsorption from the ascending limb of Henle's loop provides the primary source of osmotic work for concentrating the urine. The ascending limb must be relatively water-impermeable so that active salt reabsorption deposits a hypertonic solution in the medullary interstitium, and leaves tubular fluid less concentrated. This single effect — the creation of an osmotic pressure difference between tubular and interstitial fluids — is thought to occur along the entire length of the ascending limb. As the descending limb penetrates the medulla, its tubular fluid becomes more concentrated by equilibrating with interstitial fluid. The equilibration, which occurs by osmotic withdrawal of water and inward diffusion of solute, brings the tubular fluid to its maximum concentration as the loop turns the bend.

After it passes through the ascending limb, tubular fluid enters the distal tubule where, in the presence of antidiuretic hormone, the osmotic pressure difference generated in the ascending limb is dissipated by simple osmosis until the tubular fluid becomes isotonic. This water lost from the distal tubule to the systemic circulation is the solvent water for the solutes left behind in the medullary interstitium; its removal in the cortex also reduces volume flow into the collecting ducts, which must be small for the efficient operation of the countercurrent

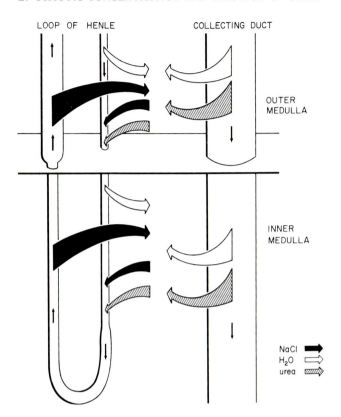

FIG. 6.   The countercurrent multiplier hypothesis as it is usually applied to tubules of the mammalian kidney. Arrows show the direction of net transtubular fluxes. The vasa recta are omitted for the sake of clarity. For details, see text.

multiplier. The tubular fluid continues down the collecting ducts through the hypertonic medullary region, and in the presence of anti-diuretic hormone, water is extracted by simple osmosis, leading to the final osmotic concentration of the urine.

The blood supply to the medulla plays an important role in the countercurrent multiplier hypothesis. Because of their high permeability to small solutes and water, the vasa recta operate as countercurrent exchangers. They supply the tissue with metabolic substrates and remove end products with minimal disturbance to the corticomedullary osmolality gradient, provided that the blood flow is kept sufficiently small.

The existence of an interstitial space common to all the tubular and vascular structures places a special responsibility on the vasa recta. In the model of Fig. 2C, water withdrawn from the collecting duct flows into the descending limb because the wall separating the two is a semi-permeable membrane; the opposite side of the descending limb is a water-impermeable membrane able to sustain the osmolality difference between the limbs of the loops. If, as in the kidney, the descending limb is separated from both collecting duct and ascending limb by an interstitial region, it cannot have radial asymmetry, as in the model. But if the descending limb has uniform permeability properties, it cannot take up water from the interstitium. For example, if the descending limb is water-permeable but salt-impermeable, it will lose water to the hypertonic interstitium. Conversely, if it is salt-permeable and water-impermeable, the influx of salt will raise the descending limb concentration, but again no water enters. These cases are the two extremes. If we consider the more reasonable position, that the descending limb is permeable to both salt and water, there still remains no possibility for extracting water from the medullary interstitium. Thus it becomes necessary to provide a route for the removal of fluid from the medulla. The ascending vasa recta are thought to provide this pathway, and the oncotic pressure difference between plasma and interstitial fluid its driving force (Gottschalk and Mylle, 1959).

Because of the high permeability of the capillary wall to small solutes, vasa recta blood concentrations can not differ much from medullary interstitial concentrations; the vasa recta remove, in effect, interstitial fluid and not water. The separation of water and solute that must occur for the medullary region to become concentrated still takes place in the loop of Henle and the distal tubule — the ascending limb deposits NaCl into the medulla and the distal tubule delivers its water load to the cortex where it is carried away into the systemic circulation.

Urea contributes significantly to the osmolality of the urine and medullary interstitial fluid. It becomes concentrated slightly in the proximal tubular fluid by solute and water reabsorption in that segment, enters the lumen of the descending limb from the interstitium of the medullary region, and becomes still more concentrated in the distal tubule and collecting duct because of osmotic withdrawal of water. The collecting duct is thought to be relatively permeable to urea, enabling it to diffuse into the medullary interstitium down a concentration gradient created by water reabsorption. Thus, urea undergoes a recirculation (Levinsky and Berliner, 1959), entering the tubular fluid in the descending limb and leaving it in the collecting duct. This arrangement has the advantage that urea is present on both sides of the collecting duct epithelium; the osmolality of the urine can be raised because of the presence of this inert, diffusable compound, which need not be balanced by an osmotically equivalent amount of NaCl in the interstitium.

B. Experimental Evidence Supporting the Countercurrent Multiplier Hypothesis

1. LOCALIZATION OF THE CONCENTRATING MECHANISM IN THE MEDULLA

If the concentrating mechanism is located in the renal medulla, and if it operates by the repetition of a single event along the corticomedullary axis, then medullary structures should all become progressively more concentrated with maximal concentrations at the tip of the papilla that correspond to the urine osmolality. Wirz, Hargitay, and Kuhn (1951) measured the osmolality of rat kidney slices cryoscopically. Their findings conformed to the prediction and were subsequently confirmed by Bray (1960). Note that the countercurrent multiplier theory depends on the maintenance of an osmotic pressure difference of some magnitude between the ascending limb and other structures. Wirz et al. (1951), and Bray (1960) found no gradient. This is probably due to the fact that ice has a substantial vapor pressure, so that even in frozen sections, small osmotic pressure differences would be expected to be obliterated by sublimation.

Subsequent work by Ullrich and Jarausch (1956) showed that the corticomedullary osmotic gradient was due almost entirely to the accumulation of NaCl and urea. In experimental circumstances where the concentrating ability of the kidney is reduced, as in water diuresis or osmotic diuresis, the corticomedullary gradient for urea disappears while that for NaCl remains, at least in the outer medulla. This result supports the proposal that active transport of NaCl is the primary driving force in the concentrating mechanism.

- The localization of the concentrating mechanism to the medulla received additional confirmation from early micropuncture work. Wirz (1953) found that vasa recta plasma had the same osmolality as collecting duct urine, and Gottschalk and Mylle (1959) showed that loop of Henle fluid also had the same osmolality as capillary plasma and urine. This isoosmolality of all fluids at the tip of the papilla was present over an extensive range of concentrations; it affirms that the concentrating mechanism involves intimate interaction between the loops, the collecting ducts, the vasa recta, and by implication, the medullary interstitium.

2. COUNTERCURRENT EXCHANGE IN THE MEDULLA

If a compound permeates a capillary endothelium readily, its rate of accumulation in most tissues should depend only on arterial blood concentration and blood flow rate. Counterflowing blood vessels and loops of Henle slow the accumulation of such compounds because counter-current exchange reduces the concentration at the arterial end of the capillary plexus fed by the descending vasa recta. The accumulation of such compounds as THO (Morel *et al.*, 1960), antipyrine, ^{85}Kr (Lassen and Longley, 1961; Thorburn *et al.*, 1963), and ^{22}Na (Maganzini and Lilenfield, 1961; Morel *et al.*, 1960) are all markedly prolonged in the renal medulla, the more diffusable compounds being slowed more. From the discussion earlier, one can predict that the rate of accumula-tion of such compounds should depend on flow rate through the count-ercurrent exchanger. Indeed, White *et al.* (1961) found that the rate of accumulation of THO was slowed by ureteral clamping, whereas Morel *et al.* (1960) showed that the rate of accumulation could be enhanced in diuretic states.

Flow rate in the vasa recta is expected to be an important factor in the ability of the medulla to generate hypertonic urine. If the flow rate is increased, countercurrent exchange becomes less efficient, and med-ullary osmolality drops as solute is lost. Support for this idea came from Thurau and Deetjen (1962). They made use of the observation that medullary circulation is not autoregulated (Kramer *et al.*, 1960), so that elevating arterial blood pressure increases medullary blood flow rate. They noted a striking dependence of urinary osmolality on arterial blood pressure; hydropenic dogs could be made to undergo water di-uresis by the simple expedient of inducing arterial hypertension.

The studies cited provide strong evidence that countercurrent ex-change is a significant feature of medullary physiology, but they have not yielded quantitative information about the properties of specific structures. The intimate contact between vasa recta in the vascular bundles allows for good exchange, but also renders it difficult to study the circulation of one medullary zone independent of the other. More-over, highly diffusible tracer compounds enter or leave the medulla in tubules as well as vasa recta, which precludes their use for measuring flow rate in one or the other class of structures. For example, Aukland and Berliner (1964) inserted platinum electrodes into the medulla of dogs receiving H_2 by breathing or by intravenous administration. If the administration of H_2 is stopped abruptly, the rate of H_2 loss from the tissue, measured with the Pt electrode should theoretically depend on blood flow. Instead, they found that H_2 disappearance was more closely correlated with flow in the collecting ducts than with loop or vasa recta flow, and they concluded that such techniques were unsuitable for blood flow measurements in the renal medulla.

Countercurrent exchange of gases and small solutes has other practical consequences. Metabolism requires substrates and O_2, yet their consumption establishes corticomedullary gradients (Kramer *et al.*, 1960; Leonhardt *et al.*, 1965; Rennie *et al.*, 1958; Ruiz-Guinazu *et al.*, 1961). The maintenance of these gradients by counterflowing loops and vasa recta is an unavoidable consequence of the medulla's physical properties; the greater the consumption rate, the more efficiently is the supply restricted. Similar difficulties beset the removal of metabolic end products. These problems are most severe for the blood gases because they penetrate cell membranes easily and diffuse rapidly through the interstitium. Thus, the pO_2 at the tip of the papilla is only one-tenth as high as in renal venous blood, during hydropenia (Rennie *et al.*, 1958). These low pO_2 values are apparently inadequate to support the work of the medulla entirely through aerobic metabolism, and anaerobic pathways provide a prominent fraction of the energy supply (Ruiz-Guinazu *et al.*, 1961). The dependence on anaerobic metabolism also minimizes the problem of tissue acidification due to the accumulation of metabolic end products. If all substrates were oxidized to CO_2, the gas would accumulate in the medulla in high concentration because of countercurrent exchange. Instead, most substrate oxidation goes only as far as lactate, which, owing to its lower penetrability, is not trapped as efficiently as CO_2.

Some aerobic metabolism does occur in the inner medulla. If the only determinants of urinary pCO_2 were the rate of CO_2 production, and flow and permeability properties of the countercurrent exchanger, one might predict that the urine pCO_2 would always exceed renal venous pCO_2. This prediction is only true when the urine is alkaline, while in very acid urines the corticomedullary gradient often reverses. Such strong pH dependence is due to the participation of CO_2 in acidification mechanisms. When the bicarbonate TM is exceeded, acidification of tubular fluid shifts the carbonic acid dehydration reaction to the right, but the reaction rate is relatively slow and the evolution of much of the CO_2 is delayed until the tubular fluid has passed deep into the medulla. The main evidence for this suggestion is the finding that administration of carbonic anhydrase, which is filtered into the tubular fluid, eliminates most of the corticomedullary pCO_2 gradient, both in urine (Ochwadt and Pitts, 1956) and in vasa recta plasma (Uhlich *et al.*, 1968). When the urine pH is low, the urinary HCO_3^- concentration is effectively zero, and the only substrate for the collecting duct acidification mechanism is CO_2 derived from metabolism or brought in the vasa recta. This CO_2 is then hydrated intracellularly, and the proton is captured by urinary buffers.

The behavior of CO_2 illustrates how additional interactions may complicate predictions based on assumed simple distributions in a countercurrent exchange system. Nevertheless, once it is understood that what has been added is either an additional source of CO_2, as in alkalinization, or an additional sink, as in acidification, the generation and maintenance of the corticomedullary CO_2 gradient follows straightforward countercurrent theory.

3. THE COLLECTING DUCT IN THE COUNTERCURRENT MULTIPLIER HYPOTHESIS

Ullrich's group (Hilger et al., 1958) localized the final concentrating step to the collecting duct. They inserted polyethylene catheters into collecting ducts of the hamster papilla and found that inulin concentrations increased two- to threefold along the length of the inner medulla. The osmolality also increased toward the tip of the papilla and from their measurements one can reasonably conclude that urine is concentrated in collecting ducts by reabsorption of a fluid hypoosmotic to the collecting duct fluid as it enters the inner medulla.

Ullrich's measurements also reveal significant solute reabsorption. A fraction of the reabsorbed solute is urea (Klümper et al., 1958), whose concentration increases in the collecting duct urine, despite its loss from the lumen. These relations are in accord with the notion that the reabsorption of urea proceeds secondary to the reabsorption of water. Gottschalk et al. (1962) reported that urea-^{14}C concentrations in collecting duct urine were 40% higher than in vasa recta plasma in hydropenic animals. This observation has been confirmed with a spectrophotometric method (Marsh, 1970b); it implies that urea reabsorption in antidiuresis is down its chemical potential gradient and so is probably passive.*

Not all the solute reabsorbed from collecting ducts is urea. Some is Na^+ and its related anions. In fact, not only is Na^+ reabsorbed from the collecting duct urine, but its concentration falls as the urine travels through the inner medulla, suggesting active reabsorption (Hilger et al., 1958). Ullrich and his colleagues estimated that 30–40% of this Na^+ reabsorption is in exchange for hydrogen and possibly K^+, but the remainder represents osmotic work in the form of net transport of NaCl.

4. THE DESCENDING LIMB IN THE COUNTERCURRENT MULTIPLIER HYPOTHESIS

Micropuncture work, primarily from Gottschalk's laboratory, and more recently from Morel's, has clarified the role of the descending limb of Henle's loop in the concentrating mechanism. As already mentioned, Gottschalk found tubular fluid from the bend of the loop to be isoosmotic with vasa recta blood and collecting duct urine from the same medullary level (Gottschalk and Mylle, 1959). He also reported an inulin tubular fluid to plasma ratio (TF/P) of 11–12 at the bend of the loop (Lassiter et al., 1961; Gottschalk et al., 1963) which is higher than at the end of the proximal tubule, and indicates significant net reabsorption of water during the descending limb's passage through the medulla.

The hypertonicity of hamster loop tubular fluid was due to high concentrations of NaCl and urea (Gottschalk et al., 1963). Urea concentrations at the bend of the loop were elevated because of net addition of urea to descending limb tubular fluid. This conclusion arose from the plausible assumption that the proximal tubule of juxtamedullary nephrons reabsorbs significant quantities of urea, while the urea load at the bend of these loops equals or exceeds the filtered load (Lassiter et al., 1961). Similar findings were reported recently by de Rouffignac and Morel (1969) who studied the desert rodent, Psammomys.

A somewhat more conclusive demonstration of the net addition of urea to descending limb fluid was obtained recently in our laboratory by inserting two pipettes into the same descending limb separated by a

---

*Considerable interest has been expressed in the possibility that urea is actively reabsorbed from collecting ducts (Truniger and Schmidt-Nielsen, 1964). When the high medullary concentrations characteristic of hydropenia are reduced, either by inducing mannitol (Bray and Preston, 1961; Clapp, 1966) or saline diuresis (Lassiter et al., 1966), or by placing the animals on a low protein diet (Clapp, 1966; Truniger and Schmidt-Nielsen, 1964; Ullrich et al., 1967) collecting duct urine concentrations fall below medullary interstitial values. There is little doubt that urea is still being reabsorbed (Clapp, 1966), and so the transport is against a concentration gradient, but that metabolic energy is expended directly on this process remains to be demonstrated. The alternative is that the contragradient flux of urea is coupled to some other flux, such as that of water, rather than requiring a separate expenditure of energy. This distinction is analogous to the differentiation made between active water transport and uphill movement of water coupled to active salt transport. It is conventionally stated that a water flux cannot raise the concentration of the entrained solute on the side of the membrane toward which the water moves (Goldberg et al., 1967), but counterexamples exist (Nims, 1961; Nims and Thurber, 1961) that could well apply to the collecting duct. A full discussion of the problem of active reabsorption of urea is beyond the intended scope of this chapter; the question remains very much an open one. The concentration differences that suggest active urea transport are small and can be uncovered only when the concentrating mechanism is seriously perturbed. If there is active urea transport, it is likely to cause only a small net flux; in the antidiuretic animal concentrating its urine normally, there is no need to invoke active transport of urea to account for its reabsorption (Gottschalk, 1964; Ullrich et al., 1967).

distance of about 1 mm (Marsh, 1970a). The inulin TF/P increased 9% while the urea concentration went up 57% as the tubular fluid flowed between the two sampling points, so that the high concentration of urea in the tubular fluid at the bend of Henle's loop results principally from net addition of urea supplied from the collecting ducts, and only to a limited extent from osmotic withdrawal of water.

The evidence is less clear in the case of NaCl. Even though salt is the main solute of loop tubular fluid, the relative concentration increase that occurs along the descending limb is much less than the corresponding increase for urea, and the load of NaCl flowing around the bend of the loop is less than the filtered load (Gottschalk et al., 1963). To decide whether there has been net addition of NaCl to descending limb fluid one must know the inulin TF/P at the end of the proximal tubule feeding the loop more accurately than is needed for a decision about urea. There are substantial differences between cortical and juxtamedullary nephrons, both in respect to size (de Rouffignac and Morel, 1967) and single nephron filtration rate (Horster and Thurau, 1968), so that extrapolation of data from cortical proximal tubules, where the inulin TF/P is known, to juxtamedullary nephrons, is not justified. Because of this difficulty, Gottschalk et al. (1963) could not decide from their data if the high salt concentration was due to salt addition or simply reflected the water lost by osmosis.

de Rouffignac and Morel (1969) compared inulin, osmolality, and sodium data from randomly selected *Psammomys* loops punctured at their bend. They found that the Na^+ concentration increased *pari passu* with osmolality but that the inulin ratio tended to increase only slightly as osmolality went up over a rather wide range. They concluded from these data that the principal reason for the high Na^+ concentration of the loop tubular fluid is net addition of Na^+, but a more direct test, with samples taken from at least two sites in the same descending limb, would make the argument more forcefully.

A limited number of such measurements were carried out in the terminal 1 mm of the hamster's descending limb (Marsh, 1970a). The Na^+ concentration rises slightly, but so does the inulin ratio, and so in this region of the hamster papilla there is no net change of the Na^+ load as tubular fluid flows toward the bend. These data do not necessarily exclude the possibility that Na^+ enters the tubular fluid from the interstitium. The corticomedullary tissue Na^+ gradient is shallow at the tip of the papilla, and the failure to find addition of NaCl might be attributable to the absence of an adequate driving force. If net addition does occur, it must take place in regions of the descending limb located more proximally where the corticomedullary gradient is steeper. The

Na^+ permeability of the descending limb appears to be high (Morgan and Berliner, 1968), and it seems probable that there is some net addition of NaCl to descending limb tubular fluid which is due to the concentration difference created when less concentrated tubular fluid flows into a medullary interstitial region made more concentrated by the operation of active salt pumping mechanisms in other tubules.

The behavior of water in the thin descending limb is particularly noteworthy. The countercurrent multiplier hypothesis posits a generally high permeability to small solutes, such as NaCl and urea, and it would then be expected that the water permeability should also be high. Perfusion experiments carried out on an *in vitro* preparation confirmed this prediction (Morgan and Berliner, 1968). As tubular fluid flows toward the bend of Henle's loop, it penetrates regions of ever increasing osmolality, which, combined with the apparent high water permeability, should lead to extensive osmotic water removal. Two lines of evidence fail to substantiate this prediction. First, micropuncture specimens taken from the bend of Henle's loop in *Psammomys* show that the inulin TF/P varies only slightly over a considerable range of osmolalities (de Rouffignac and Morel, 1969). There is a definite correlation, but the regression coefficient is much less than would be predicted on the basis of perfect adherence to the van't Hoff law. Second, comparison of proximal with distal inulin data from *Psammomys*, an animal whose cortical nephrons penetrate deeply into the inner medulla and which therefore have long thin segments, reveals a much smaller rise of the inulin concentration during traversal of the loop than in the rat (Morel *et al.*, 1969). Recall that the rat's superficial nephrons lack a thin ascending limb (Sperber, 1944). These findings suggest that minimal net transfer of water occurs across the loops' epithelial membranes regardless of the tonicity of the medullary regions. For the descending limb, the failure of the available osmotic forces to create a volume flux out of the tubule lumen must mean that these forces are relatively ineffective, which in turn implies that the osmotic reflection coefficients for NaCl and urea, the two main osmotic constituents of medullary fluids, must be much less than unity. Low reflection coefficients usually occur in membranes whose solute permeabilities are high, and so in this respect the results are consistent with the notion that the descending limb has a permeable wall which permits the accumulation of solutes in the tubular fluid by diffusion from the interstitial region.

Finally, it is a moot question as to whether the thin descending limbs are capable of active salt transport. It is tempting to speculate that all tubular epithelia transport salt, and that the descending limb is no exception. The attractions of this philosophical argument notwith-standing, there is no operational necessity for ascribing salt pumping to the descending limb since none of its properties depend for explanation on transepithelial transport. Even if active pumping did occur, the high salt permeability would probably short-circuit it sufficiently to preclude the possibility of its detection.

5. THE ASCENDING LIMB AND DISTAL TUBULE

The *sine qua non* of the countercurrent multiplier hypothesis is the requirement that the ascending limbs deliver a hypertonic reabsorbate into the interstitium. Extensive evidence exists for the application of the hypothesis to thick limbs in the outer medulla. Early distal tubular fluid invariably has a lower osmolality (Gottschalk and Mylle, 1959; Wirz, 1956) and a lower sodium concentration (Malnic *et al.*, 1966; Windhager and Giebisch, 1961) than the blood in the adjacent cortical interstitium and fluid at the end of the proximal tubule. These concentration changes occur regardless of the diuretic condition of the animal, and are always accompanied by an increase of the inulin TF/P between the late proximal and the early distal tubule (Malnic *et al.*, 1966; Ullrich *et al.*, 1963). There seems no reasonable way to account for these data except through active salt transport in the thick ascending limb of Henle's loop and the application of the countercurrent multiplier hypothesis to the outer medulla is therefore not open to serious question.

The relative inaccessibility of the thick ascending limb has hampered detailed investigation of its properties. An approach to its study has been taken by Cortney *et al.* (1966) and by Schnermann (1968) which involves perfusion from the end of the proximal tubule through to the distal tubule of individual short looped nephrons. Interpretation of these experiments is necessarily complicated because the perfusion fluid must first traverse the pars recta and thin descending limb before entering the thick ascending limb, and the composition of the medullary interstitial region is not as stable as in the cortex. Despite these restrictions, Schnermann (1968) has shown that the reabsorptive capacity of thick limbs is load-dependent in a manner reminiscent of the proximal tubule. No attempt has been made to clarify the mechanism of this load dependency, so that it remains at least as well understood as the analogous behavior of the proximal tubule.

The return of the nephron to the cortex provides an opportunity for free water generated by ascending limb salt reabsorption to leave the distal tubule by osmosis and to return to the systemic circulation. Evidence to support this view first came from Gottschalk and Mylle (1959),

C. Unresolved Questions about the Countercurrent Multiplier Hypothesis

1. REMOVAL OF THE FLUID BY THE VASA RECTA

In addition to their usual role of bringing substrates and removing metabolic end products, the medullary blood vessels must remove the volume of fluid entering the interstitial region from the descending limb of Henle's loop and from the collecting duct—no other structure remains if the ascending limb is pumping salt and is relatively water-impermeable. This hypothesis has scarcely been discussed and has never been tested. The protein concentration of vasa recta plasma at the tip of the hamster papilla is two to three times greater than in systemic plasma (Wilde *et al.*, 1963). Since the protein concentration change can be used as an index of water movement in or out of the capillary, this finding suggests that there is a net volume efflux from the descending vasa recta, and it places the entire burden of removing absorbed tubular fluid on the capillary plexus which envelops the tubules, and on the ascending vasa recta.

The driving force thought to cause fluid to move into these capillaries is the summation of the hydrostatic and oncotic pressure differences that exist across the endothelial wall. There simply are no data from which to estimate the magnitude of this driving force, and no permeability measurements from which the flow of reabsorbed fluid into the capillary lumen might then be calculated. Obviously this general area needs more detailed study.

Before leaving the subject it might be worthwhile to add yet another word of caution. Several investigators agree that the medullary albumin space exceeds the corresponding vascular space by 50% or more (Bethge *et al.*, 1962; Goldberg and Lilenfield, 1963; Pinter, 1967b; Slotkoff and Lilenfield, 1967). This albumin reaches its extravascular location by permeation through the capillary membrane, most probably through the fenestrated endothelial walls of the peritubular capillary plexus and of the ascending vasa recta. The medullary interstitial region is closely packed with many interstitial cells (Osvaldo and Latta, 1966b) and much mucopolysaccharide, and the concentration of albumin in the interstitial water might be even higher than predicted from the space measurement. It would be of no small interest to know the true value of the endothelial albumin gradient. There are obvious difficulties awaiting any experimental evaluation of the interstitial space's composition, and the need for doing so might be obviated it if could be shown that there is a net volume increase during passage of blood through the capillaries and ascending vasa recta.

who found early distal fluid to be invariably hypotonic, while late distal fluid was isotonic. Lassiter *et al.* (1961) later reported that this distal osmotic equilibration led to a fourfold rise in the inulin TF/P, which reduces the volume load presented to collecting ducts.

In certain respects, Gottschalk's choice of the rat for his experiments was very fortunate. In other species, such as dog (Clapp and Robinson, 1966) and monkey (Bennett *et al.*, 1968), and even in some strains of rats (Morell, 1966) distal fluid remains hypotonic along the entire length of the segment, and the rise of inulin TF/P is less striking than in the rat (Bennett *et al.*, 1967, 1968). To explain these results one assumes that the water-permeable segment is more distal than the region accessible on the surface. This interpretation is easily arrived at with Gottschalk's data already available; there is no telling what might have resulted had the order of discovery been reversed.

Urea measurements from distal tubules support the recirculation concept. Lassiter *et al.* (1961) found that early distal tubules from short looped nephrons of the rat had urea loads that exceeded the filtered load. Even though these loops penetrate only through the outer medulla with its modest urea gradient, there is sufficient entry of urea into loop tubular fluid to more than double the mass flow of urea. This relationship is more striking in long looped nephrons. In *Psammomys*, Morel *et al.* (1969) reported that the early distal urea load is three to four times the filtered load. In both these studies, considerably less than the filtered load was excreted, indicating that the collecting duct is a site of reabsorption, as had already been shown by Klümper *et al.* (1958).

There is evidently a large urea pool carried in constant circulation between cortex and medulla by the passage of tubular fluid, and prevented from leaving the medullary interstitium by countercurrent exchange in the vasa recta. The surprising feature of this concept is that all the urea is not lost from the distal tubule, together with water. Nevertheless, it is true that urea losses from the distal tubule are small (Lassiter *et al.*, 1961), which is attributable to low distal urea permeability (Capek *et al.*, 1966).

Most of the experiments cited thus far support the validity of the countercurrent multiplier hypothesis. Their interpretation is generally accepted, and where controversy touches them the dispute is usually on other questions not related directly to countercurrent theory. But support is not proof, and a single ugly fact can vitiate the most elegant theory. Unanswered questions about the medulla have persisted, and these lie at the core of the countercurrent multiplier model in the inner medulla.

exception. The attractions of this philosophical argument notwith-standing, there is no operational necessity for ascribing salt pumping to the descending limb since none of its properties depend for explana-tion on transepithelial transport. Even if active pumping did occur, the high salt permeability would probably short-circuit it sufficiently to pre-clude the possibility of its detection.

5. The Ascending Limb and Distal Tubule

The *sine qua non* of the countercurrent multiplier hypothesis is the requirement that the ascending limbs deliver a hypertonic reabsorbate into the interstitium. Extensive evidence exists for the application of the hypothesis to thick limbs in the outer medulla. Early distal tubular fluid invariably has a lower osmolality (Gottschalk and Mylle, 1959; Wirz, 1956) and a lower sodium concentration (Malnic et al., 1966; Windhager and Giebisch, 1961) than the blood in the adjacent cortical interstitium and fluid at the end of the proximal tubule. These concen-tration changes occur regardless of the diuretic condition of the ani-mal, and are always accompanied by an increase of the inulin TF/P between the late proximal and the early distal tubule (Malnic et al., 1966; Ullrich et al., 1963). There seems no reasonable way to account for these data except through active salt transport in the thick as-cending limb of Henle's loop and the application of the countercurrent multiplier hypothesis to the outer medulla is therefore not open to se-rious question.

The relative inaccessibility of the thick ascending limb has hampered detailed investigation of its properties. An approach to its study has been taken by Cortney et al. (1966) and by Schnermann (1968) which involves perfusion from the end of the proximal tubule through to the distal tubule of individual short looped nephrons. Interpretation of these experiments is necessarily complicated because the perfusion fluid must first traverse the pars recta and thin descending limb before entering the thick ascending limb, and the composition of the medul-lary interstitial region is not as stable as in the cortex. Despite these re-strictions, Schnermann (1968) has shown that the reabsorptive capacity of thick limbs is load-dependent in a manner reminiscent of the prox-imal tubule. No attempt has been made to clarify the mechanism of this load dependency, so that it remains at least as well understood as the analogous behavior of the proximal tubule.

The return of the nephron to the cortex provides an opportunity for free water generated by ascending limb salt reabsorption to leave the distal tubule by osmosis and to return to the systemic circulation. Evi-dence to support this view first came from Gottschalk and Mylle (1959),

Na^+ permeability of the descending limb appears to be high (Morgan and Berliner, 1968), and it seems probable that there is some net addition of NaCl to descending limb tubular fluid which is due to the concentration difference created when less concentrated tubular fluid flows into a medullary interstitial region made more concentrated by the operation of active salt pumping mechanisms in other tubules.

The behavior of water in the thin descending limb is particularly noteworthy. The countercurrent multiplier hypothesis posits a generally high permeability to small solutes, such as NaCl and urea, and it would then be expected that the water permeability should also be high. Perfusion experiments carried out on an *in vitro* preparation confirmed this prediction (Morgan and Berliner, 1968). As tubular fluid flows toward the bend of Henle's loop, it penetrates regions of ever increasing osmolality, which, combined with the apparent high water permeability, should lead to extensive osmotic water removal. Two lines of evidence fail to substantiate this prediction. First, micropuncture specimens taken from the bend of Henle's loop in *Psammomys* show that the inulin TF/P varies only slightly over a considerable range of osmolalities (de Rouffignac and Morel, 1969). There is a definite correlation, but the regression coefficient is much less than would be predicted on the basis of perfect adherence to the van't Hoff law. Second, comparison of proximal with distal inulin data from *Psammomys*, an animal whose cortical nephrons penetrate deeply into the inner medulla and which therefore have long thin segments, reveals a much smaller rise of the inulin concentration during traversal of the loop than in the rat (Morel *et al.*, 1969). Recall that the rat's superficial nephrons lack a thin ascending limb (Sperber, 1944). These findings suggest that minimal net transfer of water occurs across the loops' epithelial membranes regardless of the tonicity of the medullary regions. For the descending limb, the failure of the available osmotic forces to create a volume flux out of the tubule lumen must mean that these forces are relatively ineffective, which in turn implies that the osmotic reflection coefficients for NaCl and urea, the two main osmotic constituents of medullary fluids, must be much less than unity. Low reflection coefficients usually occur in membranes whose solute permeabilities are high, and so in this respect the results are consistent with the notion that the descending limb has a permeable wall which permits the accumulation of solutes in the tubular fluid by diffusion from the interstitial region.

Finally, it is a moot question as to whether the thin descending limbs are capable of active salt transport. It is tempting to speculate that all tubular epithelia transport salt, and that the descending limb is no

A serious but generally ignored challenge to the thesis that ascending vasa recta remove tubular reabsorbates from the medullary region came from the work of Niesel and Röskenbleck (1963b). They analyzed a model of the vasa recta in which the volume flow rates in the counterflowing limbs differed from each other. In all models previously studied, consideration had been limited to the simple case of equal flows in both limbs. Niesel and Röskenbleck concluded that if the volume flow rate of the ascending vasa recta exceeds that in the descending vasa recta, washout of the medullary interstitial solute will occur. They went on to suggest that since the vasa recta are known to be efficient countercurrent exchangers, they could not serve as the route of egress from the medulla of water reabsorbed from the tubules. These conclusions abound with subjective value judgments. If the driving forces and permeabilities are adequate to cause water withdrawal, and if their analysis is correct, it becomes necessary to rephrase the question they raise into the following form: How is it that the vasa recta can function as efficient countercurrent exchangers despite the imposition of a greater volume flow rate on the ascending blood vessel?

The model they analyzed consisted of two juxtaposed vessels separated by a membrane. Fluid entered the descending vessel as distilled water, while the ascending vessel fluid contained a solute which could penetrate the membrane. The flows from both vessels were collected and not recirculated. The basis for their conclusion that increasing ascending vasa recta volume flow rate degraded countercurrent exchanger function was the finding that the rate of solute loss leaving the system in the ascending vessel fluid increased as ascending vessel volume flow rate increased; evidently solute was being lost from the system at increasing rates.

Their model is subject to constraints that do not exist in the kidney. Fluid enters the ascending vessel of their model at constant solute concentration; only the volume flow rate may vary. This ascending fluid concentration sets the limit to which descending vessel fluid concentration can be raised, and since descending flow rate is held constant, the rate at which solute leaves the system in the descending vessel is therefore arbitrarily limited. In the steady state, any model conserves solute. They supply solute to their system in the ascending inflow, and permit it to leave in the descending and ascending outflows. If solute inflow is increased, and descending limb solute outflow held constant, the solute is forced to leave in the ascending outflow. Thus, it is not particularly informative to discuss efficiency in terms of the rate of ascending vessel solute loss. In the kidney, increased rates of solute addition can be used to raise interstitial solute concentration, and this is probably a more meaningful index of the function of the system.

Although the challenge arising from Niesel and Röskenbleck's model seems now to be less serious, it is nevertheless true that no other successful model has examined the consequences of disparate flows in the two limbs, and so we recently undertook such an analysis (Marsh and Segel, 1969). This study also provided an opportunity for examining some of the functional implications of recent morphological findings. Since the vasa recta are not simple loops randomly intermingled with medullary tubules, but descend for most of their length in separate vascular bundles (Kriz, 1967), there is no need to assume that the two classes of vasa recta have similar properties or numbers, and one can examine how differences between them influence countercurrent exchanger function.

Figure 7 shows the model. In it, the number of descending vasa recta may differ from the number of ascending vessels. The properties of

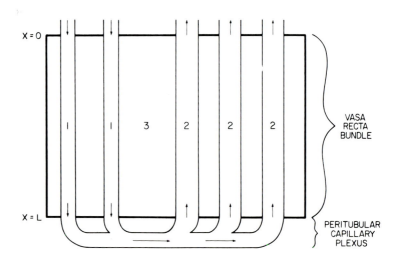

Fig. 7. A model of the vasa recta used for an analysis of countercurrent exchange. The descending and ascending vessels share an interstitial space between $X = 0$, which corresponds to the corticomedullary junction, and $X = L$, which corresponds to the tip of the papilla. They are connected by a capillary plexus which lies outside the interstitial region of the vasa recta. Solute and water are added to blood as it flows through the capillary plexus. The numbers, radii, and solute permeabilities of ascending vasa recta are permitted to differ from corresponding values for the descending vasa recta. 1 = Descending vasa recta; 2 = ascending vasa recta; 3 = interstitial space of the vasa recta bundle.

each class of blood vessels is uniform within a class, but may be different for the two classes. Addition of solute and water occurs in the capillary plexus interposed between the end of the descending and the beginning of the ascending vessels. Differential equations were derived to describe the variation of the concentration of a solute as a function of distance between $X = 0$ and $X = L$. These equations were solved and put into dimensionless form to facilitate numerical analysis. The results of this analysis show that interstitial concentration at the tip of the papilla ($X = L$) is a function of four dimensionless parameters. These are

$$\kappa = 2\pi a_D P_D L / V_D$$
$$\nu = U / n_D V_D CO$$
$$\beta = n_A V_A / n_D V_D$$
$$\rho = n_A a_A P_A / n_D a_D P_D$$

where the subscripts A and D indicate ascending vasa recta and descending vasa recta; a is a single vessel's radius; P, a single vessel's solute permeability; V, a single vessel's volume flow rate; n, a number of vessels; L, the length of the system; CO, the inflow solute concentration; and U, the rate of solute addition in the capillary plexus. The parameter κ expresses the conventional relationship among permeability, length (or, more correctly, vasa recta surface area), and volume flow rate, while ν is simply the ratio of solute input rate at the capillary plexus to solute input rate entering the descending vasa recta.

The dependence of interstitial concentration on β and ρ is shown in Figs. 8 and 9. The concentration increases significantly as ρ increases to values greater than unity. Measurements in the hamster papilla indicate that the value of ρ for Na^+ is about 4.5. This estimate was arrived at by counting the numbers of blood vessels ($n_A / n_D = 1.7$), by measuring the radii ($a_A / a_D = 1.35$), and by measuring the permeability coefficients ($P_A / P_D = 2$). Little additional benefit accrues if ρ increases beyond a value of 5. Thus, the first conclusion of this study is that inequalities between ascending and descending vasa recta enhance the exchanger function of the blood vessels. The reason for this result is that interstitial concentration is a weighted average of concentrations in the vasa recta blood. The weighting factor for descending vasa recta is

$$\frac{n_D a_D P_D}{(n_D a_D P_D + n_A a_A P_A)}$$

whereas the corresponding weighting factor for ascending vessels is

$$\frac{n_A a_A P_A}{(n_D a_D P_D + n_A a_A P_A)}$$

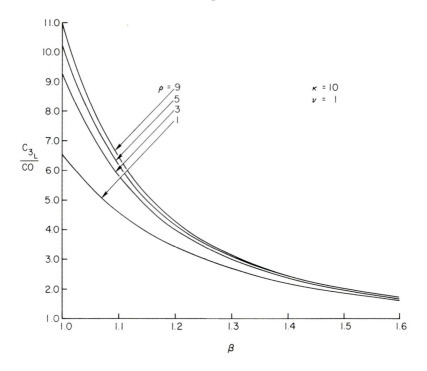

FIG. 8.   Computed results from the model of Fig. 7. Interstitial concentration of an arbitrary solute at the tip of the papilla (C_{3l}/CO) is plotted as a function of β, the ratio of ascending vasa recta volume flow rate to descending vasa recta volume flow rate, for different values of ρ, the ratio of ascending vasa recta surface area times permeability to descending vasa recta surface area times permeability. The dimensionless conductance, κ, and ν, the dimensionless rate of solute addition, are held constant.

The addition of solute that raises interstitial concentration throughout the system occurs in the capillary plexus, so that the blood returning to the vascular bundle in the ascending vasa recta will have the highest concentration of all structures within the bundle. If the ascending vasa recta is weighted more heavily, as happens when ρ exceeds unity, the effect of this high concentration is enhanced.

Interstitial concentration is quite sensitive to increasing values of β; β is the ratio of total ascending vasa recta volume flow to total descending volume flow rate, and so this result would seem at first glance to confirm the challenge raised by Niesel and Röskenbleck (1963b). This conclusion is not supported by additional analysis. The interstitial concentration rises above systemic plasma levels because the countercurrent exchanger mixes two flows: the inflowing descending vasa recta blood, and the fluid entering through the wall of the capillary plexus from the tubules. The concentration of the second fluid, the "absorbate," is the extremum which no other concentration in the system can exceed. If v, the dimensionless rate of solute addition, remains constant while β increases, the concentration of the absorbate, which is given by $v/(\beta-1)$, must decrease, and so therefore must the interstitial fluid concentration, which is limited by the value of $v/(\beta-1)$. As shown in Fig. 9, if $v/(\beta-1)$ is held constant as β increases, interstitial concentration increases toward the value of the absorbate.

In the real kidney, it is likely that the conditions in Fig. 8 will be met, since v will remain relatively constant, limited as it is by the rate of solute delivery to the ascending limbs, while β will vary depending on the diuretic circumstances. But the point of the analysis is that interstitial concentration decreases as β increases, not because the efficiency of countercurrent exchange is degraded, but because the limits imposed by the absorbate concentration are pushed down. In a certain sense exchanger efficiency is increased by increasing β, since, as can be seen clearly in Fig. 9, medullary interstitial concentration approaches the absorbate concentration more closely.

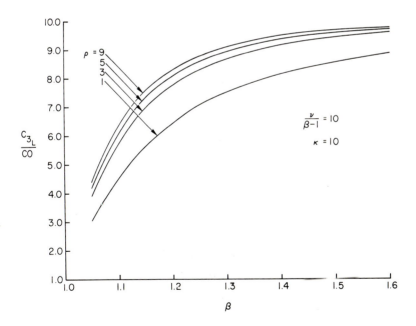

FIG. 9.   As in Fig. 8, except that v is varied to hold $v/(\beta-1)$, the dimensionless concentration of fluid absorbed from the tubules, constant.

2. ACTIVE SALT TRANSPORT BY THIN ASCENDING LIMBS

The major disagreements about the countercurrent multiplier theory center on the role of the thin ascending limb. Doubts have been expressed that this epithelium can do any active salt reabsorption at all, much less the work necessary to deliver a hypertonic reabsorbate. Evidence to sustain these doubts comes from morphologic and physiologic sources.

Although morphologic arguments are not often convincing to physiologists, the issue was first joined by Homer Smith (1959) when he accepted the countercurrent multiplier hypothesis in principle, but expressed doubts that the thin limbs could so drastically change their properties simply by turning the bend. At that time it was still impossible to differentiate between the descending and thin ascending limbs. Although modern electron microscopy has revealed some differences between the two limbs, these are relatively minor, and Smith's question still deserves an answer. Figures 10–12 are electron micrographs of descending, thin ascending, and thick ascending limbs. As can be seen, of all three structures the thin ascending limb is the simplest and least well differentiated, although the differences between descending and thin ascending limbs are not striking.

The morphological criticism of the countercurrent multiplier has three basic components.

(1) There is no morphologic substrate for the requirement that the thin ascending limbs are water-impermeable. In answer, it should be noted that virtually all plasma membranes show a typical trilamellar, unit membrane appearance, despite wide variations in water permeability. Moreover, there is now increasing evidence that the electron micrographic evidence supporting the paucimolecular theory of cell membranes gives an oversimple view of their real structure (Korn, 1966). We may conclude that there is no reliable way of learning about water permeability from electron micrographs and if there is no reason from microscopy to support the water permeability requirements of the countercurrent multiplier hypothesis, at least there is no reliable reason from this source for doubting it.

(2) Thin limbs contain few mitochondria which should be needed to generate ATP for the work of active transport. This criticism can be answered in part by pointing out that mitochondrial enzymes are primarily concerned with generating high energy phosphate bonds from aerobic metabolism. Medullary pO_2 is substantially less than that of the renal venous blood and there is evidence that much of the metabolism of the inner medulla is anaerobic. Since the enzymes supporting glyco-

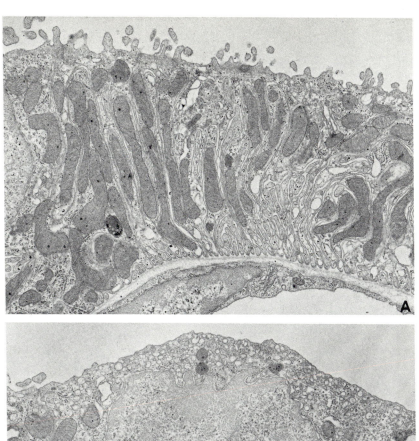

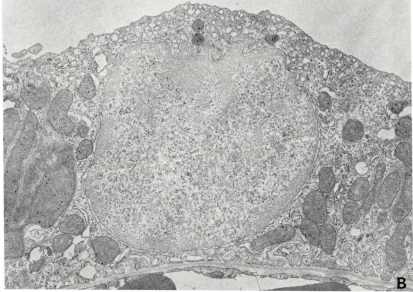

Fig. 10. (A) Electron micrograph of a thick ascending limb in the outer medulla. There are many infolded plasma membranes and interdigitations of cell processes extending to a high level in the cell. The interdigitation often extends to the lumen, ending there in a tight junction. Mitochondria are prominent, × 8,470. (B) Thick ascending limb. Cytoplasmic bodies and a number of vesicles lie above and to the right of the nucleus. × 9,240. (Reprinted, with permission, from Osvaldo and Latta, 1966a.)

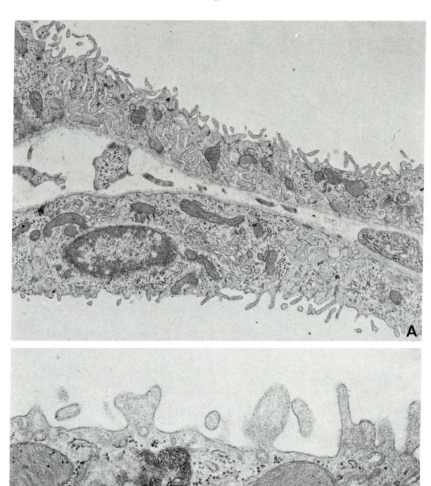

Fig. 11. (A) Electron micrograph of two descending thin limbs. The limb at the top shows the microvilli and the abundant basal and lateral small cell projections. The thin limb at the bottom shows that no basilar infoldings or projections are usually seen near the nucleus. × 8,470. (B) Descending thin limb, at higher magnification. (Reprinted, with permission, from Osvaldo and Latta, 1966a.) × 37,730.

lytic pathways are dissolved in the cytoplasm, there is a lesser need for mitochondria to support the work of the inner medullary tubules. Nevertheless, it is true that the thick ascending limb of the outer medulla operates in a region of lower pO_2, albeit not quite as low as in the inner medulla. There is no doubt about the ability of the thick ascending limb to reabsorb salt by active transport. The corticomedullary oxygen

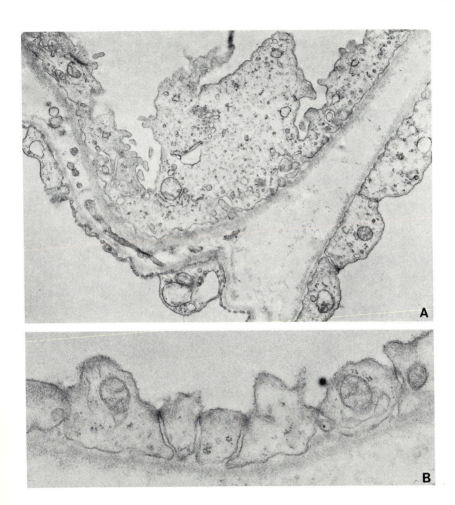

FIG. 12. (A) Thin limbs in inner medulla. The descending thin limb is above, an ascending thin limb to the right, and a capillary to the lower left. × 6,160. (B) Ascending thin limb. The cell processes have a simple structure and project irregularly into the lumen. The attachment zones are quite short. (Reprinted, with permission, from Osvaldo and Latta, 1966a.) × 27,720.

gradient appears to be smooth, with no discontinuity at the junction between the inner and outer medullas, and since the thick limbs have mitochondria in abundance, the reason for the sharp morphological boundary, if there is no functional distinction between the thin and thick ascending limbs, remains unclear.

(3) The cells of the thin ascending limb form a relatively flat, nondifferentiated epithelium, in contrast to the tall, differentiated cells of the thick ascending limb. Thus, if the thick ascending limbs use their structure to generate hypertonic reabsorbates, should not the thin ascending limbs have difficulty fulfilling the same function? This argument can be made to cut both ways. If one were to design an epithelium to reabsorb hypertonically, the most efficient plan would call for the flattest possible epithelium, so that the transported salt could diffuse readily away from the cells and minimize the transepithelial osmotic pressure difference created by the transport process. In many epithelia, the presence of long intercellular channels provides an opportunity for isotonic equilibration of the absorbate (Diamond, 1964; Diamond and Bossert, 1967). In at least this respect, the thin ascending limb appears admirably designed to produce a hypertonic reabsorbate. Nevertheless, the thick ascending limb reabsorbs hypertonically, its long intercellular channels notwithstanding. Thus, the differentiation argument cannot reasonably be interpreted without phenomenological observations on the function of the epithelia.

In summary, we can draw no definite conclusion from morphology. But the differences between thin and thick ascending limbs are more striking than between thin ascending and descending limbs, whereas the countercurrent multiplier hypothesis must have it just the other way, at least in regard to function. If we cannot make any definitive criticism of the hypothesis from microscopy, neither can we comfortably support it, and so we are still forced to wonder.

Direct tests of the transport capabilities of thin limbs provide the strongest challenge to the application of the countercurrent multiplier theory in the inner medulla. Stopped flow microperfusion experiments, originally developed for mammalian tubules by Gertz (1963), permit isolation of perfusion solutions between oil columns in the tubular lumen so that solutes and water are free to exchange between perfusate and interstitium. This procedure permits an evaluation of the transport capability of an epithelium with various test solutions and is independent of the delivery of glomerular filtrate and the operations of more proximal regions of the tubule on it. As is shown in Fig. 13, when saline is isolated between oil columns in the lumen of the prox-

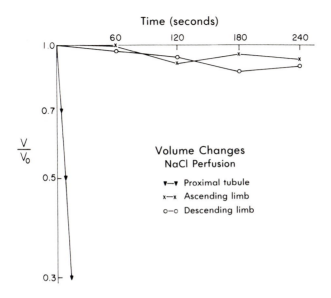

FIG. 13. Results of stopped flow microperfusion experiments in thin limbs compared with results of similar experiments in proximal tubule. Perfusion with NaCl solutions: 150 mM in proximal tubule, 450 mM in loops.

imal tubule, it is reabsorbed with a half-time of 10 seconds. Marsh and Solomon (1965) performed similar experiments in thin ascending and descending limbs in the hamster papilla and found no reabsorption of the saline test droplet over prolonged periods of time (the longest observation was 4 hours, during which time the test droplet remained at the same volume).

Since it had been postulated that the thin ascending limb is water-impermeable, the failure to find reabsorption of a saline droplet could result either from a lack of active salt transport or from water impermeability. Two different sets of experiments were done to decide between these possibilities. In one, the saline perfusates were put into place, permitted to equilibrate with the interstitial fluid, and then reaspirated for analysis; vasa recta blood from adjacent capillaries provided a measure of interstitial fluid composition. There was no osmolality difference between perfusate and interstitial fluid, and so the question of water impermeability was judged to be irrelevant because there was no osmotic gradient to cause water movement. The electrochemical potential differences for both Na^+ and Cl^- were zero across both limbs in these saline microperfusion experiments. Neither the volume of the droplets nor their concentrations were changing at the time of the measurements, so that the net flux of salt was zero when the electro-chemical potentials were zero. The condition for equilibrium was there-fore fulfilled and we concluded that there is no metabolic force capable of moving either Na^+ or Cl^- against their respective electrochemical potential gradients in either ascending or descending thin limbs.

In another set of experiments, isotonic raffinose was used as the test solution. There was no salt in the perfusion solution and so there was a relatively large concentration gradient down into the lumen. In the proximal tubules such experiments lead to a rapid influx of salt, drag-ging water with it. A qualitatively similar result occurred in both de-scending and thin ascending limbs. Hence, water appeared to cross the epithelium when an appropriate driving force was present, so the failure to observe reabsorption of the saline test droplet could not be due to water impermeability of either epithelium. The most reasonable and self-consistent explanation for these results is that both epithelia lack the capability for active salt reabsorption.*

This experimental approach is the most direct test yet devised of what a tubular epithelium can do; if the results are correct, the coun-tercurrent multiplier theory can not work in the medulla and some other mechanism for concentrating the urine in this region must be sought. To decide on the validity of the result, one must turn to other experimental designs.

One such test was provided by the experiments of Jamison *et al.* (1967). They used a partial nephrectomy technique developed to pro-vide greater exposure of the rat inner medullary surface than is pos-sible by simple excision of the renal pelvis (Sakai *et al.*, 1965). Their main result is shown in Fig. 14. They compared specimens taken from adjacent descending and thin ascending limbs and found the osmolality of ascending limb fluid to be significantly and consistently lower than

---

*Gottschalk (1964) has reported confirmation of the volume measurements in the as-cending limb when using saline as the test solution. He interprets these results to indicate water impermeability of the thin ascending limb, but this interpretation is contradicted by the results of raffinose experiments and by the isoosmolality of perfusion solution and vasa recta plasma, both of which he also confirmed. He also reported a volume increase with raffinose solutions in the thin descending limb, but in contrast to the results of Marsh and Solomon, found a volume decrease with saline as the perfusion solution in the descending limbs. His results can be reproduced when the tubule is damaged by exces-sive distention induced by injecting large quantities of oil, which raises pressure in the tubule (Marsh and Solomon, 1965). The reabsorption is due to elevated hydrostatic pres-sure differences made more effective by damage to the tubule wall. In any event, the sig-nificance of Gottschalk's results cannot be evaluated because he has never published them in full; he mentioned them in passing in a review article published 4 years ago, followed by a recital of the technical difficulties encountered during their performance.

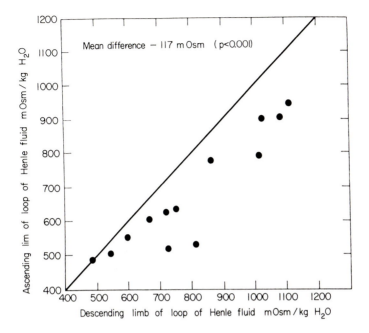

Fɪɢ. 14.   This figure compares tubular fluid osmolalities from rat thin ascending limbs with those from adjacent descending limbs. (Reprinted, with permission, from Jamison *et al.*, 1967.)

descending limb fluid. They also showed that 91% of this osmolality difference could be accounted for by a difference of NaCl concentrations. This result is predictable from the countercurrent multiplier hypothesis since the hypertonic reabsorption of NaCl by thin ascending limbs should bring its tubular fluid osmolality and NaCl concentrations to values lower than in adjacent descending limbs which are equilibrating with the interstitial fluid.

But if these results are consistent with the countercurrent multiplier hypothesis, they do not prove it, for several reasons. For example, a concentration difference between two points along a tubule might result either from the removal of solute or from the addition of water. The thin ascending limb moves through a region of ever decreasing osmolality, and if solute and water movements are governed solely by concentration gradients across its wall, net influx of water into its lumen would be expected. Second, to ascribe significance to an osmolality difference between two limbs at the same level requires the assumption that both make contact with the same interstitial region. Recent anatomical findings, discussed earlier, suggest that this requirement is not fulfilled (Kriz, 1967). Recall that descending limbs run with the vasa recta in bundles, whereas the ascending limbs are partitioned into a separate region along with collecting ducts. Thus it needs to be proved that the interstitial fluid of both spaces is the same in a given plane of the medulla. No such proof exists. Finally, the loop penetrates a medullary interstitial region whose NaCl and urea concentrations increase steadily toward the papillary tip. Thus, NaCl concentrations in the thin descending limb must first increase before they can start to decrease in the ascending limb, and some urea will be added to the tubular fluid. Until it becomes possible to separate the changes occurring in the two segments of the loop, no particular significance can be attached to the fact that most of the solute concentration between the two limbs is provided by a difference of NaCl concentration.

Two reports subsequently appeared which should have clarified some of these points. Jamison (1968) found that inulin concentrations were, on average, higher in thin ascending limbs than in descending limbs. This result would seem to exclude the possibility of a net volume influx anywhere along the thin limb, but Horster and Thurau (1968) obtained the opposite result in a study designed to examine some other aspects of flow dynamics in juxtamedullary nephrons. The experimental design in both was apparently identical. And both suffer from the same defect. Specimens were taken from random loops in different animals, with no effort to match ascending to descending limb collections. The composition of the medullary interstitial fluid is simply too variable from animal to animal, and even from time to time in the same animal, for random collections productively to be referred to each other.

To avoid these pitfalls, I recently performed a series of experiments in which paired collections were made at separate sites from single thin ascending limbs (Marsh, 1970a). Figure 15 shows the paired inulin data from these experiments. There was no detectable change of the inulin TF/P along the first 750–1000 μ of thin ascending limb, which is approximately 20% of the total length of this segment in the hamster. This result refutes the suggestion that the function of the thin ascending limbs is to remove water from the medulla. Figure 16 compares these inulin data with values for osmolality, sodium, and urea, measured in the same specimens. There is, on average, net reabsorption of solute from the thin ascending limb in antidiuresis, and the main solute reabsorbed is NaCl. Since there is virtually no water movement from a segment which is reabsorbing NaCl, it follows that these loops reabsorb salt hypertonically, as required by the countercurrent multiplier hypothesis. Note that the reabsorption of solute is more than

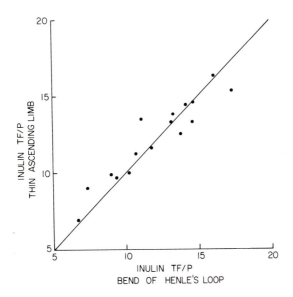

FIG. 15.   A comparison of inulin TF/P values from hamster thin ascending limbs with those from the bend of the same loop of Henle (Marsh, 1970a).

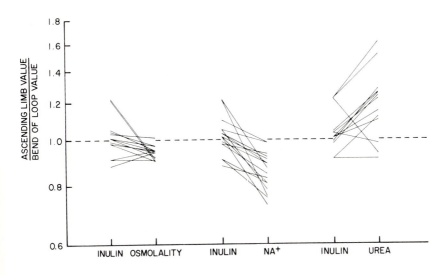

FIG. 16.   Results of paired collections from sites 0.75–1.0 mm apart in single thin ascending limbs. The lines connect values for inulin ratios with the corresponding values for osmolality, Na^+, and urea. Negative slopes indicate net reabsorption between the two collection sites, positive slopes show net entry into tubular fluid (Marsh, 1970a).

accounted for by the reabsorption of NaCl. The apparent discrepancy is due to net influx of urea from the interstitial region into the tubular fluid.

By themselves these results permit no conclusion about the mechanism of the reabsorption. The thin ascending limb crosses the corticomedullary solute gradient as it returns toward the cortex, so that the tubular fluid always comes from a region of higher NaCl concentration, a circumstance which could readily create a concentration gradient favoring the efflux by diffusion of NaCl from the lumen. Hence, the observed reabsorption might simply reflect passive movement of NaCl in response to existing gradients. If this were true, these results would be compatible with the stopped flow microperfusion data, which failed to show evidence of active NaCl reabsorption. Tempting though it may be to adopt this interpretation to reconcile two apparently conflicting sets of data, I will now attempt to show the difficulties inherent in such a course.

Assume for the moment that the results of this last study are due to passive movement of NaCl across the thin ascending limb epithelium. If the loops do no osmotic work, some other structure must be responsible for the production of the corticomedullary solute gradient. It has been argued that the collecting duct is such a structure (Marsh, 1966), and indeed there is little question that the collecting duct performs osmotic work in the form of active salt transport. However, for this work to be harnessed to the urinary concentration mechanism, certain stringent requirements must be met. The reabsorbate generated by the collecting ducts must be hypotonic with respect to the collecting duct luminal contents. An isotonic reabsorbate will simply transfer volume but cause no change of concentration, and hypertonic reabsorption might concentrate the interstitial region, but would leave the urine more dilute. Thus, only if the reabsorbate is primarily hypotonic, and then, only if some mechanism exists for the removal of this hypotonic solution from the interstitial region can collecting duct salt transport serve to concentrate both the urine and the medullary interstitium. The data of Fig. 15 exclude the loops of Henle from consideration as the route of water removal from the medulla, and it is difficult to conceive that the vasa recta have the permeabilities needed to accomplish this task. Thus, these results, while only consistent with the active participation of the loops of Henle as countercurrent multipliers, actually argue more strongly for countercurrent multiplication because they exclude the participation of the loops in a collecting duct mechanism.

To decide finally whether the thin ascending limbs act on the interstitium or the interstitium on the ascending limbs, we must know the composition of the interstitial fluid adjacent to the thin ascending limb. If tubular fluid NaCl concentration is lower than interstitial fluid the results will compel adoption of the countercurrent multiplier hypothesis; but if it is higher, the hypothesis must be rejected. Since the two limbs run in separate spaces, no measurements in the descending limb–vascular space can tell us the interstitial concentration in the ascending limb collecting duct space.

But we may ask under what circumstances the vasa recta–descending limb space might have the highest osmolality of any other space in a given plane perpendicular to the corticomedullary axis. The answer can be formulated in a general way: The region where the osmotic work is done will have the highest concentration. For the vasa recta–descending limb space to be at the highest concentration requires that blood vessels or descending limbs be the locus of the single effect.

Although the properties of vasa recta have not been extensively studied, there is no reason to believe that they or any other capillaries are capable of osmotic work. Moreover, active secretion of NaCl into the lumen of the descending limb, which could undoubtedly work as the single effect in the countercurrent multiplier, is unsupported by the slightest shred of evidence, might actually leave the descending limb–vascular bundle interstitial region less concentrated rather than more concentrated than in other regions, and is inelegant, because it requires that salt be pumped in a direction it never takes elsewhere in the nephron. Thus, by a process of exclusion, we are left with active salt reabsorption from the thin ascending limb as the primary supplier of work for the urinary concentrating mechanism in the inner medulla. The conclusion is insecure because it is not rigorously proved, and because there are conflicting data from the stopped flow microperfusion studies. Free flow collections are more standard, and inherently more trouble-free, easier to perform, and easier to control, than stopped flow microperfusion. For these reasons, and because purely passive behavior of the thin ascending limb leads to an apparently unresolvable dilemma about the origins of the corticomedullary solute gradient, I conclude that the stopped flow microperfusion result is in error, for reasons that are not at all apparent.

There are additional data consistent with countercurrent multiplication in the inner medulla. Morgan and Berliner (1968) excised the inner medulla of rats, placed it in a bath of Ringer's solution, and perfused single tubules on the surface of the excised tissue. They found that the descending limb Na^+ and water permeabilities were several times higher than corresponding values in the thin ascending limbs. The urea permeability was essentially the same in both segments.

These results, particularly with respect to Na$^+$ and water, are exactly those required by the countercurrent multiplier hypothesis, since they would permit rapid equilibration of descending limb tubular fluid with the interstitial space and prevent back flux of water and NaCl into the thin ascending limb lumen during formation of a hypertonic reabsorbate. Unfortunately, the validity of these results is clouded by the fact that the authors could not find the least vestige of active salt transport in any epithelium in this tissue, not even in the collecting ducts where there is no dispute about its presence during life. Active salt transport is such a fundamental process that its absence may be a rather elegant way of demonstrating that the tissue under study is dead. What the effects of tissue death on epithelial permeability might be is a matter of conjecture. On the other hand, it would be surprising if the relationships among the permeabilities established by these studies did not bear at least some qualitative resemblance to what is present *in vivo*.

Another set of results bearing on the question of thin ascending limb function comes from measurements of electrical potential differences. Windhager (1964) found that in antidiuretic hamsters, the descending limb lumen is isopotential with the interstitial fluid, whereas the thin ascending limb is 9–11 mV negative. These results were confirmed by Marsh and Solomon (1965). Windhager ascribed the ascending limb negativity to active salt transport, in analogy with the behavior of anuran epithelia (Leaf *et al.*, 1958; Ussing and Zerahn, 1951), the distal tubule (Windhager and Giebisch, 1965), and what was then thought to be the electrical behavior of the proximal tubule (Windhager and Giebisch, 1965). In support of this interpretation, he showed that the perfusion of thin ascending limbs with Ringer solution produced the same result as was found in free flow conditions, while substitution of Na$^+$ by choline, which presumably permeates less well than Na$^+$, led to a reversal of the potential, with the lumen becoming positive. This result was purported to show that the development of the potential found during free flow depended on having Na$^+$ in the lumen. While there can be no quarreling with such a conclusion, it does not follow that the Na$^+$ is needed to support active transport, since the elimination of Na$^+$ from the lumen establishes a diffusion gradient across the epithelial wall and creates a diffusion potential where none normally exists.

Windhager also perfused the thin ascending limb lumen with a saline solution containing a mixture of sodium cyanide and sodium iodoacetate, to study the metabolic dependence of the electrical potential difference. The inhibitors eliminated the potential, which seems to support the notion that the potential depends on metabolic energy and so is related to active transport. Marsh and Solomon confirmed these results, but when they perfused with higher concentrations of inhibitors, found that the potential reversed and the lumen became positive. The inhibitor anions are present only in the lumen, creating large gradients for them across the tubule wall. Thus, it is at least conceivable that the apparent inhibition found by Windhager is really due to the establishment of a diffusion potential of countersign, particularly owing to the presence of cyanide, a highly mobile anion. Whether this is possible depends on the transference numbers for the various ions, and these values are not known.

Marsh and Solomon (1965) eliminated the possibility that the ascending limb electrical potential difference found during free flow in antidiuresis could be due to diffusion processes by showing that there were no concentration gradients for any of the major ions, and suggested that the potential might be due to electrokinetic phenomena—a streaming potential. This suggestion was strengthened by preliminary indications that there might be an influx of water into the lumen of the thin ascending limb (Thurau and Henne, 1963). These findings were not confirmed by more standard techniques involving measurement of inulin TF/P ratios in thin ascending limbs (Marsh, 1970a). In the absence of a demonstrable water flux, the streaming potential hypothesis becomes untenable, and the electrical potential measurements must therefore be considered as consistent with active salt reabsorption from the thin ascending limb.

However, Marsh and Solomon (1965) also found that the electrical potential difference of the ascending limb disappeared during mannitol diuresis. If this potential is due to active salt reabsorption it is hard to understand why it should disappear when the Na^+ concentration is still 200–300 meq/liter. Its disappearance cannot be attributed to the development of a diffusion potential of countersign since it could be shown that there were no concentration gradients of sufficient magnitude to produce a counterpotential. This observation remains as a puzzling inconsistency.

V. Alternatives to the Countercurrent Multiplier Theory

The evidence available to date seems on balance to support the application of the countercurrent multiplier hypothesis in the inner medulla. Because this evidence has been slow in accumulating and often conflicting, there have been several attempts to provide alternatives to the countercurrent multiplier hypothesis which do not depend on salt pumping by the thin ascending limb. Although each of these attempts suffers serious defects, it is useful for historical reasons to review them here. They may be put into two groups: (1) those that use work performed away from the inner medulla, and (2) those that depend on work performed directly in the inner medulla itself.

A. Sources of Work Not in the Inner Medulla

Two models have been proposed that depend on work performed outside the inner medulla to concentrate this region. The first depends on hydrostatic pressure; in effect the heart provides the work (Lever, 1965). However, when Hargitay and Kuhn (1951) used a hydrostatic pressure multiplier, as in Fig. 2A, to illustrate the operation of a countercurrent multiplier model, they recognized that pressures available from vascular structures were inadequate to account for the osmotic concentration routinely observed in dehydrated mammals, even those that need only concentrate to osmotic U/P's of 3 or 4. Their calculation of the maximum osmolality that could be obtained from a hydrostatic multiplier was based on the assumption that the membrane separating the two limbs discriminates perfectly between solute and solvent. If the membrane does not discriminate well, i.e., if the osmotic flow entrains solute and carries it across by solvent drag, the efficiency of such a multiplier suffers. For small solutes such as NaCl and urea, capillaries generally have vanishingly small osmotic reflection coefficients, (a useful index of the membrane's ability to discriminate between solute and solvent), making it even less likely that a hydrostatic multiplier could be solely responsible for the concentrating mechanism.

On the other hand, it has been suggested that a hydrostatic multiplier could provide an important fraction of the work (Lever, 1965). For example, assume that the countercurrent multiplier operates in the outer medulla where urine is concentrated to 700–800 mosmols. The available hydrostatic pressures could produce an additional increase of 600–700 mosmols in the inner medulla, but only if there is perfect solute–solvent discrimination. The more realistic assumption, that discrimination is almost totally absent, renders even this more restricted hydrostatic multiplier inadequate. Moreover, there are many species that concentrate the urine to osmolalities greatly in excess of 2000–3000 mosmols, clearly beyond the capability of hydrostatic pressure multipliers working with available vascular pressures. One is compelled to argue that the same basic concentrating mechanism operates in all mammals, which leads to the conclusion that hydrostatic pressure cannot be contributing significantly to osmotic concentration in the inner medulla. Hydrostatic pressure available to tubules is lower than in blood vessels. Thus, in principle, hydrostatic pressure can furnish a fraction of the work necessary for increasing urinary osmolality, but it is likely to be an insignificant factor, whether it operates with the loops or vasa recta, or even both, as the site of multiplication.

Pinter and Shohet (1963; Shohet and Pinter, 1963) suggested that countercurrent multiplication limited to the outer medulla provides work that could be distributed into the inner medulla by the descending limbs of Henle's loops and the vasa recta. They analyzed this model with an analog computer and concluded that it could indeed account for the corticomedullary gradient seen in antidiuresis. Unfortunately, their formulation of the mathematical problem was inconsistent, as pointed out by Stephenson (1966) and by Kelman *et al.* (1966) whose results prove that the maximal interstitial osmolality can occur only in the outer medulla if salt pumping is limited to that zone. The best that can be hoped from their model is that the inner medullary interstitial concentration does not decrease, but remains constant over the length of the corticomedullary axis. If any conclusion can be drawn from this work, it is that some source of osmotic work located directly in the inner medulla is necessary to generate the inner medullary concentration gradients.

Pinter and Shohet's error arose in their treatment of a discontinuity in the curve of interstitial concentration vs. length which occurred at the junction of the inner and outer medulla. The discontinuity originates in their decision to neglect longitudinal diffusion in the interstitial space, certainly a justifiable choice in view of the fact that its effect on the concentration profile is trivial (Marsh *et al.*, 1967) and that to deal with it would require introduction of a second order equation into their system of first order equations. They simply smoothed the discontinuity by imposing the artificial boundary condition that the interstitial concentration was the same on both sides of the junction. Their system then became overdetermined, and their incorrect conclusion emerged.

After the dust had settled on this issue, Marumo *et al.* (1967) reported on an analog computer simulation of the medulla in which they claim that active salt pumping restricted to the outer medulla could raise inner medullary interstitial NaCl concentrations. Their model differs from Pinter and Shohet's by including a collecting duct, and by considering the behavior of urea as well as NaCl. Their equation describing the interstitial NaCl profile is exactly the same as Pinter and Shohet's, yet their results show no discontinuity, nor do they comment on the problem. From their computer program, it appears that they use a single amplifier to compute interstitial NaCl concentrations for both inner and outer medulla. This places the same erroneous constraint on the inner medullary interstitial concentration that led Pinter and Shohet into trouble; the correct way to deal with this problem is to compute interstitial curves for the two zones independently of each other.

B. Sources of Work in the Inner Medulla

Three mechanisms have been proposed as sources of osmotic work in the inner medulla. Pinter (1967a) recently noted that mucopolysaccharides, which abound in the medullary interstitium, are normally heavily hydrated. This hydration water is not a solvent for most other solutes, and so the removal of the hydrated hyaluronic acid by the circulation would serve to dehydrate the interstitial region. This is a provocative idea which is difficult to evaluate on the basis of present information. It would be necessary to have some estimate of the rate of hyaluronic acid production and the extent of its hydration before it could be decided whether this hypothesis is feasible.

A somewhat older variant of this idea is that the oxidation of glucose to lactate produces two osmotically active particles for each one consumed and that the countercurrent arrangement of the loops and vasa recta serves to amplify the hyperosmolality this effect produces (Niesel and Röskenbleck, 1963a). It would be necessary to have some idea of the rate at which this reaction or similar ones proceed to provide a quantitative estimate of the concentrating effect that could result. A prediction of this hypothesis is that the osmotic increase of the medulla is due largely to Na^+ and an anion such as lactate or bicarbonate. The difference between medullary and systemic plasma Na^+ concentrations is accounted for almost perfectly by chloride, while the bicarbonate concentration does not differ in the two regions (Uhlich et al., 1968). It is unlikely that this hypothesis could provide the major driving force for the hyperosmolality of the inner medullary fluids, although again it might provide some fraction of the work.

Collecting ducts are capable of active salt reabsorption, as first became apparent from the microcatheterization work of Hilger et al. (1958). Ullrich et al. (1963), Malnic et al. (1966), and Landwehr et al. (1967) confirmed this conclusion when they showed that under most experimental circumstances, the fraction of salt excreted is significantly less than the fraction of the filtered Na^+ passing through the distal tubule. Thus, the collecting ducts are capable of osmotic work. Although several authors had suggested in passing that collecting duct salt reabsorption could contribute to inner medullary concentrating processes, the most detailed exposition was made by Marsh and co-workers (1967; Marsh, 1966) who termed the proposal the lineal multiplication mechanism.

In this hypothesis, the countercurrent multiplier was thought to operate only in the outer medulla. The single effect in the inner medulla occurred in the collecting duct, whose salt transport mechanism was required to generate a primary hypotonic reabsorbate. It should be appreciated that in order for collecting duct urine to be concentrated by any mechanism, the fluid reabsorbed from its lumen must be hypoosmotic with respect to the luminal contents, but in this proposal the hypoosmolality was attributed to transport processes occurring in the epithelial wall itself, rather than to simple osmosis, as in the countercurrent multiplier hypothesis. Repetition of this collecting duct hypotonic reabsorption along the length of the corticomedullary axis would generate a collecting duct urine of increasing osmolality towards the tip of the papilla, provided that the osmolality of the reabsorbate was always governed by the collecting duct fluid osmolality, and hypotonic to it.

At first glance, it would seem that the transfer of a more dilute solution into the interstitial fluid should dilute the interstitial space, whereas it is well known that the medullary interstitial fluid becomes more concentrated toward the tip of the papilla. There are two answers to this problem. First, the reabsorbate itself would become progressively more concentrated towards the tip of the papilla, thereby providing the element of stratification needed to initiate the concentrating mechanism in the interstitial region. Second, to maintain a steady state in which the concentration at any given level in the papilla remains constant with time, there must be some route by which this dilute fluid can leave the medulla, and the proposal was made that the ascending limb might be the route of water removal. It was further proposed that this water movement could be coupled to solute diffusion into the lumen as the thin ascending limb ran through the stratified reabsorbate from the collecting ducts, an idea that would have assigned a passive albeit essential role to the thin loops.

Thus, the lineal multiplication mechanism has two requirements, (a) that the collecting duct reabsorb hypotonically and (b) that the thin ascending limb remove a hypotonic fluid. Experimental evidence for the first came from microperfusion experiments in an *in vitro* isolated papilla preparation (Marsh, 1966). These initial results were obtained along with other data suggesting that collecting ducts perfused under these circumstances were capable of active salt transport. It later became impossible to sustain active salt reabsorption in this preparation, and once the ability to perform active work was lost, hypotonic reabsorption disappeared. The reasons for the initial success and subsequent failure have never been discovered. Subsequently, Morgan *et al.* (1968) were also unable to show active salt transport in a similar preparation. Thus, the question of the absorbate tonicity and its concentration dependence remains open. Although hypotonic reabsorption had never been demonstrated for any other epithelium, at least two groups of investigators predicted from theoretical arguments (Curran and MacIntosh, 1962; Patlak *et al.*, 1963; Diamond, 1962) that it might occur, particularly at high salt concentrations such as occur in the medulla.

The second part of the hypothesis, having to do with the removal from the medulla of a hypotonic fluid by the thin ascending limbs, was supported by dye injection measurements of volume flow rates in the loops (Marsh, 1968; Thurau and Henne, 1963). Because it requires that volume flow rate be calculated from linear flow velocity and the cross sectional area of the tubule, this technique relies critically on accurate measurements of tubule radius. The available optical instruments lack a sufficiently large numerical aperture to provide the resolution needed of this parameter, and the results of such studies are open to question. More recent results (Marsh, 1970a), described above, which use more conventional inulin measurements, fail to show a volume influx into the lumen of the thin ascending limb. This hypotonic volume influx is an essential precondition for the operation of the lineal multiplication mechanism. Since the most reliable measurements show that it does not occur in thin ascending limbs, and since there is no reason to believe that vasa recta possess the selectivity required to generate anything but an isotonic absorbate, it is necessary to discard the lineal multiplication mechanism.

VI. Water Diuresis

When the levels of antidiuretic hormone in the circulating plasma drop, the urine flow rate increases and the urine becomes less concentrated than systemic plasma. Both glomerular filtration rate and sodium excretion remain unchanged (Brooks and Pickford, 1958), although the latter may undergo transient fluctuations. The most generally accepted explanation of these phenomena is that the absence of ADH causes the water permeability of the distal tubule and collecting ducts to decrease; osmotic gradients first created by the hypertonic reabsorption of NaCl from the thick ascending limb cannot be dissipated in the more distal segments. The water permeabilities do not fall to zero without ADH, and some water reabsorption probably occurs, but the low osmolality of the tubular fluid is maintained by active salt reabsorption from the lumen of the distal nephron. The behavior of the proximal tubule is thought to be unaffected by the hormone.

Experimental support for some of the more important assumptions of this model have recently come from several groups of investigators. Ullrich *et al.* (1964) measured the water permeability of proximal and distal tubules in normal rats and in rats with diabetes insipidus induced by anodal hypothalamic lesions. Distal tubule water permeabilities were ten times greater in antidiuresis than in water diuresis. Grantham and Burg (1966) showed that outer medullary collecting ducts also respond to ADH and to cyclic AMP when studied with an elegant isolated perfused collecting tubule preparation they developed. Gardner and Maffly (1964) demonstrated that ADH increased the water permeability of inner medullary collecting ducts in an isolated perfused papilla, while Morgan *et al.* (1968) also observed an effect of ADH on perfused collecting ducts in an *in vitro* inner medullary preparation. However, these investigators were unable to maintain the viability of the active transport systems known to be present *in vivo* in these structures. Since active salt transport invariably exerts a strong frictional effect on water fluxes across epithelia, their observation must be accepted with reservation.

Finally, the nonparticipation of the proximal tubule in the formation of dilute urine was shown by Gertz *et al.* (1964), who found that proximal tubular reabsorptive capacities measured with the split-drop technique were unchanged in diabetes insipidus rats as compared with normals; by Davis *et al.* (1967) who found that proximal inulin TF/P's in dogs undergoing water diuresis were the same as in antidiuretic proximal tubules; and by Schnermann *et al.* (1969), who also found that end proximal inulin TF/P in rats with hereditary diabetes insipidus did not change after ADH administration.

There are some unresolved questions in water diuresis. Although the mode of action of ADH on renal tubules is fairly well understood (Orloff and Handler, 1964), there appears to be at least one difference between its effects on distal and collecting tubules on the one hand, and on frog skin, toad bladder, and inner medullary collecting ducts on the other. ADH increases the permeability of the latter group to urea (Orloff and Handler, 1964), but does not affect the urea permeability of the rat distal tubule (Capek *et al.*, 1966) or the perfused rabbit collecting tubule (Grantham and Burg, 1966). Whether this difference reflects fundamental dissimilarities in the mode of action of the hormone, or whether it is a secondary effect arising out of the local geometry, is not known. For example, unstirred layers adjacent to a membrane can lead to underestimation of permeability coefficients (Dainty and House, 1966). This interference arises because there are concentration gradients through the unstirred layer and the concentration of penetrating solute at the membrane differs from the concentration in the bulk phase. Mixing minimizes this error because it accelerates transport through the unstirred layer by convection. Unstirred layers abound in frog skin (Dainty and House, 1966) and toad bladder (Lichtenstein and Leaf, 1965), but operationally they cannot exist in the lumen of mammalian renal tubules because diffusion distances across the tubule are too short to sustain significant concentration gradients (Friedlander and Walser, 1965; Kelman, 1962). The effect of ADH on urea permeability in the frog skin and toad bladder could be due to increased convection (because of the stimulation of Na transport) through a dense unstirred layer. Similar, although not identical suggestions, have been made by Lichtenstein and Leaf (1965) and by Hays (1968). The inner medullary collecting ducts have a considerably larger cross sectional area than the cortical tubules, and so the possibility of unstirred layers is not excluded.

Antidiuretic hormone causes an increased short-circuit current in frog skin (Ussing and Zerahn, 1951) and toad bladder (Leaf *et al.*, 1958) indicating that the rate of active Na$^+$ transport is increased. The usual explanation for this observation is that the rate of active transport is determined by the availability of Na$^+$ to the pump, and that this availability is in turn governed by the permeability of the ADH-responsive area. One would therefore expect to find decreased Na reabsorption in water diuresis, but in practice salt excretion remains at antidiuretic levels (Brooks and Pickford, 1958). This apparent contradiction will not be resolved until the effects of the hormone on salt reabsorption in individual tubule segments are studied.

Another important question in water diuresis has to do with the composition of the medullary interstitial fluid. Bray (1960) measured medullary osmolality with the cryoscopic technique first used by Wirz *et al.* (1951) in antidiuresis. Bray confirmed Wirz's findings and also showed that the corticomedullary gradient in the inner medulla disappears during water diuresis although outer medullary hypertonicity is virtually the same in both conditions. Boylan and Asshauer (1962) made similar observations. When viewed in the context of the countercurrent multiplier theory this behavior of the inner medullary gradient is surprising. As discussed earlier, a countercurrent multiplier generates the highest concentrations when it is not required to extract water from other tubules. In the absence of ADH one would expect less water to enter the medullary region from the collecting duct and so the countercurrent multiplier should be able to raise medullary interstitial concentrations even higher than in antidiuresis.

Two different phenomena have been invoked to explain this apparent paradox. First, it has been asserted that more water is actually reabsorbed from collecting ducts in water diuresis than in antidiuresis (Berliner and Davidson, 1957). This assertion was based on inferences drawn from clearance experiments; it is not substantiated by recent micropuncture experiments on rats with diabetes insipidus (D.I.). In D.I. due to hypothalamic lesions, the middistal inulin TF/P is the same as in normal antidiuretic animals, whereas the inulin U/P is, of course, much lower in D.I. (Gertz et al., 1964). In rats with hereditary diabetes insipidus, the distal inulin TF/P was actually higher than in the same animals given antidiuretic hormone (Schnermann et al., 1969). In this latter study, ADH greatly increased the urinary inulin U/P but had no effect on GFR; the volume reabsorbed between the distal collection site and the final urine increased threefold after the hormone was given.

The possibility remains that some of this fluid is reabsorbed from the late distal and early collecting tubules of antidiuretic rats so that the actual load presented to the collecting ducts entering the medullary rays is not as great as suggested by these data. However, it should be recalled that the water efflux which leads to the return to isotonicity in the distal tubules does not occur invariably in this segment; in the antidiuretic dog (Bennett et al., 1967) and monkey (Bennett et al., 1968) this takes place beyond the distal tubule, presumably in the early collecting tubules which may already have entered the medullary rays, which are a functional part of the outer medulla. Until there is some way of making measurements in the collecting tubules of intact animals, no definitive answer to this problem can be given. At present, the available evidence does not support the suggestion that the diminished medullary osmolality observed in water diuresis is due to a paradoxical increase in the amount of water entering the medullary region from the collecting ducts.*

The second explanation for the diminished medullary tonicity is that

---

*The suggestion of increased collecting duct water reabsorption in water diuresis has been made because reduction of GFR by arterial constriction in dogs undergoing a water diuresis led to the excretion of hypertonic urine, suggesting that the water permeability of collecting ducts in the absence of antidiuretic hormone was not zero (Berliner and Davidson, 1957). Since there is a sizeable osmolality gradient between collecting duct urine and medullary interstitial fluid in water diuresis, but not in antidiuresis, it was then assumed that the apparent larger gradient present in water diuresis could more than compensate for the diminished water permeability. The inferences drawn from the collecting duct transmural gradient seem to me to be incorrect; there is little or no gradient in antidiuresis because osmotic water flow has already occurred in response to it. Osmotic flow cannot occur in water diuresis because of the lower permeability, and the gradient is uncovered. To evaluate the effective osmotic gradient, one should compare the osmolality of fluid entering the collecting ducts from the distal tubule, about 300 mosmols, with the osmolality of the interstitial fluid at the tip of the papilla, about 2000–3000 in commonly used laboratory animals in antidiuresis. In water diuresis the entering collecting duct fluid has an osmolality of 100–200 mosmols, and the medullary interstitial tip, 500–600 mosmols. Hence, the effective gradient is larger in antidiuresis and not in water diuresis.

medullary blood flow increases in water diuresis. (Recall that counter-current exchange efficiency varies inversely with flow.) Thurau *et al.* (1960) studied this problem by placing photoresistive elements on the surface of the inner medulla of the dog kidney and a light source in the renal parenchyma. They injected Evans blue and recorded vascular transit times, from which regional blood flow can be calculated if tissue blood volume is known. Induction of water diuresis led to a progressively shortened vascular transit time and administration of ADH lengthened it again. The transit time acceleration followed the same time course as the U/P osmolality decrease. Assuming that blood volume remained constant, their measurements indicate that inner medullary flow increased about 75% in water diuresis.

However, Aukland (1968) followed the washout kinetics of H_2 from the outer medulla and found no difference between antidiuretic and water diuretic dogs. He concluded that vasopressin showed no effect on medullary blood flow. Although the measurements in these two studies were made in different medullary areas, there is no reason to believe that their blood supplies are under different control, and the results may be in conflict. One way to reconcile them is to assume that the blood flow is effected by the local osmolality. The osmolality of the inner medulla decreases substantially when ADH is withdrawn; the outer medulla changes scarcely at all. Blood flowing through the vasa recta should undergo a volume reduction because of osmotic extraction of water, which is "shunted" across the top of the vascular loops. If the corticomedullary gradient is reduced, as in water diuresis, less water will be shunted, but we are then left without an explanation for the diminished inner medullary tonicity. Increased blood flow cannot be both cause and effect.

As alternatives to explain reduced inner medullary osmolality, two possibilities deserve mention. First, vasa recta to the inner medulla may be under vascular control by ADH. The hormone is a potent vasoconstrictor at supranormal concentrations, and the arterioles of juxtamedullary nephrons might be hypersensitive. This idea is appealing; there are no data from which it might be evaluated. Second, ADH might have an effect on thin ascending limb NaCl reabsorption, either as it does in frog skin (Ussing and Zerahn, 1951) and toad bladder (Leaf *et al.*, 1958), or by controlling the rate of NaCl delivery to thin limbs. The latter suggestion is a corollary of the idea that ADH has a vasoconstrictor action on arterioles of juxtamedullary nephrons. If the hormone has such an action, and if its locus is the efferent arteriole, single nephron filtration rate will fall in water diuresis because the lower vascular resistance of the vasa recta will reduce hydrostatic pressures in glomerular capillaries. Reduced filtration rate in water diuresis would lead to a reduced NaCl load delivered to thin-limb pumping sites. These ideas are frankly speculative. That ADH might have an effect on salt reabsorption is a suggestion that comes from studies on anuran epithelia; in the mammalian kidney, ADH has no effect on NaCl reabsorption by thick ascending limbs (Schnermann *et al.*, 1969), or on overall Na$^+$ excretion by the dog kidney, all of whose nephrons have thin ascending limbs. Evidently, the behavior of the inner medulla in water diuresis is not well understood.

REFERENCES

Aukland, K. (1968). Vasopressin and intrarenal blood flow distribution. *Acta Physiol. Scand.* **74**, 173–182.

Aukland, K., and Berliner, R. W. (1964). Renal medullary countercurrent system studied with hydrogen gas. *Circulation Res.* **15**, 430–442.

Bennett, C. M., Clapp, J. R., and Berliner, R. W. (1967). Micropuncture study of the proximal and distal tubule in the dog. *Am. J. Physiol.* **213**, 1254–1262.

Bennett, C. M., Brenner, B. M., and Berliner, R. W. (1968). Micropuncture study of nephron function in the rhesus monkey. *J. Clin. Invest.* **47**, 203–216.

Berliner, R. W., and Davidson, D. G. (1957). Production of hypertonic urine in the absence of pituitary antidiuretic hormone. *J. Clin. Invest.* **36**, 1416–1427.

Berliner, R. W., Levinsky, N. G., Davidson, D. G., and Eden, M. (1958). Dilution and concentration of the urine and the action of antidiuretic hormone. *Am. J. Med.* **24**, 730–744.

Bethge, H., Ochwadt, B., and Weber, R. (1962). Der scheinbare Verteilungsraum von [131]J-albumin in verschiedenen Schichten der Niere bei Diurese und Antidiurese. *Arch. Ges. Physiol.* **276**, 236–241.

Boylan, J. W., and Asshauer, E. (1962). Depletion and restoration of the medullary osmotic gradient in the dog kidney. *Arch. Ges. Physiol.* **276**, 99–116.

Bray, G. A. (1960). Freezing point depression of rat kidney slices during water diuresis and antidiuresis. *Am. J. Physiol.* **199**, 915–918.

Bray, G. A., and Preston, A. S. (1961). Effect of urea on urine concentration in the rat. *J. Clin. Invest.* **40**, 1952–1959.

Brodsky, W. A., Rehm, W. S., Dennis, W. H., and Miller, D. G. (1955). Thermodynamic analysis of the intracellular osmotic gradient hypothesis of active water transport. *Science* **121**, 302.

Brooks, F. P., and Pickford, M. (1958). The effect of posterior pituitary hormones on the excretion of electrolytes in dogs. *J. Physiol. (London)* **142**, 468–493.

Capek, K., Ruchs, G., Rumrich, G., and Ullrich, K. J. (1966). Harnstoffpermeabilität der corticalen Tubulusabschnitte von Ratten in Antidiurese und Wasser diurese. *Arch. Ges. Physiol.* **290**, 237–249.

Clapp, J. R. (1966). Renal tubular reabsorption of urea in normal and protein-depleted rats. *Am. J. Physiol.* **210**, 1304–1308.

Clapp, J. R., and Robinson, R. R. (1966). Osmolality of distal tubular fluid in the dog. *J. Clin. Invest.* **45**, 1847–1853.

Cortney, M. A., Nagel, W., and Thurau, K. (1966). A micropuncture study of the relationship between flow-rate through the loop of Henle and sodium concentration in the early distal tubule. *Arch. Ges. Physiol.* **287**, 286–295.

Curran, P. F., and MacIntosh, J. F. (1962). A model system for biological water transport. *Nature (London)* **193**, 347.

Dainty, J., and House, C. R. (1966). "Unstirred layers" in frog skin. *J. Physiol. (London)* **182**, 66-78.

Davis, B. B., Knox, F. G., and Berliner, R. W. (1967). Effect of vasopressin on proximal tubule sodium reabsorption in the dog. *Am. J. Physiol.* **212**, 1361-1364.

de Rouffignac, C., and Morel, F. (1967). Etude par microdissection de la distribution et de la longueur des tubules proximaux dans le rein de cinq especes de rongeurs. *Arch. Anat. Microscop. Morphol. Exptl.* **56**, 123-132.

de Rouffignac, C., and Morel, F. (1969). Micropuncture study of water, electrolyte, and urea movements along the loops of Henle in Psammomys. *J. Clin. Invest.* **48**, 474-486.

Diamond, J. M. (1962). The mechanism of water transport by the gallbladder. *J. Physiol. (London)* **161**, 503-527.

Diamond, J. M. (1964). The mechanism of isotonic water transport. *J. Gen. Physiol.* **48**, 15-42.

Diamond, J. M., and Bossert, W. H. (1967). Standing-gradient osmotic flow—a mechanism for coupling of water and solute transport in epithelia. *J. Gen. Physiol.* **50**, 2061-2083.

Friedlander, S. K., and Walser, M. (1965). Some aspects of flow and diffusion in the proximal tubule of the kidney. *J. Theoret. Biol.* **8**, 87-96.

Gardner, K. D., and Maffly, R. H. (1964). An *in vitro* demonstration of increased collecting tubular permeability to urea in the presence of vasopressin. *J. Clin Invest.* **43**, 1968-1975.

Gertz, K. H. (1963). Transtubuläre Natriumchloridflüsse und Permeabilität für Nichtelektrolyte im proximalen und distalen Konvolut der Rattenniere. *Arch. Ges. Physiol.* **276**, 336-356.

Gertz, K. H., Kennedy, G. C., and Ullrich, K. J. (1964). Mikropunktionsuntersuchungen über die Flüssigkeitsrückresorption aus den einzelnen Tubulusabschnitten bei Wasserdiurese. *Arch. Ges. Physiol.* **278**, 513-519.

Goldberg, A. H., and Lilenfield, L. S. (1963). Effect of hypertonic mannitol on accumulation rate and distribution of albumin in the renal papilla. *Proc. Soc. Exptl. Biol. Med.* **113**, 795-798.

Goldberg, M., Wojtszak, A. M., and Ramirez, M. A. (1967). Uphill transport of urea on the dog kidney: effects of certain inhibitors. *J. Clin. Invest.* **46**, 388-399.

Gottschalk, C. W. (1964). Osmotic concentration and dilution of the urine. *Am. J. Med.* **36**, 670-685.

Gottschalk, C. W., and Mylle, M. (1959). Micropuncture study of the mammalian urinary concentrating mechanism: evidence for the countercurrent hypothesis. *Am. J. Physiol.* **196**, 927-936.

Gottschalk, C. W., Lassiter, W. E., and Mylle, M. (1962). Studies of the composition of vasa recta plasma in the hamster kidney. *Proc. Intern. Union Physiol. Sci., 22nd Intern. Congr., Leiden* **1**, 375-376.

Gottschalk, C. W., Lassiter, W. E., Mylle, M., Ullrich, K. J., Schmidt-Nielsen, B., O'Dell, R., and Pehling, G. (1963). Micropuncture study of composition of loop of Henle fluid in desert rodents. *Am. J. Physiol.* **204**, 532-535.

Grantham, J. J., and Burg, M. B. (1966). Effect of vasopressin and cyclic AMP on permeability of isolated collecting tubules. *Am. J. Physiol.* **211**, 255-259.

Hargitay, B., and Kuhn, W. (1951). Das Multiplikationsprinzip als Grundlage der Harn Konzentrierung in der Niere. *Z. Elektrochem.* **55**, 539-558.

Hays, R. M. (1968). A new proposal for the action of vasopressin, based on studies of a complex synthetic membrane. *J. Gen. Physiol.* **51**, 385–398.

Hilger, H. H., Klümper, J. D., and Ullrich, K. J. (1958). Wasserrückresorption und Ionentransport durch die Sammelrohrzellen der Säugertierniere. *Arch. Ges. Physiol.* **267**, 218–237.

Horster, M., and Thurau, K. (1968). Micropuncture studies on the filtration rate of single superficial and juxtamedullary glomeruli in the rat kidney. *Arch. Ges. Physiol.* **301**, 162–181.

Jamison, R. L. (1968). Micropuncture study of segments of thin loop of Henle in the rat. *Am. J. Physiol.* **215**, 236–242.

Jamison, R. L., Bennett, C. M., and Berliner, R. W. (1967). Countercurrent multiplication by the thin loops of Henle. *Am. J. Physiol.* **212**, 357–366.

Kelman, R. B. (1962). A theoretical note on exponential flow in the proximal part of the mammalian nephron. *Bull. Math. Biophys.* **24**, 303–317.

Kelman, R. B., Marsh, D. J., and Howard, H. C. (1966). Nonmonotonicity of solutions of linear differential equations occurring in the theory of urine formation. *SIAM (Soc. Ind. Appl. Math.) Rev.* **8**, 463–478.

Klümper, J. D., Ullrich, K. J., and Hilger, H. H. (1958). Das Verhalten des Harnstoffs in den Sammelrohren der Säugertierniere. *Arch. Ges. Physiol.* **267**, 238–243.

Korn, E. D. (1966). Structure of biological membranes. The unit membrane theory is reevaluated in light of the data now available. *Science* **153**, 1491–1498.

Kramer, K., Thurau, K., and Deetjen, P. (1960). Hämodynamik des Nierenmarks. I. Mitteilung. Capilläre Passagezeit, Blutvolumen, Durchblutung, Gewebshämatokrit und O$_2$-Verbrauch des Nierenmarks in situ. *Arch. Ges. Physiol.* **270**, 251–269.

Kriz, W. (1967). Der architektonische und funktionelle Aufbau der Rattenniere. *Z. Zellforsch. Mikroskop. Anat.* **82**, 495–535.

Kuhn, W., and Ramel, A. (1959). Aktiver Salztransport als möglicher (und wahrscheinlicher) Einzeleffekt bei der Harnkonzentrierung in der Niere. *Helv. Chim. Acta* **42**, 628–660.

Kuhn, W., and Ryffel, K. (1942). Herstellung konzentrierter Lösungen aus verdünnten durch blosse Membranwirkung: Ein Modellversuch zue Funktion der Niere. *Z. Physiol. Chem.* **276**, 145–178.

Landwehr, D. M., Klose, R. M., and Giebisch, G. (1967). Renal tubular sodium and water reabsorption in the isotonic sodium chloride-loaded rat. *Am. J. Physiol.* **212**, 1327–1333.

Lapp, H., and Nolte, A. (1962). Vergleichende elektronenmikroskopische Untersuchungen am Mark der Rattenniere bei Harnkonzentrierung und Harnverdünnung. *Frankfurter Z. Pathol.* **71**, 617–633.

Lassen, N. A., and Longley, J. B. (1961). Countercurrent exchange in vessels of renal medulla. *Proc. Soc. Exptl. Biol. Med.* **106**, 743–748.

Lassiter, W. E., Gottschalk, C. W., and Mylle, M. (1961). Micropuncture study of net transtubular movement of water and urea in nondiuretic mammalian kidney. *Am. J. Physiol.* **200**, 1139–1146.

Lassiter, W. E., Mylle, M., and Gottschalk, C. W. (1966). Micropuncture study of urea transport in rat renal medulla. *Am. J. Physiol.* **210**, 965–970.

Leaf, A., Anderson, J., and Page, L. P. (1958). Active sodium transport by the isolated toad bladder. *J. Gen. Physiol.* **41**, 657–668.

Leonhardt, K. O., Landes, R. R., and McCauley, R. T. (1965). Anatomy and physiology of intrarenal oxygen tension: preliminary study of the effects of anesthetics. *Anesthesiology* **26**, 648–658.

Lever, A. F. (1965). The vasa recta and countercurrent multiplication. *Acta Med. Scand. Suppl.* **434**.

Lever, A. F., and Kriz, W. (1966). Countercurrent exchange between the vasa recta and the loop of Henle, Lancet i, 1057–1060.

Levinsky, N. G., and Berliner, R. W. (1959). The role of urea in the urine concentrating mechanism. *J. Clin. Invest.* **38**, 741–748.

Lichtenstein, N. S., and Leaf, A. (1965). Effect of amphotericin B on the permeability of the toad bladder. *J. Clin. Invest.* **44**, 1328–1342.

Longley, J. B., Banfield, W. G., and Brindley, D. C. (1960). Structure of the rete mirabile in the kidney of the rat as seen with the electron microscope. *J. Biophys. Biochem. Cytol.* **7**, 103–109.

Maganzini, H. C., and Lilenfield, L. S. (1961). Demonstration of countercurrent diffusion exchange in the vasa recta of the renal medulla. *Proc. Soc. Exptl. Biol. Med.* **107**, 872–875.

Malnic, G., Klose, R. M., and Giebisch, G. (1966). Micropuncture study of distal tubular potassium and sodium transport in rat nephron. *Am. J. Physiol.* **211**, 529–547.

Marsh, D. J. (1966). Hypo-osmotic reabsorption due to active salt transport in perfused collecting ducts of the rat renal medulla. *Nature (London)* **210**, 1179–1180.

Marsh, D. J. (1968). Solute and water flows in thin ascending Henle's loop in the hamster. *Federation Proc.* **27**, 2693.

Marsh, D. J. (1970a). Solute and water flows in thin limbs of Henle's loop in the hamster kidney. *Am. J. Physiol.* **218**, 824–831.

Marsh, D. J. (1970b). Unpublished observations.

Marsh, D. J., and Segel, L. A. (1969). Analysis of countercurrent exchange properties of vasa recta. *Federation Proc.* **28**, 3165.

Marsh, D. J., and Solomon, S. (1965). Analysis of electrolyte movement in thin Henle's loops of hamster papilla. *Am. J. Physiol.* **208**, 1119–1128.

Marsh, D. J., Kelman, R. B., and Howard, H. C. (1967). The theory of urine formation in water diuresis with implications for antidiuresis. *Bull. Math. Biophys.* **29**, 67–89.

Marumo, F., Oshikawa, Y., and Koshikawa, S. (1967). A study on the concentration mechanism of the renal medulla by mathematical model. *Japan. Circulation J. (Engl. Ed.)* **31**, 1309–1317.

Moffat, D. B., and Fourman, J. (1963). The vascular pattern of the rat kidney. *J. Anat.* **97**, 543–553.

Morel, F. (1966). Current concepts in renal physiology. *Proc. 3rd Intern. Congr. Nephrol., Washington, D.C.* **1**, 1–17.

Morel, F., Guinnebault, M., and Amiel, C. (1960). Mise en evidence d'un processus d'-echange d'eau par contrecourant dans les regions profondes du rein de hamster. *Helv. Physiol. Acta* **18**, 183–192.

Morel, F., de Rouffignac, C., Marsh, D., Guinnebault, M., and Lechene, C. (1969). Etude par microponction de l'eboration de l'urine chez le *Psammomys* non diuretique. Nephron, **6**, 533–570.

Morgan, T., and Berliner, R. W. (1968). Permeability of the loop of Henle, vasa recta, and collecting duct to water, urea, and sodium. *Am. J. Physiol.* **215**, 108–115.

Morgan, R., Sakai, F., and Berliner, R. W. (1968). In vitro permeability of medullary collecting ducts to water and urea. *Am. J. Physiol.* **214**, 574–581.

Niesel, W., and Röskenbleck, H. (1963a). Möglichkeiten der Konzentrierung von Stoffen in biologischen Gegenstromsystemen. *Arch. Ges. Physiol.* **276**, 555–567.

Niesel, W., and Röskenbleck, H. (1963b). Die Bedeutung der Stromgeschwindigkeiten in den Gefässsystemen der Niere und der Schwimmblase für die Aufrechterhaltung von Konzentrationsgradienten. *Arch. Ges. Physiol.* **277**, 302-315.

Nims, L. F. (1961). Steady state material transfer through biological barriers. *Am. J. Physiol.* **201**, 987-994.

Nims, L. F., and Thurber, R. E. (1961). Ion distribution patterns in stationary state systems. *Am. J. Physiol.* **201**, 995-998.

Ochwadt, B. K., and Pitts, R. F. (1956). Effects of intravenous infusion of carbonic anhydrase on carbon dioxide tension of alkaline urine. *Am. J. Physiol.* **185**, 426.

Orloff, J., and Handler, J. S. (1964). The cellular mode of action of antidiuretic hormone. *Am. J. Med.* **36**, 686-697.

Osvaldo, L., and Latta, H. (1966a). The thin limbs of loop of Henle. *J. Ultrastruct. Res.* **15**, 144-168.

Osvaldo, L., and Latta, H. (1966b). Interstitial cells of the renal medulla. *J. Ultrastruct. Res.* **15**, 589-613.

Patlak, C. S., Goldstein, D. A., and Hoffman, J. F. (1963). The flow of solute and solvent across a two-membrane system. *J. Theoret. Biol.* **5**, 426-442.

Pinter, G. G. (1967a). A possible role of acid mucopolysaccharides in the urine concentrating process. *Experientia* **23**, 100-101.

Pinter, G. G. (1967b). Distribution of chylomicrons and albumin in dog kidney. *J. Physiol. (London)* **192**, 761-772.

Pinter, G. G., and Shohet, J. L. (1963). Origin of sodium concentration profile in the renal medulla. *Nature (London)* **200**, 955-958.

Plakke, R. K., and Pfieffer, E. W. (1964). Blood vessels of the mammalian renal medulla. *Science* **146**, 1683-1685.

Rennie, D. W., Reeves, R. B., and Pappenheimer, J. R. (1958). Oxygen pressure in urine and its relation to intrarenal blood flow. *Am. J. Physiol.* **195**, 120-132.

Rollhäuser, H., Kriz, W., and Heinke, W. (1964). Das Gefäss-system der Rattenniere. *Z. Zellforsch. Mikroskop. Anat.* **64**, 381-403.

Ruiz-Guinazu, A., Pehling, G., Rumrich, G., and Ullrich, K. J. (1961). Glucose-und Milchsäurekonzentration an der Spitze des vascularen Gegenstromsystems im Nieremark. *Arch. Ges. Physiol.* **274**, 311-317.

Sakai, F., Jamison, R. L., and Berliner, R. W. (1965). A method for exposing the rat renal medulla in vivo: micropuncture of the collecting duct. *Am. J. Physiol.* **209**, 663-668.

Schmidt-Nielsen, B., and O'Dell, R. (1961). Structure and concentrating mechanism in the mammalian kidney. *Am. J. Physiol.* **200**, 1119-1124.

Schnermann, J. (1968). Microperfusion study of single short loops of Henle in rat kidney. *Arch. Ges. Physiol.* **300**, 255-282.

Schnermann, J., Valtin, H., Thurau, K., Nagel, W., Horster, M., Fischbach, H., Wahl, M., and Liebau, G. (1969). Micropuncture studies on the influence of antidiuretic hormone on tubular fluid reabsorption in rats with hereditary hypothalamic diabetes insipidus. *Arch. Ges. Physiol.* **306**, 103-118.

Shohet, J. L., and Pinter, G. G. (1963). Derivation of the partial differential equations utilized in a model describing the Na concentration profile in the renal medulla. *Nature* **204**, 689-690.

Slotkoff, L. M., and Lilenfield, L. S. (1967) Extravascular renal albumin. *Am. J. Physiol.* **212**, 400-406.

Smith, H. W. (1959). The fate of sodium and water in the renal tubules. *Bull. N.Y. Acad. Med.* **35**, 293-316.

Sperber, I. (1944). Studies on the mammalian kidney. *Zool. Bidrag., Uppsala* **22**, 249-435.

Stephenson, J. L. (1966). Concentration in renal counterflow systems. *Biophys. J.* **6**, 539–551.

Thorburn, G. D., Kopald, H. H., Herd, J. A., Mollenberg, M., O'Morchoe, C. C. C., and Barger, A. C. (1963). Intrarenal distribution of nutrient blood flow determined with krypton[85] in the unanesthetized dog. *Circulation Res.* **13**, 290–307.

Thurau, K., and Deetjen, P. (1962). Die Diurese bei arteriellen Drucksteigerungen. *Arch. Ges. Physiol.* **274**, 567–580.

Thurau, K., and Henne, G. (1963). Dynamik des Harnstromes in der Henleschen Schleife der Goldhamsterniere, *Arch. Ges. Physiol.* **278**, 45.

Thurau, K., Deetjen, P., and Kramer, K. (1960). Hämodynamik des Nierenmarks. II. Mitteilung. Wechselbeziehung zwischen vasculärem und tubularen Gegenstromsystem bei arteriellen Drucksteigerungen, Wasserdiurese und osmotischer Diurese. *Arch. Ges. Physiol.* **270**, 270–285.

Truniger, B., and Schmidt-Nielsen, B. (1964). Intrarenal distribution of urea and related compounds: effects of nitrogen intake. *Am. J. Physiol.* **207**, 971–978.

Uhlich, E., Baldamus, C. A., and Ullrich, K. J. (1968). Verhalten von CO_2-Druck and Bicarbonat im Gegenstromsystem des Nieremarks. *Arch. Ges. Physiol.* **303**, 31–48.

Ullrich, K. J., and Jarausch, K. H. (1956). Untersuchungen zum Problem der Harnkonzentrierung und Harnverdünnung. Uber die Verteilung von Elektrolyten (Na, K, CA, Mg, Cl, anorganischem Phosphat.) Harnstoff, Aminosäuren und exogenem Kreatinin in Rinde und Mark der Hundeniere bei verschiedenen Diuresezuständen. *Arch. Ges. Physiol.* **262**, 537–550.

Ullrich, K. J., Schmidt-Nielsen, B., O'Dell, R., Pehling, G., Gottschalk, C. W., Lassiter, W. E., and Mylle, M. (1963). Micropuncture study of composition of proximal and distal tubular fluid in rat kidney. *Am. J. Physiol.* **204**, 527–531.

Ullrich, K. J., Rumrich, G., and Fuchs, G. (1964). Wasserpermeabilität und transtubulärer Wasserfluss corticaler Nephronabschnitte bei verschiedenen Diuresezuständen. *Arch. Ges. Physiol.* **280**, 99–119.

Ullrich, K. J., Rumrich, G., and Schmidt-Nielsen, B. (1967). Urea transport in the collecting duct of rats on normal and low protein diet. *Arch. Ges. Physiol.* **295**, 147–156.

Ussing, H. H., and Zerahn, K. (1951). Active transport of sodium as the source of electric current in the short-circuited isolated frog skin. *Acta Physiol. Scand.* **23**, 110–127.

von Kügelgen, A., and Braunger, B. (1962). Quantitative Untersuchungen über Kapillaren und Tubuli der Hundeniere. *Z. Zellforsch. Mikroskop. Anat.* **57**, 766–808.

White, H. L., Rolf, D., and Tosteson, D. C. (1961). Water and sodium exchange in renal tubule fluid. *Am. J. Physiol.* **200**, 591–600.

Wilde, W. S., Thurau, K., Schnermann, J., and Prchal, K. (1963). Countercurrent multiplier for albumin in renal papilla. *Arch. Ges. Physiol.* **278**, 43.

Windhager, E. E. (1964). Electrophysiological study of renal papilla of golden hamsters. *Am. J. Physiol.* **206**, 694–700.

Windhager, E. E., and Giebisch, G. (1961). Micropuncture study of renal tubular transfer of sodium chloride in the rat. *Am. J. Physiol.* **200**, 581–590.

Windhager, E. E., and Giebisch, G. (1965). Electrophysiology of the nephron. *Physiol. Rev.* **45**, 214–244.

Wirz, H. (1953). Der osmotische Druck des Blutes in der Nierenpapilla. *Helv. Physiol. Acta* **11**, 20–29.

Wirz, H. (1956). Der osmotische Druck in den corticalen Tubuli der Rattenniere. *Helv. Physiol. Acta* **14**, 353–362.

Wirz, H., Hargitay, B., and Kuhn, W. (1951). Lokalisation des Konzentrierungsprozesses in der Niere durch direkte Kryoskopie. *Helv. Physiol. Acta* **9**, 196–207.

3 | SODIUM EXCRETION

Mackenzie Walser

127

I. Introduction

The renal mechanism of sodium transport and the manner in which renal regulation of sodium balance is achieved have probably been studied more intensively than any other function of the kidney. Nevertheless, the complexities of the problem continue to defy a coherent synthesis, as this review will testify. Perhaps because of its phylogenetic importance, renal sodium transport is characterized by an extensive system of interdependent variables and overlapping regulatory responses. Not only is transport in any given segment subject to many hydrodynamic and chemical influences, but also each segment is dependent upon the performance of other segments, by virtue of the anatomy of the nephron and its vascular supply. While two segments sufficed for describing renal function a generation ago, at least nine distinct functional entitites possessing different characteristics with respect to salt and water transport can now be distinguished. Mathematically, such an interlinked system cannot be described usefully without a vast amount of information, much of which seems to be almost inaccessible.

A particular problem, more pertinent to excretion of sodium than most other constituents, is the relationship between "load," defined as the product of water flow and sodium concentration at any point in the nephron, and local reabsorptive rate. Since only a minute fraction of the filtered sodium is excreted under ordinary circumstances, such relationships not only must exist but are likely to be critical in determining sodium balance. Nevertheless, these relationships continue to lack clear theoretical or experimental basis.

In recent years, several novel techniques have been added to the classical armamentarium of clearance techniques and free-flow micropuncture. These include the stop-flow method and its modifications, microperfusion of individual nephrons *in situ*, the split oil-drop technique, measurements of luminal, cellular, and peritubular electrical potentials, the occlusion time method, perfusion of the isolated kidney or of isolated single nephrons, measurement of passage time, microperfusion of peritubular capillaries, and many others. A discussion of the technical aspects of these methods and their limitations is beyond the scope of this review but has been ably summarized in a recent monograph by Windhager (1968).

II. Characteristics of Individual Segments with Respect to Sodium Transport

A. Glomerular Filtration

The functional and morphological characteristics of the glomerular filter have been reviewed in other chapters (Vol. I, Chapters 2,4; Vol. III, Chapter 1). Since the fluid elaborated is essentially an ultrafiltrate of plasma containing only traces of protein, it is to be expected that the concentration of sodium in the filtrate is nearly equal to that in whole plasma. This circumstance results from approximately equal and opposite effects of the water content of plasma (some 93%) and the Donnan factor (approximately 0.95). Classical micropuncture studies (Walker *et al.*, 1941; Bott, 1943) confirmed this expectation, as have more recent observations with more refined techniques (e.g., Khuri *et al.*, 1963). The quantity of sodium filtered is the product of the concentration of sodium in the filtrate and the filtration rate. Normal values for the total glomerular filtration rate (GFR) in various species are given elsewhere (Smith, 1951). Average single nephron filtration rates may be estimated as the quotient of GFR by the number of nephrons (Vol. I, Chapter 2). The result of this calculation yields values of about 50 nl/minute in dog and rat and 65 nl/minute in man according to Holliday and Egan (1962). However, directly measured filtration rates in superficial nephrons of the rat are considerably lower (Landwehr *et al.*, 1968), whether calculated from flow and inulin concentration as measured in proximal or in distal tubules. This discrepancy may be in part attributable to the pronounced differences between cortical and juxtamedullary glomeruli. The latter comprise 22% of the total in the rat, and have larger glomerular tufts with higher filtration rates (Vol. I, Chapter 2; Baines and de Rouffignac, 1969; Horster and Thurau, 1968). The fact that a lesser fraction of the plasma supplying the deeper portions of the cortex is filtered than of the plasma supplying the superficial portions (Nissen, 1966) is not inconsistent with this observation, because it may indicate the existence of arteriovenous communications which bypass the glomeruli (see Chapter 1). As noted below, this heterogeneity of glomerular function may play an important role in the homeostasis of sodium excretion.

B. Proximal Convoluted Tubule

In normal circumstances, the concentration of sodium remains constant at the plasma level throughout the portion of the proximal convolution accessible to micropuncture (Walker *et al.*, 1941; Bott, 1943). The tubular fluid-to-plasma (TF/P) ratio of osmolality also remains at unity or very slightly below (Cortney *et al.*, 1965). These observations reflect the isosmotic nature of proximal salt reabsorption. When perfused with isotonic mixtures of mannitol and saline, proximal tubules of *Necturus* exhibit proportionate efflux of water and sodium (Fig. 1) (Windhager *et al.*, 1959). This could be most readily explained by a high degree of osmotic permeability to water, which would then prevent the persistence of any osmotic gradients between plasma and tubular fluid created by the reabsorption of salt. However, the rate of movement of water alone across the tubular membrane, in response to imposed osmotic gradients, is insufficient (Ullrich *et al.*, 1964). Consequently, some form of codiffusion of salt and water must be involved. The mechanism of this process is a central question in ion transport, since it applies not only to the proximal tubule but to transepithelial movement of salt and water generally (see below).

A constant rate of salt and water reabsorption with length, i.e., $v = 1 - kx$ (where v is flow at a point x, expressed as a fraction of filtration rate, and x is distance along the nephron), would be manifested by a curvilinear increase in inulin concentration with length, given by $TF/P = 1/v = 1/(1 - kx)$. The available data indicate that water reabsorption is

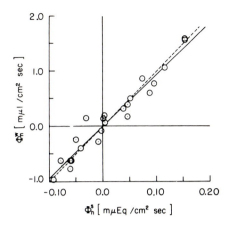

FIG. 1. Net water flux (Φ_n^w) is proportional to net solute flux (Φ_n^s) in proximal tubules perfused with solutions of varying salt concentrations made isosmotic with mannitol. When salt concentration is low, net flux of water and salt into the lumen occurs. At an intermediate value, water and salt flux both cease. The linear relationship shows that water movement is uniformly coupled to salt transport in either direction. Reprinted by permission from Windhager *et al.* (1959).

greater in the early portions of the proximal convolution than in the middle, so that TF/P for inulin tends to rise more or less linearly with length. The reason for this change in absorptive characteristics is obscure. The possibility that flow velocity might itself affect reabsorption seems unlikely for reasons considered below. No obvious change in the morphological properties of the proximal convolution with length have been found (Vol. I, Chapters 2 and 5). Accumulation of a poorly reabsorbable solute which inhibits salt reabsorption might be a conceivable explanation but tubules microperfused *in situ* show the same phenomenon (Fig. 2) (Wiederholt *et al.*, 1967). However, isolated proximal tubules perfused *in vitro* apparently do not exhibit this characteristic (Burg and Orloff, 1968), although the critical experiments have yet to be performed.

The fraction of the filtrate reabsorbed in the proximal convolution is about 50% in the dog (Clapp *et al.*, 1963; Bennett *et al.*, 1967) as well as the rat (Cortney *et al.*, 1965; Landwehr *et al.*, 1968; Horster and Thurau, 1968). The rate of reabsorption in relation to tubular length can be calculated (1) simply from the TF/P inulin ration and length, (2) from this ratio and the simultaneously measured transit time to the same point, or (3) from the rate of disappearance of a drop of fluid injected into a luminal oil column. The first and third techniques both yield values averaging 3.6 nl mm^{-1} min^{-1}. The second technique gives a

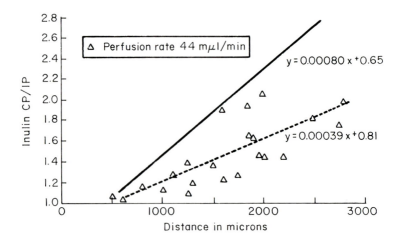

FIG. 2.   Fluid reabsorption, expressed as inulin concentration ratio between collected fluid and perfusate, as a function of tubular length in microperfused proximal nephrons of the rat. The solid line represents the results at low and at intermediate perfusion rates. The triangles and dotted line show the results at higher rates of perfusion. The apparent inhibition of fractional reabsorption at higher rates could be overcome by further tubular dilatation achieved by ureteral clamping. Reprinted by permission from Wiederholt *et al.* (1967).

lower value, as pointed out by Burg and Orloff (1968). The diameter of the lumen under free-flow conditions is about 22 μ (Burg and Orloff, 1968).

Although it was generally accepted for many years that a significant transepithelial electrical potential difference (PD) exists across the proximal tubule, recent data indicate that these earlier observations may have been artifacts, at least in the rat (Frömter and Hegel, 1966; Frömter *et al.*, 1967). The position of the electrode tip, even when by microscopic inspection seen to be in the lumen, often was in fact within tubular cells. By means of fluid ejection, the electrode can be made to penetrate the lumen, with the simultaneous disappearance of the PD. This finding has so far been made conclusively only in the rat. In the rabbit, a small (<4 mV) PD may be present (Burg, 1969). In *Necturus*, a PD of −15 to −20 mV does exist even when precautions are taken to avoid this artifact (Boulpaep, 1967). The electrical resistance of the proximal tubule is comprised of transcellular plus intercellular pathways. The latter have a much lower resistance than the former (Windhager *et al.*, 1967), and doubtless account for most of the large passive backflux of sodium in this segment (Oken *et al.*, 1963; Bentzel *et al.*, 1968). In the rat, the overall wall resistance is 5 Ωcm² of surface area or 602 Ωcm of tubular length (Hegel *et al.*, 1967). The partial conductance of sodium, chloride, and potassium measured from unidirectional fluxes, sum to a value which corresponds closely to the measured electrical conductance.

Thus, the movement of sodium against an electrical gradient across the proximal tubular epithelium has not been clearly established in mammalian species. However, movement against a chemical gradient has been demonstrated repeatedly. During diuresis promoted by infusion of nonelectrolytes, or following instillation of a nonelectrolyte solution in the tubule, a minimal TF/P ratio of sodium concentration is reached, at which sodium efflux and influx become equal. This value is 0.66 to 0.80 in the rat (Kashgarian *et al.*, 1963; Giebisch *et al.*, 1964a Hierholzer *et al.*, 1965; Windhager and Giebisch, 1965; Malnic *et al.*, 1966b; Hayslett *et al.*, 1968; Ullrich *et al.*, 1963). By measuring water reabsorption from perfused solutions containing varying proportions of NaCl, NaHCO$_3$, and sucrose, Rector *et al.* (1966a) estimated the reflection coefficient of NaCl to be 0.36. This coefficient expresses the degree to which a given membrane permits a specific solute to exert its full osmotic pressure across the membrane. A solute with a reflection coefficient of 1 exerts its full theoretical osmotic pressure across the membrane. A substance with a reflection coefficient of zero induces no osmotic water flux. The low value obtained by Rector *et al.* (1966a) raised the possibility that salt reabsorption was passive (due to solvent drag) in the proximal tubule, the driving force for water movement being derived from transport of some other solute (such as glucose or bicarbonate). Using somewhat different techniques, Ullrich (1967) obtained a considerably higher reflection coefficient, 0.68, as did Bentzel *et al.* in *Necturus* (1968). Unfortunately, there is no theoretical or experimental reason to believe that this coefficient is in fact a constant under the conditions prevailing in the nephron during these experiments.

C. The Loop of Henle

The straight portion of the proximal tubule, which constitutes the first portion of the loop of Henle, is inaccessible to micropuncture, and little is known of its function. By inference from measurements in the segments which precede and follow, its rate of salt and water reabsorption appears to be considerably smaller than in the convoluted portion. Lengths of tubules from this region isolated and perfused *in vitro* reabsorb water at a rate half as great as do proximal convoluted tubules (Burg and Orloff, 1968). There are also characteristic differences in its morphology (Vol. I, Chapters 2 and 5).

The thin loop of Henle plays a major (though perhaps passive) role in the countercurrent mechanism of urinary concentration (Chapter 2). It is now well established that the total osmolality of the fluid in this segment rises as the papillary tip is approached. Less certain are the relative roles of water removal and solute entry in determining the increase in concentrations along the descending limb. Marsh and Solomon (1965) found no water reabsorption from thin loops of hamster kidneys perfused with saline, unless distension was produced. Raffinose solutions increased in volume, suggesting influx of salt as well as water. Jamison (1968) demonstrated removal of water and sodium between descending and ascending limbs in the rat. Morgan and Berliner (1968) could not detect active sodium out-pumping in this segment, but observed an influx of sodium in the descending limb, as did de Rouffignac and Morel (1969) in the desert animal *Psammomys*. Attempts to infer thin loop function by comparing late proximal or early distal measurements of sodium and inulin with inulin values from loop fluid are questionable, because of the profound differences between cortical nephrons, which usually have short loops, and juxtamedullary nephrons, which give rise to the long loops accessible to micropuncture. De Rouffignac and Morel (1969) have emphasized that sodium added in the descending limb may be reabsorbed in the ascending limb. Such medullary recycling of sodium renders difficult a quantitative assessment of the net contribution of the thin loop to overall sodium reabsorption.

Significant transepithelial PD has been observed in the ascending, but not the descending limb of the thin loop (Windhager, 1964; Marsh and Solomon, 1965). This finding could reflect either active sodium transport or electroosmosis.

Indirect observations of sodium permeability in various portions of the nephron, made with the aid of radioactive sodium, have been interpreted as indicating the existence of a high rate of transtubular flux in this region (de Rouffignac and Morel, 1967; Foulkes and Banks, 1968).

The thick ascending limb, which represents the first portion of the distal tubule (Vol. I, Chapter 2) differs from the thin loop in having a low permeability to water and an unequivocal capacity to bring about net transport of sodium (Gottschalk, 1961). As a result, early distal fluid is invariably hypotonic (Walker *et al.*, 1941; Wirz, 1956; Gottschalk and Mylle, 1959; Windhager and Giebisch, 1965; Rector and Clapp, 1962; Ullrich *et al.*, 1963; Clapp and Robinson, 1966; Malnic *et al.*, 1966a,b; Landwehr *et al.*, 1967).

By comparison of late proximal with early distal samples, it is possible to make an estimate of the net sodium reabsorption in the loop as a whole (as opposed to the thin loop). In the rat, this amounts to $\frac{1}{4}$ of the quantity filtered (Cortney et al., 1965).

D. Distal Convoluted Tubule

In general, the distal convolution reabsorbs both sodium and water, but the magnitudes of these two processes vary considerably between species. In the rat and dog some 10% of filtered sodium is reabsorbed in the distal convolution (Cortney et al., 1965; Bennett et al., 1967; Wiederholt and Wiederholt, 1968). In the presence of antidiuretic hormone (ADH), water reabsorption equals or exceeds sodium reabsorption, so that tubular fluid sodium concentration may rise along the course of this segment (Gottschalk and Mylle, 1959; Landwehr et al., 1968) or remain constant (Malnic et al., 1966a; Landwehr et al., 1967; Clapp and Robinson, 1968). In the absence of ADH, water reabsorption in this segment is greatly reduced (Chapter 2), and tubular fluid sodium concentration consequently falls (Fig. 3) (Clapp and Robinson, 1966; Wiederholt and Wiederholt, 1968). In terms of reabsorptive rate per unit length of tubule, the difference between the distal and proximal convolution is less apparent, since the length of the distal convolution is only a small fraction of the length of the proximal (Vol. I, Chapter 2). Nevertheless, Ullrich (1967) found the net isotonic efflux of sodium from isotonic saline instilled in the distal tubule to be far less than in the proximal.

A large difference exists, however, in the passive permeability of this segment to sodium, in comparison with the proximal tubule (Ullrich, 1967). The TF/P ratio at which influx and efflux become equal is about 0.3 (Ullrich et al., 1963; Hierholzer et al., 1965; Malnic et al., 1966b; Maude et al., 1966; Landwehr et al., 1967; Hayslett et al., 1968). This large chemical gradient can be maintained despite a large electrical gradient. Transepithelial PD in this segment is 35–60 mV under normal circumstances (Frömter and Hegel, 1966; Giebisch et al., 1966; Malnic et al., 1966b; Maude et al., 1966). Studies of isotopic sodium influx have confirmed the low permeability to sodium (de Rouffignac and Morel, 1967). The apparent absence of intercellular shunt pathways may be responsible (Giebisch, 1968).

The relative contributions of sodium, potassium, and chloride conductances to distal PD, as well as the role of luminal and peritubular cell membranes are discussed in this volume, Chapter 6.

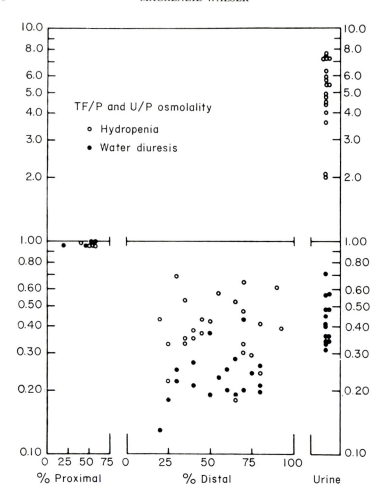

FIG. 3. Distal tubule fluid osmolality is higher during hydropenia than during water diuresis, but still hypotonic. Reprinted by permission from Clapp and Robinson (1966).

E. Collecting Duct

Reabsorption of salt in the collecting duct was first demonstrated by Hilger et al. (1958). The contribution of this process to overall sodium reabsorption is quantitatively small but unique in that it is here that the concentration of sodium is reduced to the extremely low values ($<10^{-4}$ M) which may be observed in the urine during salt deprivation. As might be anticipated, the reflection coefficient for NaCl in this segment is nearly unity (Morgan et al., 1968), and the transepithelial electrical resistance is high, 2700 Ωcm^2 (Burg et al., 1968). The existence of a definite transepithelial PD of 14 to 25 mV (Windhager, 1964; Marsh and Solomon, 1965; Burg *et al.*, 1968), considered in light of this resistance, suggests a "short-circuit current" of 10 $\mu A/cm^2$, but the net rate of sodium transport *in vivo* is probably lower than this value would suggest, particularly because of the low permeability to sodium and chloride which presumably characterizes this membrane.

III. Energy Sources for Sodium Transport

A. Oxygen Consumption

A considerable portion of renal oxygen consumption is directly related to sodium reabsorption (Kramer and Deetjen, 1960; Lassen *et al.*, 1961; Fujimoto *et al.*, 1964; Bálint and Forgács, 1966; Knox *et al.*, 1966; Torelli *et al.*, 1966). A relatively fixed ratio of 29 or 30 equivalents of sodium reabsorbed per mole of oxygen consumed is seen during spontaneous or volume-induced variations in sodium excretion, during ethacrynic acid diuresis (Knox *et al.*, 1966), or during hypothermia (Boylan and Hong, 1966). Basal oxygen consumption—that portion apparently unrelated to sodium transport, calculated by extrapolation—amounts to only 100 μmoles gm^{-1} hr^{-1} (Fig. 4) (Torelli *et al.*, 1966). Mannitol diuresis, by contrast, reduces the ratio of sodium reabsorbed to oxygen consumed (Bálint and Forgács, 1966; Knox *et al.*, 1966) and also reduces the pO_2 of the urine (Aukland and Krog, 1961; Washington and Holland, 1966). The presumptive explanation is that increased sodium influx proximally, promoted by the large sodium gradient, effectively increases the load of sodium presented to the ascending limb for reabsorption (Kiil *et al.*, 1961). Acute hypoxia did not inhibit sodium reabsorption (Ullman, 1961; Arcila *et al.*, 1968), but it is conceivable that renal oxygen consumption was unaffected by the procedures employed in these experiments. Hypoxia does, however, accentuate the inhibition of tubular sodium reabsorption produced by cyanide (Arcila *et al.*, 1968), which is associated with a proportionate reduction in oxygen consumption, at least in nonhypoxic animals (Fujimoto *et al.*, 1964).

B. Aerobic vs. Anaerobic Metabolism

A large body of evidence indicates that anaerobic glycolysis plays a major role in medullary sodium transport (e.g., Martinez-Maldonado *et al.*, 1969). But, in general, inhibitors of aerobic metabolism are more effective in blocking sodium reabsorption than are inhibitors of anaer-

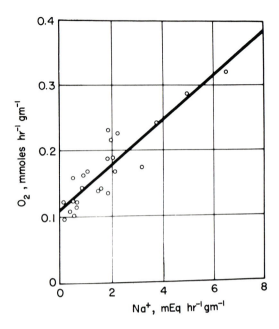

FIG. 4.   Oxygen consumption by the rabbit kidney as function of sodium reabsorption. A basal oxygen consumption independent of sodium reabsorption is present; increments in sodium reabsorption are accompanied by an increase of 1 mole of oxygen consumed for every 30 equivalents of sodium reabsorbed. Reprinted by permission from Torelli *et al.* (1966).

obic metabolism (Herms and Malvin, 1963; Strickler and Kessler, 1963). Dinitrophenol, an inhibitor of ATP synthesis, has little (Chertok *et al.*, 1966) or no (Strickler and Kessler, 1963) saluretic action at doses which augment oxygen consumption (Fujimoto *et al.*, 1964) and reduce cortical ATP concentration (Kessler, 1969). This may indicate that utilization of ATP as an energy source for sodium transport is facultative, rather than obligatory. Further evidence for this view is the poor correlation between effects on sodium excretion and on the rate of incorporation of radiophosphate into ATP seen with other agents such as *p*-chloromercuribenzoate, chlorothiazide, and dichlorphenamide (Fig. 5) (Kessler *et al.*, 1968). Cannon *et al.* (1968) find that the common diuretic drugs all increase the corticomedullary gradient for lactate, suggesting that they may act by inhibiting oxidative metabolism. Further aspects of the metabolic effects of individual diuretic agents are discussed below.

C. Sodium and Potassium Stimulated Adenosine Triphosphate Splitting Enzyme System (Na-K-ATPase)

This enzyme system, discovered in crab nerve by Skou (1957), is now believed to play a major role in homocellular as well as transcellular transport of sodium and potassium. Evidence for this view has been reviewed recently by Skou (1965) and others (Katz and Epstein, 1967, 1968). The specific role of this enzyme system in renal tubular reabsorption of sodium is not yet clear. The levels of enzymatic activity in renal tissue are high, particularly in the ascending limb and distal convolution; activity in the proximal convolution is relatively low (Hendler *et al.*, 1969; U. Schmidt and Dubach, 1969). The increase in glomerular filtration rate and tubular reabsorption of sodium which follows unilateral nephrectomy, high protein intake, or corticosteroid administration in rats is associated with an increase in the activity of this enzyme in relation to protein content of a cortical microsome fraction (Katz and Epstein, 1967). This finding could represent an increase in enzyme levels or a decrease in nonenzyme protein in this fraction; however, tissue levels of other enzymes changed much less than did Na-K-ATPase. The effect of adrenalectomy on enzyme levels is less clear. In the first 2 weeks, following extirpation in rats, Na-K-ATPase

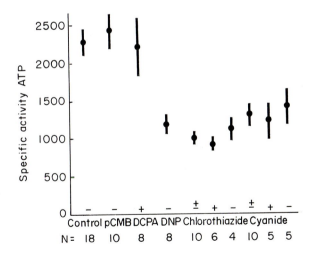

FIG. 5.   A comparison between diuretic activity (indicated by + and −) and inhibition of radiophosphate incorporation into ATP of cortical tissue for several compounds. No correlation is seen. pCMB, *p*-Chloromercuribenzoate; DCPA, dichlorphenamide; DNP, 2,4 dinitrophenol. Reprinted by permission from Kessler *et al.* (1968).

may fall (Chignell and Titus, 1966; Katz and Epstein, 1967), but there is evidence to suggest that this response is secondary to the accompanying changes in plasma sodium and potassium concentrations (Ebel *et al.*, 1968; Jorgensen, 1968).

The correlation between saluretic action of drugs and their ability to inhibit Na-K-ATPase is generally poor, with some exceptions. Cardiac glycosides inhibit tubular reabsorption of sodium and activity of this enzyme at comparable concentrations, but among most other agents examined to date, the hypothesis that natriuresis is attributable to inhibition of Na-K-ATPase cannot be supported (see Section VIII,B).

Thus, the evidence pertaining to the role of ATP is analogous to that pertaining to the role of Na-K-ATPase; in both, this mechanism of transport may be a major but not exclusive one, whose role can to some extent be replaced by other biochemical processes. The nature of other sources of chemical energy for sodium transport in the kidney is as yet unknown.

IV. Effect of Discrete Hydrodynamic Factors on Sodium Reabsorption

Attempts to study such phenomena as isolated variables are, of course, fraught with difficulty, since a change in flow, pressure, or resistance in the vascular or tubular system is likely to be accompanied by changes in all of these variables. Nevertheless, useful information has been obtained from experiments designed to examine these factors more or less independently. In nearly every instance, a contribution of intrarenal humoral mechanisms cannot be excluded with certainty (see Section X, A, 4).

A. Glomerular Filtration Rate (GFR)

Primary reduction of GFR has been examined chiefly by reducing arterial pressure, and is considered below. Lindheimer *et al.* (1967) recently examined in dogs the effect of increasing GFR, in the apparent absence of changes in renal arterial pressure, by means of administering a high-protein intake, dexamethasone, or dopamine. Care was taken to avoid any increase in extracellular fluid volume. Despite increments in GFR of about 30%, salt excretion was unaffected. Pretreatment with mineralocorticoids or with spironolactone plus salt did not alter the results. Behrenbeck and Reinhardt (1967) have also observed a postprandial increase in renal hemodynamic parameters without change in sodium excretion. If one accepts the premise that the change was primarily in GFR and secondarily in tubular reabsorption [rather than the reverse, as Bojesen (1954) and Leyssac (1963) might suggest], and that no humoral or nervous influences on sodium reabsorption were brought into play, one would conclude that intrinsic renal mechanisms alter the absolute rate of tubular reabsorption *pari passu* in response to increments in filtration. This phenomenon is discussed further in Section X, A.

B. Renal Arterial Pressure

Selkurt (1951) and Thompson and Pitts (1952) clearly demonstrated that reduction of renal arterial pressure profoundly reduces sodium excretion, and that the percentage excretion of filtered sodium likewise falls. Neither adrenalectomy nor surgically induced diabetes insipidus prevented these responses. A number of recent studies have examined the mechanism of these effects, with somewhat conflicting results. In adequately hydrated, nondiuretic rats, constriction of the aorta above the renal arteries leads to reduced GFR and may lead to increased (Gertz et al., 1965; Brenner et al., 1968; Landwehr et al., 1968), unchanged (Glabman et al., 1965; Rector et al., 1966b), or decreased (Wahl et al., 1968) fractional reabsorption of salt and water in the proximal tubule. Gottschalk and Leyssac (1968) found constancy of fractional reabsorption until GFR fell below 0.7 ml/minute gm kidney wt; further reduction in aortic pressure and GFR led to a fixed minimal rate of proximal transport and hence progressively increasing fractional reabsorption. Clearly the phenomenon of autoregulation, i.e., constancy of renal hemodynamic parameters in the face of varying arterial pressure, was not occurring in these experiments—and is not readily shown in the rat kidney.

The rat distal tubule exhibits higher sodium concentration during hypotension, as assessed by free-flow micropuncture or by perfusion of Henle's loop (Schnermann et al., 1966). In the hemoperfused kidney, however, distal sodium transport, as estimated by the stop-flow minimum in sodium concentration, is impaired at higher perfusion pressure (Tobian et al., 1964).

In the dog, autoregulation is more prominent, and hypotension induced by phentolamine may not alter the GFR. Under these circumstances fractional reabsorption in the proximal tubule is unchanged (Liebau et al., 1968). Larger reductions in blood pressure, whether induced by phentolamine (Liebau et al., 1968), or arterial clamping (Dirks et al., 1965; Watson, 1966) lower GFR, but fractional reabsorption still remains constant in this species. Clearance data, however, lead to the opposite conclusion: fractional distal delivery of sodium, estimated as plasma/urine inulin ratio during water diuresis, falls during renal artery constriction, implying that fractional sodium reabsorption proximally must have increased (R. M. Stein *et al.*, 1965).

In both dog and rat, hypotension induced by arterial constriction fails to alter the pressure in proximal tubules or peritubular capillaries (Thurau and Wober, 1962; Leyssac, 1964; Martino and Earley, 1968).

Acutely induced hypertension augments sodium excretion (Cort and Lichardus, 1963a), even in the absence of change in GFR (Selkurt *et al.*, 1965) or in the perfused kidney (Mills, 1968). An accompanying fall in negative free water clearance and an increase in the distal minimum sodium concentration seen in stop-flow experiments (Tobian *et al.*, 1964; Wilkins *et al.*, 1965) suggest that part of the effect is distal. Carotid ligation in rats induces hypertension which is accompanied by increased GFR and diminished proximal sodium reabsorption, despite tubular dilatation (Koch *et al.*, 1968). In the dog, however, autoregulation may prevent change in total or cortical nephron GFR following carotid ligation, and proximal sodium reabsorption may remain unaltered (Liebau *et al.*, 1968). When autoregulation has been abolished by pharmacological means, pressor agents augment the percentage of filtered sodium excreted (Earley and Friedler, 1966; Earley *et al.*, 1966).

C. Renal Vascular Resistance and Renal Blood Flow

Vasodilators injected into the renal artery increase renal blood flow but have little effect on glomerular filtration rate; sodium excretion regularly increases (Fig. 6). Inhibition of sodium reabsorption in this manner has been demonstrated with acetylcholine (Pinter *et al.*, 1964; Earley and Friedler, 1965a; Willis *et al.*, 1968), arecoline (Williams *et al.*, 1965), prostaglandin, bradykinin (Daugharty *et al.*, 1968), kallidin (Webster and Gilmore, 1964), and bacterial pyrogen (Brandt *et al.*, 1956), as well as other agents. A direct tubular effect is suggested by the fact that saluresis is produced in chickens by infusing arecoline (May and Carter, 1967) or acetylcholine (Parmelee and Carter, 1968) into the renal portal system, which perfuses the tubules but not the glomeruli. However, when the augmentation of renal blood flow is prevented by arterial constriction in dogs, natriuresis does not occur (Willis *et al.*, 1968). The effects of both of these agents are blocked by atropine (Williams *et al.*, 1965; Parmelee and Carter, 1968). Inhibition of proximal rather than distal reabsorption following acetylcholine is suggested by the observation that urine flow (during water diuresis) rises as much as does sodium clearance (Daugharty *et al.*, 1968). Intrarenal hydro-

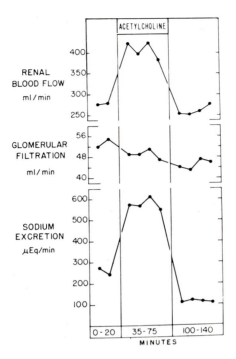

FIG. 6. Effect of unilateral renal vasodilatation produced by infusing acetylcholine into one renal artery of a dog. Renal blood flow and sodium excretion rise abruptly, on the infused side only. Reprinted by permission from Earley (1966).

static pressure increases, as a result of "greater transmission of renal perfusion along the intrarenal circulation" (Martino and Earley, 1968). These authors suggest that capillary uptake of sodium may be impaired following renal vasodilatation. The detailed mechanism of this response remains to be elucidated, but it is probably related to the intrarenal mechanisms involved in autoregulation of vascular resistance (see Chapter 1). Earley and Friedler (1965a) have summarized the evidence for the conclusion that these vasodilators augment sodium excretion through an effect on vascular resistance as opposed to direct pharmacologic effects on tubular transport, including their own observation that little or no effect is seen when sodium excretion has already been greatly increased by saline diuresis, with associated vasodilatation.

D. Renal Venous Pressure

Early observations on the inhibitory effect of elevated renal venous pressure on sodium excretion were generally interpreted as being attributable to accompanying reduction in GFR (Winton, 1952). Alternatively, changes in effective extracellular fluid volume secondary to vena cava constriction (J. O. Davis and Ball, 1958; Cirksena *et al.*, 1966) or to negative pressure applied to the lower half of the body (Gilbert *et al.*, 1966) could lead to responses attuned to volume rather than to venous pressure per se. Recently, efforts towards clarifying a more direct effect of venous pressure on tubular reabsorption have appeared. Partial renal venous occlusion augments peritubular capillary pressure as well as proximal intratubular pressure (Gottschalk, 1958; Lewy and Windhager, 1968) and might impair capillary absorption of tubular reabsorbate by altering the balance of Starling forces. Lewy and Windhager (1968) have provided evidence for this view from measurements of proximal reabsorptive capacity in rat kidneys during partial renal venous occlusion. Both from measurements of lissamine green passage time and from observation of the half-time of reabsorption by the split oil drop technique, they found proximal reabsorption to be impaired (Fig. 7). GFR fell owing to increased intratubular pressure and decreased renal blood flow, but the results with the split oil drop technique should be independent of this change. They suggest that expanded interstitial volume, brought about by the elevated capillary pressure, may impair the transfer of salt and water from tubules to capillaries, a concept proposed in a more general context by Martino and Earley (1967a) (see preceding section).

Wathen and Selkurt (1969) found that the response to partial venous occlusion in the dog depended upon the diuretic state of the animal; in oliguric dogs, sodium excretion rose in association with a fall in renal vascular resistance and virtually unchanged GFR and renal blood flow. In saline-loaded animals, by contrast, sodium excretion, GFR, and renal blood flow fell, with a rise in renal vascular resistance. Their results in nondiuretic dogs lend support to a mechanism such as that proposed by Lewy and Windhager (1968); the explanation for reduced GFR exclusively in diuresing animals is not clear.

An oft-neglected factor which may play a critical role in these experiments is lymphatic uptake of sodium, which increases considerably in response to elevated venous pressure (Cockett *et al.*, 1968).

E. Intratubular Pressure

Just as it is extremely difficult to assess separately the effects of changes in renal vascular resistance and in arterial pressure on sodium reabsorption, so it is equally difficult to examine independently the

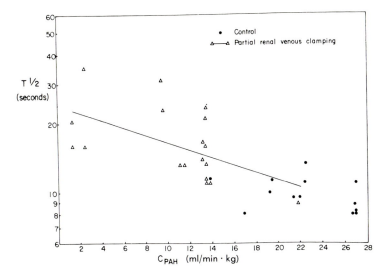

FIG. 7. Relationship between reabsorptive half-time observed in split drop experiments and renal blood flow during control observations and partial clamping of the renal vein. The results suggest that capillary uptake of reabsorbate from the proximal tubule may be rate-limiting under these conditions. Reprinted by permission from Lewy and Windhager (1968).

roles of intratubular pressure and tubular diameter. The hydraulic conductivity of the proximal and distal tubules is small (Ullrich, 1967), but the possibility that pressure might exert an effect on coupled transport of salt and water is hard to exclude. Nutbourne (1968) has described such an effect in frog skin, apparently unrelated to stretch. However, these results have not been confirmed (von Stackelberg, 1969). Transmural pressure gradients evidently exert profound effects on intestinal transport of water and solute (Hakim and Lifson, 1969). On the other hand, sodium transport in the toad bladder, as measured by short-circuit current, is little affected by the direction or magnitude of the transepithelial pressure gradient (in the absence of changes in stretch) (Walser, 1969).

Obstruction to the outflow of tubular fluid leads to tubular dilatation along with increased intratubular pressure, and is considered in the section which follows.

A distinctly different form of interdependence of tubular pressure and reabsorption is envisaged in the concept championed by Leyssac (1963), in which changes in reabsorption bring about parallel changes in filtration as a result of altered filtration pressure across the glomerular membrane. This view was advanced earlier by Bojesen (1954), but Leyssac (1963) provided more supporting evidence by showing that occlusion time depended on the GFR immediately before occlusion (Fig. 8). Later work in his laboratory has shown that proximal pressure is unaltered during spontaneous variations in GFR or following partial clamping of the aorta (Leyssac, 1964; Bojesen and Leyssac, 1969), and has reinforced his view that an intrarenal humoral mechanism is responsible for altering GFR.

F. Tubular Diameter

Gertz *et al.* reported in 1965 that the reabsorptive half-time for isotonic saline, as measured by the split oil drop technique, remained constant despite spontaneous variations in tubular diameter, implying a linear dependence of reabsorption on tubular volume. Several groups of investigators subsequently confirmed that proximal reabsorption is proportional to luminal volume during spontaneous variations in GFR (Nagel *et al.*, 1966; Wahl *et al.*, 1967; Levine *et al.*, 1968; Schnermann *et al.*, 1968), during varying rates of microperfusion *in vivo* (Wiederholt *et*

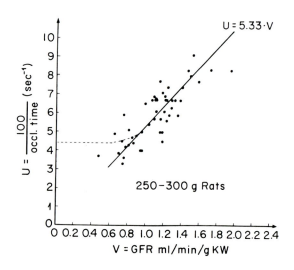

Fɪɢ. 8.   Reciprocal occlusion time of rat proximal tubules as a function of GFR at spontaneously varying rates of filtration. There is a close correlation between the time to tubular collapse following aortic clamping and the GFR which existed immediately beforehand. At lower rates of filtration, achieved by partial clamping, a different relationship is seen (dotted line). Reprinted by permission from Leyssac (1965).

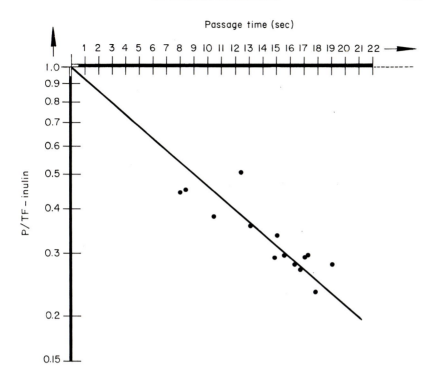

FIG. 9. Relationship between water reabsorption measured at various points in the rat proximal nephron, and the passage time of dye from the glomerulus to the same point. The fractional reabsorption of filtered water, measured as plasma-to-tubular-fluid inulin ratio, increases as the passage time becomes longer. Reprinted by permission from Gertz *et al.* (1965).

al., 1967) or *in vitro* (Maude, 1968), following hemorrhagic hypotension (Steinhausen *et al.*, 1965), aortic constriction, or ureteral occlusion (Brunner *et al.*, 1966; Rector *et al.*, 1966b).

Further evidence given by Gertz for his hypothesis was the identity of reabsorptive rate per unit of tubular volume whether measured by the split oil drop technique or by combined measurements of lissamine green transit time and TF/P inulin ratios during free flow (Gertz *et al.*, 1965) (Fig. 9). Since the tubule is distended during the split oil drop measurements, similar results by these independent measurements also support the view that reabsorption is proportional to tubular volume. This scheme would provide a convenient explanation for proximal glomerulotubular balance, i.e., the ability of the tubule to adapt reabsorption to altered filtration with unchanged fractional reabsorption.

A possible model for stimulation of reabsorption with stretching is seen in the toad bladder, where sodium transport is reversibly stimulated by stretch (Walser, 1969). This response is not dependent on increased chloride conductance, nor on increased access of oxygen or glucose to the mucosal epithelium. It may be dependent on increased passive permeability to sodium in response to stretch. It is inhibited by high oxygen tension and by actinomycin D.

Other data, however, have brought into question the dependence of reabsorptive rate or tubular diameter found by Gertz. Brenner et al. (1968) found a poor correlation between tubular volume and reabsorptive rate in rats subjected to aortic or ureteral constriction, and raised the possibility that previously published findings to the contrary may have suffered from contamination of proximal micropuncture samples by distal fluid during the elevated intratubular pressure brought on by ureteral obstruction. Others (Baines et al., 1968; Lewy and Windhager, 1968; Wahl et al., 1968) have also failed to confirm the correlation between luminal volume and reabsorptive rate during arterial clamping. Alterations in downstream resistance may fail to produce proportionate changes in reabsorption and tubular volume, according to Schnermann et al. (1969) and Steinhausen (1967a,b). Technical questions have also been raised concerning the identical significance of reabsorptive rate measurements based on transit time, occlusion time, TF/P inulin ratios, and split-drop half-times (Wahl et al., 1967; Burg and Orloff, 1968; Schnermann et al., 1968).

A more direct test of the Gertz hypothesis was provided by Burg and Orloff (1968) in isolated perfused proximal tubules. When outflow resistance was increased, the tubules dilated but reabsorption remained unchanged. Unless the environment of the tubule in these experiments differed in some crucial way from the environment of the tubule *in vivo*, the conclusion that dilatation has no effect on transport seems inescapable. However, proximal tubules in the rat kidney slices perfused *in vitro* continue to exhibit a proportionality between reabsorption and the square of diameter, so that the peritubular circulation cannot be the crucial factor (Maude, 1968).

G. Velocity of Tubular Flow

Intuitively, it might appear that reabsorption would be diminished by increasing the velocity of the flow of tubular fluid, because each element of filtrate would then be exposed to reabsorbing epithelium for a shorter period of time. This is a misconception based on considering

the history of each element of filtrate rather than the steady-state rate of reabsorption. Although the fraction of filtered salt and water reabsorbed would indeed decrease in this simple intuitive scheme, the absolute rate of reabsorption would not be altered. If the tubular epithelium were continuously exposed to fluid of unchanging composition, there is no obvious reason why the velocity of flow should have any relation to the rate of reabsorption. Although this point has been made repeatedly, the concept dies hard.

At a more sophisticated level, Kelman (1962, 1965) proposed that proximal reabsorption might be velocity-dependent in the same manner that reaction velocity in a catalytic flow reactor is dependent on flow rate under certain conditions. The basis of this proposal was a survey of published data on TF/P inulin ratios with length in the proximal nephron, which the author felt to be best described by an exponential function. As noted above (Section II,B), a linear function comes as close as any other, and an exponential one is probably a less good fit. Nevertheless, this idea provoked an examination of possible similarities between proximal reabsorption and flow-dependent reaction rate. Robinson (1954) had previously examined theoretically the possibility of radial gradients in sodium concentration. Although he used an abbreviated mathematical model and somewhat inappropriate diffusion constants, his conclusion that no appreciable radial gradient for sodium could exist was substantiated in a more complete treatment by Friedlander and Walser (1965). This analysis took into account the radial as well as axial components of fluid velocity, in a general form similar to that given by Macey (1963, 1965), but required the assumption of constant sodium concentration at the mucosal surface. In view of the present uncertainty as to the mechanism of coupled transport of salt and water across such epithelia, the conclusion of these workers that velocity should not affect sodium reabsorption cannot be considered as final. It is interesting to note that their analysis does predict a substantial radial gradient for protein concentration, which might conceivably play a role in salt and water reabsorption (see below).

Experimental tests of the role of velocity of tubular fluid flow as a discrete variable are few. The work of Burg and Orloff (1968), studying the isolated proximal tubule, and of Wiederholt et al. (1967), in which microperfusion in situ was employed, has been cited above. In preliminary reports of in vivo microperfusion studies, Morgan and Berliner (1969a,b) indicate that the absolute rate of fluid reabsorption is uninfluenced by perfusion rate in the proximal convolution, but rises with perfusion rate in the distal convolution.

V. Effects of Discrete Changes in the Composition of Blood and Tubular Fluid on Sodium Reabsorption

A. Hematocrit

Two groups of investigators have recently reexamined the question of whether alterations in the relative volumes of plasma and red cells perfusing the kidney, with constant total blood volume, lead to alterations in renal sodium transport. Bahlmann *et al.* (1967a), working with intact dogs, found that reduction of the hematocrit regularly increased filtration rate but inconsistently increased sodium excretion. Knox *et al.* (1968) found that the same maneuver reduced the filtration fraction and led to increased fractional sodium reabsorption in the proximal tubule, but that nevertheless little or no change in sodium excretion ensued. Thus, it would appear that the hematocrit level does affect the filtration rate and thereby the rate of proximal sodium reabsorption but that compensatory adjustments in more distal portions of the nephron limit or prevent any resultant change in sodium excretion.

B. Oncotic Pressure

A primary role of the transtubular oncotic pressure gradient in bringing about proximal reabsorption of salt and water was proposed by Malvin *et al.* (1958) but has been discounted because it could not lead to reabsorption of sodium against a chemical gradient, as occurs in osmotic diuresis. Furthermore, the water permeability of the tubule is sufficient to account for only a minute rate of water reabsorption if driven by the transtubular oncotic pressure gradient (Whittembury *et al.*, 1959).

However, it has been observed repeatedly that reduction of the colloid osmotic pressure of the blood perfusing the kidney inhibits sodium reabsorption and induces natriuresis (e.g., Bojesen, 1954; Vereerstraeten and Toussaint, 1969), while adding additional colloids leads to a decrease in sodium excretion (e.g., Welt and Orloff, 1951; Keck *et al.*, 1969). Such results could be secondary to changes in the oncotic pressure gradient across the peritubular capillary or across the tubular epithelium itself. The latter possibility has been excluded by instilling protein-containing solutions into the tubules and observing the rate of water reabsorption, in comparison with reabsorption of saline alone; no inhibition occurs (Whittembury *et al.*, 1959; Kashgarian *et al.*, 1963; Giebisch *et al.*, 1964a).

The oncotic pressure gradient across the peritubular capillary is one of the Starling forces determining the net rate of movement of salt and water from the interstitial space into the bloodstream; if capillary uptake of salt and water were a limiting factor in proximal reabsorption, peritubular plasma oncotic pressure and rate of sodium reabsorption should be directly related. A tubular locus of action of albumin infusion in reducing sodium excretion is supported by its efficacy when infused into the chicken renoportal venous system (Vereerstraeten and Toussaint, 1965). Proximal rather than distal action is indicated by the equivalent changes which are produced in sodium clearance and urine flow during water diuresis in dogs (Daugharty et al., 1968), and also by direct measurement of increased fractional reabsorption in superficial proximal tubules (Howards et al., 1968). Compensatory changes in distal reabsorption presumably account for the occasional failure of sodium excretion to respond (Fig. 10) (Howards et al., 1968; Schrier et al., 1968). Windhager et al. (1969) have recently succeeded in perfusing peritubular capillaries with solutions containing varying concentrations of dextran and have clearly demonstrated the dependence of proximal reabsorption on oncotic pressure. The absence of extrarenal hormonal or nervous influences in mediating the effects of albumin is also shown by their occurrence in the isolated perfused kidney (Rosenfeld et al., 1965; Nizet, 1968). Thus, all of the available evidence is consistent with the view that peritubular capillary oncotic pressure may affect proximal sodium reabsorption by altering the rate of uptake of reabsorbed salt and water from the interstitial space. The manner in which this response is mediated remains to be clarified.

An additional factor may be the altered distribution of renal blood flow which accompanies acute elevation of plasma oncotic pressure. Elpers and Selkurt (1963) showed that extraction of PAH by the kidney is considerably reduced coincident with the increase in renal plasma flow.

C. Plasma Sodium Concentration

The renal response to infusion of hypertonic saline has been examined repeatedly in clearance experiments, with an aim to elucidating the relationship between the filtered load of sodium and its reabsorptive rate. Such experiments usually entail expansion of the extracellular fluid volume as well as increase in plasma sodium concentration, and the resulting changes in sodium reabsorption are, thus, the summated effects of at least two variables. GFR often rises too, probably as a result

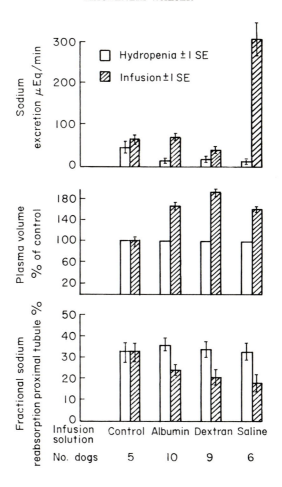

Fig. 10. Sodium excretion, plasma volume, and fractional sodium reabsorption by the proximal tubule during hydropenia and after infusion of albumin, dextran, or saline in dogs. All three solutions expanded plasma volume and inhibited proximal reabsorption, but only saline leads to substantial natriuresis. Reprinted by permission from Howards *et al.* (1968).

of expansion. Attempts to eliminate this change by partial clamping of the renal artery do not counteract completely the natriuretic effect of expansion, as has been repeatedly demonstrated in isotonic saline loading experiments (see below).

By analogy with the kinetics of simple enzyme systems, one would anticipate that increase in the sodium concentration in the tubular fluid would augment the absolute rate of sodium reabsorption, but less than proportionately, so that sodium excretion would also increase. Filtered

load should have no direct effect on reabsorption, although it obviously is a major determinant of excretion. Some, though by no means all, clearance experiments support this conclusion. Bresler (1960), Kamm and Levinsky (1964), and Bálint and Forgács (1966) found that, at any given GFR, sodium reabsorption varied directly with plasma sodium concentration in dogs infused with hypertonic saline. However, when the increase in filtered load of sodium fails to occur (Levy and Ankeney, 1952), or is prevented by arterial clamping, sodium reabsorption may be inhibited (Blythe and Welt, 1963; Kamm and Levinsky, 1964). Furthermore, some clearance experiments have shown reduced sodium reabsorption (Baldwin *et al.*, 1950; Papper *et al.*, 1955). Although this might be attributed to the accompanying expansion of extracellular fluid volume, Kamm and Levinsky (1965a) have presented evidence against this conclusion: when hypertonic saline was infused directly into the renal artery and filtered load controlled by clamping, sodium reabsorption was again inhibited. Selkurt and Post (1950) had shown earlier that infusion of hypertonic saline into the renal artery led to unchanged or increased sodium reabsorption.

The assumption that hypertonic saline infusion plus clamping permits examination of the discrete effect of plasma sodium concentration on sodium reabsorption may not be warranted. Renal perfusion pressure is reduced by clamping, as is the distribution of renal blood flow, and under some conditions this maneuver leads to decreased fractional reabsorption of salt and water in the proximal tubule (see Sections II, A and XI, D).

Micropuncture samples obtained from the proximal convolution during hypertonic saline administration in rats have shown unaltered fractional reabsorption except under the most vigorous natriuresis (Giebisch *et al.*, 1964b; Lassiter *et al.*, 1964), indicating that at least in this portion of the nephron sodium reabsorption increases in direct proportion to sodium concentration until high levels are reached. Even at high rates of natriuresis, no evidence for inhibition of the absolute rate of sodium reabsorption is found; enhancement of sodium reabsorption occurs at all levels of diuresis (judging from the whole kidney GFR and fractional rate of water reabsorption). In the dog, however, hypertonic saline reduces absolute as well as fractional sodium reabsorption proximally (Dirks *et al.*, 1965). In the rat distal nephron, the absolute rate of sodium reabsorption appears to be unaffected (Lassiter *et al.*, 1964; recalculated by Cortney *et al.*, 1965; Giebisch *et al.*, 1964b). On the other hand, indirect evidence obtained by observing free water reabsorption during hypertonic saline infusion suggests augmented sodium reabsorption in the diluting segment of the distal nephron (Goldberg *et al.*, 1965; Friedler and Earley, 1966).

Acute reduction of plasma sodium concentration is also difficult to examine as a discrete variable, because changes in extracellular fluid volume or GFR often occur concomitantly. When a nonreabsorbable electrolyte such as mannitol is infused in order to reduce plasma sodium concentration, interpretation becomes further clouded. Water loading may have the additional effect of inhibiting antidiuretic hormone secretion. Blythe and Welt (1965) found that hyponatremia produced by infusing a dextrose solution into dogs previously loaded with saline, in whom filtered load of sodium was kept constant by the simultaneous release of an aortic clamp, responded with increased sodium reabsorption. Again, the inevitable change in renal perfusion pressure resulting from clamping may have played a role, though the effects are the opposite of those seen in the experiments of Kamm and Levinsky (1965a). The explanation may be that glucose itself can facilitate sodium reabsorption (Bloom, 1962; Renschler *et al.*, 1969). Goldsmith *et al.* (1962) observed that chronic hyponatremia inhibited the natriuretic effect of mannitol infusion but acute hyponatremia did not.

The resolution of these problems is of considerable importance to our understanding of the kinetics of sodium reabsorption and also to the question of the role of antidiuretic hormone in sodium balance, since plasma sodium concentration is regulated not by tubular sodium reabsorption but rather by free water reabsorption under the influence of ADH and by thirst.

D. Plasma Potassium Concentration

Infusion of potassium salts generally leads to natriuresis. This effect cannot be attributed to alterations in the filtered load of sodium, and must indicate an alteration in tubular transport. Conversely, mild potassium depletion may be associated with sodium retention (Wesson, 1969).

On the other hand, saline diuresis in the isolated perfused dog kidney is partially dependent on the reduced potassium concentration of the perfusate and is blunted if hypokalemia is prevented (Nizet, 1967).

E. Plasma Calcium Concentration

Numerous reports have documented an increase in sodium excretion and diminution in sodium reabsorption in response to hypercalcemia (e.g., Levitt *et al.*, 1956; Freedman *et al.*, 1958; Beck *et al.*, 1959). Fülgraff and his associates (1968a; Fülgraff and Heidenreich, 1967) have demonstrated that high calcium concentration reduces sodium reabsorption in the proximal tubule. In the absence of calcium, the capacity of the collecting ducts to establish a transtubular sodium gradient is impaired (Uhlich *et al.*, 1969).

F. Plasma Magnesium Concentration

Intravenous infusion of magnesium salts also induces natriuresis (Chesley and Tepper, 1958; Kelly *et al.*, 1960; Samiy *et al.*, 1960; Wiswell, 1961; Ardill *et al.*, 1962; Knippers and Hehl, 1965), but often only transiently (Pritchard, 1955; Barker *et al.*, 1959).

G. Plasma Anionic Composition

Sodium reabsorption must be accompanied by equivalent reabsorption of anions or secretion of potassium or hydrogen ions. The former process is quantitatively far greater than the latter. In the mammalian proximal tubule, the apparent absence of a significant electrical potential, recently established (see above), necessitates a reappraisal of the traditional view that chloride is reabsorbed passively in response to the electrostatic drag established by sodium reabsorption. Even in the distal nephron, passive forces are inadequate to account for the extremely low concentrations of chloride (10^{-4} M) seen in some micropuncture samples (Rector and Clapp, 1962) or in the urine (Walser and Rahill, 1965a, 1966a). Consequently, it seems necessary to postulate active transport mechanisms for chloride, possibly coupled to sodium in the proximal tubule if not in the distal.

The results of numerous comparisons of the simultaneous fractional reabsorptive rates of small monovalent anions are kinetically consistent with passive reabsorption of nearly the entire filtered quantities. When chloride reabsorption becomes nearly complete, independent distal reabsorptive processes become apparent (Kruhoffer, 1950; Saugman, 1957; Walser and Rahill, 1963, 1965a,b, 1966a,b; Wesson, 1969). If passive reabsorption does indeed play a major role, the extent of restraint on sodium reabsorption imposed by small monovalent anions will be determined by the summated products of concentrations of individual anions in the glomerular filtrate, and their permeabilities. This sum should be proportional to the total transmural flux in response to a uniform driving force at the tubular wall, whether the force be electrical potential or coupling with sodium reabsorption. The chloruretic and natriuretic effects of nitrate infusion (Rapoport and West, 1950), for example, can be explained in this manner, as can the absence of a natriuretic or chloruretic effect of thiocycanate (Saugman, 1957).

A distinctly different type of anionic restraint is imposed by the presence of increased quantities of multivalent anions or large monovalent anions (e.g., Vogel and Stoeckert, 1966) in the glomerular filtrate. The quantity of these substances which appears in the urine is close to the amount filtered, and must be accompanied by an equivalent amount of cations. This type of restraint on sodium reabsorption is often manifested by increased transepithelial PD in the distal nephron (Rector and Clapp, 1962), with consequent effects on hydrogen and potassium transport in this segment (Chapters 4,6). In the presence of such anions, potassium and hydrogen secretion may predominate, especially at low GFR (Lauson and Thompson, 1958).

Bicarbonate does not fit clearly into either of these categories of anion. The effect on chloride and sodium reabsorption of varying concentrations of bicarbonate and hydrogen ion is considered in Chapter 4.

H. Osmotic Diuretics

Poorly absorbed nonelectrolytes, infused intravenously, lead to natriuresis despite the resulting hyponatremia (Wesson, 1969). Fractional reabsorption of sodium falls in the proximal tubule (Dirks et al., 1966) but may increase somewhat distally (Malnic et al., 1966a). The accumulation of the nonreabsorbable solute downstream in the proximal tubule, as isotonic salt solution is reabsorbed, is balanced by an osmotically equivalent reduction in sodium concentration. Because the proximal tubule is limited in its capacity to maintain a transtubular gradient for sodium (see Section II,B) sodium reabsorption is impaired.

This traditional explanation of the natriuresis which follows isotonic mannitol infusion is not entirely satisfying. It appears to predict greater and greater natriuresis as plasma mannitol level is increased, but this is clearly wrong because filtered sodium is progressively falling at the same time. Integration of pump and leak kinetics for sodium reabsorption in an isosmotic segment can be examined theoretically with the aid of the computer (Walser, 1966). Maximal natriuresis occurs when the nonreabsorbable solute comprises one-fourth of the total osmotically active solute in the filtrate (Fig. 11). If passive permeability to sodium is relatively low (despite a limiting gradient of 80 mM), little or no natriuresis occurs. The minimal permeability necessary to achieve substantial natriuresis is 6×10^{-4} mm/sec, which corresponds closely to the value measured in vivo (Gertz, 1963). The inference that increased backflux of sodium is chiefly responsible for the natriuresis of isotonic mannitol infusion is in accord with the earlier suggestion of Kiil et al. (1961), referred to above (Section III,A).

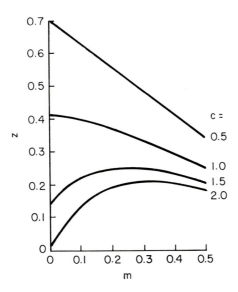

FIG. 11.   Computer-generated model of osmotically induced natriuresis. Salt excretion (z), expressed as a fraction of the total filtered solute, is plotted as a function of the un-reabsorbable fraction of filtered solute (m), for a uniform isosmotic segment. Solute reabsorption is assumed to follow "pump and leak" kinetics, i.e., $dz/dx = -a/(1 + b/y) + c(w - y)$, where x is distance, y and w salt concentration in tubular fluid and peritubular plasma, respectively. The constants a, b, and c were chosen so that influx equals efflux when the tubular fluid sodium concentration is reduced by 60 mM. Curves are shown for various values of c, the passive permeability to salt. Note that salt excretion increases appreciably with osmotic diuresis only if permeability is relatively high. Maximal natriuresis is seen when about one-fourth of the filtered solute is unreabsorbable. Reprinted by permission from Walser (1966).

Osmotic diuresis frequently depresses GFR, evidently by increasing proximal tubular pressure. Since the applied tubular pressure required to bring out total cessation of glomerular filtration is not affected, the glomerular capillary pressure is apparently unchanged (Koch *et al.*, 1967).

VI. Effects of Other Physiological Variables on Sodium Excretion

A. Nutrients

Starvation has long been known to be associated with renal loss of sodium, perhaps attributable in part to the resulting acidosis. However, bicarbonate supplements fail to alter the negative sodium balance (Veverbrants and Arky, 1969), as does ammonium chloride, if some carbohydrate is provided (Katz *et al.*, 1968). Carbohydrate or protein feeding inhibits the sodium loss, while fat aggravates it. The effect of glucose is cited above (Section V, C).

B. Environmental Temperature

Hypothermia reduces renal hemodynamic parameters but impairs sodium reabsorption even more, with resulting natriuresis (Segar *et al.*, 1956; Boylan and Hong, 1966). The distal minimum in sodium concentration seen in stop-flow experiments persists, suggesting that proximal reabsorption may be more profoundly affected.

VII. Hormones

A. Antidiuretic Hormone (ADH)

Vasopressin release is primarily attuned to the osmolality of the body fluids, and its actions are primarily on the formation or reabsorption of solute-free water in the kidney (Chapter 2). This mechanism therefore plays a major role in regulation of plasma sodium concentration, by virtue of its effect upon water balance. Its actions on sodium balance are much less prominent. Normal animals are secreting vasopressin most of the time; consequently, it is not surprising that neither Pitressin nor purified vasopressin, given in physiological doses, has a consistent effect on electrolyte excretion. During maximal antidiuresis, it may increase urine flow (Macfarlane *et al.*, 1967), evidently by inhibiting sodium reabsorption. When administered to hydrated subjects, however, both agents usually increase sodium excretion (Anslow and Wesson, 1955; Brooks and Pickford, 1958). This response is exaggerated in the presence of overhydration; in this instance, suppression of aldosterone secretion by the expanded extracellular fluid volume is partly responsible (Leaf *et al.*, 1953; Bartter *et al.*, 1956; Chan and Sawyer, 1961).

Water loading has minor and inconsequential effects on sodium excretion, following brief natriuresis attributable to washout of more concentrated urine from the tubules and collecting system and the loss of some medullary sodium (Barclay *et al.*, 1947; Crutchfield and Wood, 1948; Dicker, 1948; Coxon and Ramsay, 1967; Massry *et al.*, 1968). Another factor contributing to the initial natriuresis following oral water loading may be an initial rise in plasma sodium which precedes the later fall (Blomhert, 1951). When distal sodium transport is blocked by diuretics, administration of water may inhibit sodium reabsorption (Martino and Earley, 1967b).

The relatively mild effects of vasopressin or water diuresis on sodium excretion seem surprising, in view of the known stimulatory action of the hormone on sodium transport in amphibian membranes (Ussing and Zerahn, 1951; Leaf *et al.*, 1958). Furthermore, the increase in sodium concentration in the distal portions of the nephron which results from vasopressin might be expected to lead to increased sodium reabsorption. The fact that sodium retention does not occur suggests that sodium transport is not concentration-dependent distally and that access of sodium to the pump mechanism may not be limiting in the nephron as a whole. Passive permeability to sodium in the collecting duct is greatly increased (Uhlich *et al.*, 1969).

An initial report that sodium reabsorption in the proximal tubule might be stimulated by vasopressin in the dog (Clapp *et al.*, 1963) was not supported by more detailed study (B. B. Davis *et al.*, 1967). In dogs, distal tubular fluid osmolality is lower during water diuresis than during antidiuresis (Fig. 3) (Clapp and Robinson, 1968), but in the rat with diabetes insipidus it is also reduced (Gertz *et al.*, 1964).

B. Oxytocin

This hormone may increase sodium excretion by raising GFR, but otherwise has only a minor natriuretic action (Wesson, 1969). However, it may play a role in the release of natriuretic factors from the central nervous system (Chan and Sawyer, 1968).

C. Adrenocortical Hormones

1. Effect of Adrenocortical Insufficiency

The classic work of Harrop *et al.* (1933) and Loeb *et al.* (1933) established that impaired renal conservation of sodium was characteristic of adrenal insufficiency. Since the filtered load of sodium is usually reduced, both by virtue of hyponatremia and reduced GFR, tubular reabsorption is clearly impaired. However, when extracellular fluid volume is restored to normal by salt loading, a defect in sodium reabsorption cannot be demonstrated by clearance techniques (Wesson, 1969). Furthermore, untreated patients with Addison's disease can maintain sodium balance despite a gradual quadrupling of normal salt intake, apparently without appreciable change in GFR (Fig. 12) (Burnett *et al.*, 1953). The diuretic response to saline is unaltered in magnitude, though delayed in onset (Kellogg and Burack, 1954). Faced with a low salt intake, however, the adrenalectomized animal continues to excrete sodium despite hypovolemia and hyponatremia. It is worth noting that only a fraction of the sodium which disappears from the extracellular

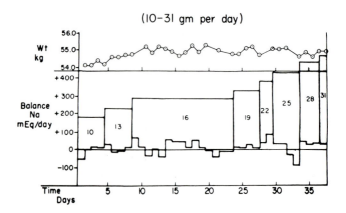

FIG. 12. Sodium balance during varying oral salt intake in a patient with Addison's disease on no hormonal therapy. Salt intake was increased from 10 to 31 gm/day over a 37-day period. Weight increased only 1 kg and glomerular filtration rate did not increase. Thus sodium balance was achieved by a mechanism not involving the adrenal cortex or GFR. Reprinted by permission from Burnett *et al.* (1953).

fluid during the development of full-blown adrenal insufficiency appears in the urine. Thus, the renal defect in sodium transport is only one manifestation of a more generalized disturbance.

The tubular localization of the defect in sodium reabsorption has been the subject of intensive study in recent years. Results of stop-flow experiments suggested that proximal tubular impairment occurred early after adrenalectomy, reduced distal reabsorption appearing later (Williamson *et al.*, 1961). Micropuncture studies by Hierholzer and associates (1965) in adrenalectomized rats indicated that the tubule's ability to establish a sodium gradient was reduced distally but unimpaired proximally. But when proximal reabsorption was assessed by the split oil drop technique, it too was reduced (Wiederholt *et al.*, 1964). Both of these observations can be interpreted in the usual pump and leak kinetic model as indicating coincident decreases in the velocity constant of the pump mechanism and in the passive permeability to sodium.

The accompanying fall in GFR further complicates the picture. As noted above (Section III, B), proximal glomerulotubular balance tends to be maintained when GFR falls as a result of hypotension. In adrenalectomized rats with reduced GFR, fractional reabsorption of sodium in the proximal nephron may be greater than normal (Hierholzer *et al.*, 1966) or normal (Cortney, 1969), but is evidently not decreased. Thus, a proximal defect exists, but apparently does not contribute to the failure of sodium conservation.

In addition to the distal impairment in establishing a sodium gradient, net reabsorption of sodium in the distal convolution is reduced in adrenalectomized animals (Hierholzer et al., 1966; Cortney, 1969). Since sodium concentration in the earliest accessible portion of the distal tubule is not as low as in normal animals, it is reasonable to infer a similar defect in the ascending limb (Windhager, 1968). Collecting duct reabsorption, which is normally responsible for removal of the last traces of sodium from the tubular fluid during salt deprivation, is reduced too, apparently owing to an abnormally high passive permeability to sodium (Cortney, 1969; Uhlich et al., 1969).

The biochemical lesions responsible for this defect in tubular reabsorption of sodium are uncertain. Activity of many enzymes in the kidney falls following adrenalectomy, including condensing enzyme, isocitrate dehydrogenase, aspartate aminotransferase, glutamate dehydrogenase, glyceraldehydephosphate dehydrogenase, and others (Kinne and Kirsten, 1968); aldosterone restores these to normal. Sodium-potassium-stimulated ATPase activity is also reduced (Chignell and Titus, 1966; Landon et al., 1966), but evidently only as a consequence of the associated alterations in plasma potassium and sodium concentrations (Ebel et al., 1968; Jorgensen, 1968).

2. MINERALOCORTICOIDS

In normal animals, aldosterone or desoxycorticosterone administration is regularly followed, within about half an hour, by a reduction in sodium excretion, with little or no change in GFR (Garrod et al., 1955; Ganong and Mulrow, 1958). Adrenalectomized animals are much more sensitive than normals. Hypophysectomy, however, reverses the response: sodium excretion rises. According to Lockett and Roberts (1963), a substance which modifies the renal actions of the hormone is released from the adrenal gland after hypophysectomy; the liberation of this substance involves a mechanism which can be interrupted by lesions in the brainstem.

Continued administration of mineralocorticoids induces retention of a modest quantity of sodium—about 200 mEq (Clinton and Thorn, 1943; August et al., 1958); thereafter, no further increase in sodium balance occurs. The point at which this "escape" phenomenon develops is dependent upon many factors, including the sympathetic nervous system. For example, adrenergic blockade with guanethidine reduces the degree of sodium retention at which escape appears (Gill et al.,

1964). The mechanism is probably similar to that of saline diuresis, considered below. GFR may (J. O. Davis and Howell, 1953) or may not be increased (August *et al.*, 1958). The presence of functioning adrenals is not necessary for escape to occur (August and Nelson, 1959). As in saline diuresis, proximal reabsorption of sodium is reduced. Nevertheless, saline administration in this setting leads to further proximal rejection (Wright *et al.*, 1969a).

Although mineralocorticoids promote potassium secretion, their net effects on total excretion of cations cannot be described simply as the replacement of a moiety of urinary sodium by an equal quantity of potassium. The sum of sodium plus potassium excretion falls (Yunis *et al.*, 1964). Furthermore, the effect on potassium excretion is obliterated if aldosterone is administered during salt deprivation (Finn and Welt, 1963).

Chronic salt loading inhibits aldosterone secretion and provides an opportunity to examine the proximal tubular action of the hormone by its absence: under these circumstances proximal reabsorption diminishes, whether measured from free-flow inulin concentrations or the split oil drop technique. Both changes are reversed by the hormone. In this situation, the proximal effect is more prominent than the distal (Stumpe and Ochwadt, 1968).

The mechanism of action of the mineralocorticoids in promoting sodium reabsorption is evidently similar to that by which they increase sodium transport in the toad bladder (Porter *et al.*, 1964), namely, stimulation of the synthesis of a protein involved in the transport mechanism. Thus, actinomycin D, an inhibitor of DNA-directed RNA synthesis, blocks aldosterone-induced antinatriuresis if given before the hormone (Williamson, 1963) but not when given after hormonal action has commenced (Ludens *et al.*, 1967). Actinomycin D has no influence on proximal or distal sodium reabsorption in adrenalectomized rats, as measured by the split oil drop technique, but reduces reabsorptive rate in both segments in normal rats or in adrenalectomized rats treated with aldosterone (Wiederholt, 1966). Coincident with the onset of antinatriuresis, RNA synthesis in the kidney is increased (Castles and Williamson, 1967; Fimognari *et al.*, 1967). The concentration of ATP in renal tissue is unaltered (Feldman *et al.*, 1961).

The role of sodium and potassium-stimulated ATPase is less clear. Actinomycin fails to inhibit the kaliuretic action of aldosterone (Williamson, 1963; Fimognari *et al.*, 1967), suggesting that the promotion of sodium-potassium exchange might occur by a mechanism distinct from the RNA-mediated one described above. Renal tissue levels of this ATPase change in the expected direction with administration of aldosterone or its antagonists, but the available evidence is consistent with the interpretation that these responses are secondary to altered plasma concentrations of sodium and potassium (Chignell and Titus, 1966; Landon *et al.*, 1966; Jorgensen, 1968).

3. Glucocorticoids

The familiar sodium-retaining action of the natural and synthetic corticoids resembles the action of aldosterone, but there are important differences. The amount of sodium retained before escape occurs is often greater, though this seems to be variable between individuals and between species. In rabbits, for example, cortisone may cause anasarca, while desoxycorticosterone leads to much less salt retention (Robb *et al.*, 1968). In normal hydropenic man, hydrocortisone may increase potassium excretion more than it diminishes sodium excretion, in contrast to aldosterone (Yunis *et al.*, 1964). Negative free water formation is increased by methylprednisolone, but unaffected by aldosterone (Jick *et al.*, 1965). In addition, glucocorticoids can restore the depressed glomerular filtration and impaired water diuresis of adrenal insufficiency more effectively than can the mineralocorticoids alone (Garrod *et al.*, 1955).

Wiederholt *et al.* (1966) and Wiederholt and Wiederholt (1968) have shown that dexamethasone, which has little or no sodium-retaining capacity in intact subjects, does not affect the intrinsic sodium reabsorptive capacity of the proximal tubule but, by virtue of its ability to restore the impaired GFR of adrenal insufficiency, can lead secondarily to decreased fractional reabsorption of sodium. In the distal segment, effects on water permeability are demonstrable, but not on sodium reabsorption.

Changes in renal Na-K-ATPase after glucocorticoids are similar to those following aldosterone, but less pronounced (Chignell and Titus, 1966; Jorgensen, 1968). There is a proportionate increase in the protein content of a membrane fraction rich in this enzyme, from which Manitius *et al.* (1968) conclude that the quantity of membrane per cell rises.

VIII. Diuretics

This term is used to identify a group of drugs which have the ability to increase the renal excretion of salt and are used clinically for that purpose. Generally, these compounds also increase water excretion, hence the term "diuretic" is not inappropriate; their characteristic action, however, is natriuresis.

A. Localization of Diuretic Action

Extensive investigation of the renal actions of these drugs has been carried out, not only because they are so widely employed clinically, but also in hopes of clarifying the mechanisms of sodium transport in various segments of the nephron. Selective action of individual diuretics on one segment of the nephron, without effects on others, might have provided a powerful tool to shed light on these problems. Although many efforts to establish such selective action have been made, further study has generally led to the conclusion, more likely on *a priori* grounds, that some degree of inhibition of transport occurs throughout the nephron. Nevertheless, clear distinctions between some of these compounds have emerged.

The interpretation of micropuncture data pertinent to the sites of action of diuretic agents is complicated by the intrinsic relationships between the rate of salt reabsorption, the velocity of tubular flow from glomerulus to final urine, and the varying diameter of each segment. The roles of diameter and velocity, considered as independent variables, are discussed below (Section X, A). A special problem in interpreting diuretic action arises from the fact that inhibition of reabsorption in distal portions of the nephron may be expected to augment downstream resistance and, hence, lead to proximal tubular dilatation. If, as suggested by Gertz (see Section IV, F), this stimulus is sufficient in itself to increase proximal reabsorption of salt and water, then an inhibitory effect of a drug on the proximal segment could be counterbalanced, and proximal reabsorption might remain unaltered. Thus, an unchanging fractional reabsorption rate in the proximal tubule following any saluretic agent may point to inhibition of proximal reabsorption, or more precisely, to an inhibition by the agent of the usual response to tubular dilatation.

Rector *et al.* (1966c), Dirks and Seely (1969), Bank (1968), Levine *et al.* (1968), and others have suggested that the "contact time of fluid with the epithelium" (as measured by the mean transit time of lissamine green, which often increases when the tubule dilates) may also influence reabsorption independently of any effects of dilatation *per se*. This is a misinterpretation of the work of Gertz and others, and reflects the intuitive but erroneous concept of velocity dependence discussed above (Section IV, G). The fallacy is most readily revealed by considering whether in fact the epithelium is bathed with tubular fluid for a shorter time. Clearly it is exposed to tubular fluid continuously, before or after a diuretic is given, and irrespective of the velocity of flow. The relationship

$$\log \mathrm{TF}/\mathrm{P}_{In} = CT/2.3\pi r^2$$

where C is reabsorptive rate, T passage time, and r tubular radius, merely states the inevitable relationship between these variables (given the assumptions on which the measurements are based), and yields no information as to whether changes in T affect C. When T and TF/P increase without change in C or r, the explanation is clearly that GFR has fallen, fractional reabsorption has increased, but absolute reabsorption has remained constant. The problem of whether velocity of tubular fluid flow independently affects reabsorption is a different question to which a final answer has yet to be given.

B. Cellular Mechanism of Action of Diuretic Drugs

Many of the compounds listed below exert specific effects on biochemical processes within the kidney which are pertinent to their mechanism of action. These are described under the individual drugs. In addition, there are some alterations in renal metabolism which are common to a number of diuretics and are considered here. The question of interest is whether inhibition of a specific reaction or group of reactions may underly the natriuretic action of several drugs.

1. Inhibition of Na-K-ATPase

The importance of this enzyme system in homocellular and transcellular sodium transport makes it a likely locus of action of diuretic drugs. Several groups of workers (e.g., Taylor, 1963; Hook and Williamson, 1965a; Nechay et al., 1967) have noted a poor correlation between inhibition of this enzyme and natriuretic activity among the more common diuretics such as organomercurials, thiazides, furosemide, and ethacrynic acid. The last-named authors have critically reviewed this problem. Some of the points which led them to conclude that this hypothesis could not be unequivocally supported were as follows.

(1) Certain organomercurials may inhibit the enzyme in vitro and become bound to the enzyme in vivo at inhibitory concentrations and yet fail to produce natriuresis.

(2) Mercaptomerin, a highly effective drug, fails to inhibit the enzyme in vivo. However, mercaptomerin (as well as ethacrynic acid) is less than additive with ouabain in producing natriuresis.

(3) During diuresis induced by hydrochlorothiazide, ouabain is still effective in further inhibiting sodium reabsorption.

(4) Ethacrynic acid, although inhibitory to the enzyme in vitro, is insufficiently bound to the enzyme in vivo to achieve inhibitory levels.

This has been borne out by studies reported by Ebel et al. (1969).

In addition, there is evidence that inhibition of homocellular sodium transport (as reflected in the intracellular sodium concentration) is poorly correlated with inhibition of sodium reabsorption, for example, following ouabain administration (Maude, 1969; Whittembury and Fishman, 1969).

On the other hand, medullary (but not cortical) ATP concentration is increased by furosemide or ethacrynic acid, suggesting impaired utilization (Kessler, 1969), and Na-K-ATPase activity is reduced in microdissected ascending limbs (although curiously unaffected in the distal convolution) (Dubach and Schmidt, 1969).

In conclusion, it appears that inhibition of this enzyme is often a feature of drug-induced diuresis, but evidence that such inhibition accounts for the natriuresis is lacking.

2. Inhibition of Oxidative Metabolism

Kessler *et al.* (1968) have examined the effect of a variety of metabolic inhibitors, including chlorothiazide and dichlorphenamide, on sodium reabsorption and on the rate of incorporation of radioactive phosphate into ATP; the correlation was poor. However, furosemide, ethacrynic acid, hydrochlorothiazide, and chlormerodrin all appear to inhibit oxidative metabolism, as measured either by oxygen consumption or by the corticomedullary gradient for lactate (Vorburger, 1964; Cannon *et al.*, 1968). As noted above (Section III, B), the inference that ATP is not the exclusive energy source for transport of sodium is worthy of further study.

3. Additivity of Diuretic Effects

The view that a common biochemical locus of action is involved in the action of the major diuretics is indirectly supported by the observation that administration of one agent during diuresis induced by another produces effects on sodium excretion which are less than additive. Thus, ethacrynic acid and furosemide are no more effective together than given separately (Hook and Williamson, 1965b; Le Zotte *et al.*, 1966). Furosemide and hydrochlorothiazide, furosemide and organomercurials (Hook and Williamson, 1965b) are less than additive. However, a competitive antagonist of hydrochlorothiazide fails to modify the natriuretic response to furosemide (Small and Cafruny, 1967).

This approach to mechanism of action is rather unreliable, as has been pointed out by Peters and Roch-Ramel (1969a). For example, the maximal response to intravenous hydrochlorothiazide in the rat may appear to be increased by oral hydrochlorothiazide, or vice versa, depending upon the time of observation. Competition for excretion, protein-binding, or metabolism could also obscure the results of such studies.

C. Specific Diuretic Drugs

1. AMMONIUM CHLORIDE

Though rarely used alone, this substance is often employed in conjunction with other diuretics, especially organomercurials (see below). By itself it is only mildly natriuretic. Why it is natriuretic at all is still uncertain, but the answer to this question is fundamental to the integration of acid–base regulation with sodium homeostasis. Clearly the acidosis which ensues after metabolism of the ammonia moiety is responsible in some way for inhibiting tubular reabsorption of sodium. Hyperchloremia may be essential, since respiratory acidosis, with associate hypochloremia, is less effective (Wesson, 1969).

Study of tubular fluid bicarbonate and chloride concentrations under various experimental conditions, summarized in this volume (Chapter 4), have led to the suggestion (Kashgarian et $al.$, 1965) that this natriuresis may be an example of altered anion restraint, i.e., that chloride is less readily reabsorbed than bicarbonate and, therefore, "restrains" sodium reabsorption to a greater degree. NH_4Cl natriuresis would, thus, be analogous to the natriuresis which results from the replacement of some of plasma chloride by a less well reabsorbed anion such as nitrate (Greene and Hiatt, 1955). The detailed mechanism of this restraint cannot be clarified until the extent of coupling between proximal sodium reabsorption, anion reabsorption, and hydrogen secretion is established and the nature of the driving force for anion transport is identified.

2. XANTHINES

Caffeine, theobromine, and theophylline are all natriuretic. Theophylline, the most potent, is often administered as the ethylenediamine salt (aminophylline). The effect of these agents on vascular smooth muscle evidently plays a role in the resulting diuresis, but whether it is exclusively responsible is uncertain. GFR usually rises but may fail to do so despite diuresis (Wesson, 1969), indicating an inhibitory effect of the drug on tubular reabsorption. Simultaneous administration of organomercurials, thiazides, or carbonic anhydrase inhibitors leads to additive or even synergistic effects on sodium excretion (Herrman and

Decherd, 1937; Weston *et al.*, 1952; Nechay, 1964), suggesting a mechanism of action distinct from those of such compounds. A predominantly proximal site of action is indicated by the observation that free water clearance rises when the drug is administered during combined water and mannitol diuresis (Porush *et al.*, 1961).

3. ORGANOMERCURIALS

Although highly effective, these compounds are being used less frequently since the advent of less toxic drugs with equal or greater efficacy. Owing to their preeminence among the diuretics in clinical use for almost 50 years, a large body of literature has accumulated concerning the effects and actions of these compounds on the kidney. For a more complete survey of this literature, see Mudge and Weiner (1957–58). Cafruny *et al.* (1966), Heidenreich (1969), and Wesson (1969).

All of the clinically useful compounds in this class have the general formula $RCH_2CH(OY)CH_2HgX$, in which R, X, and Y are a variety of substituents. Mercuric salts of inorganic anions or of cysteine are also diuretic but have greater cardiovascular toxicity. After administration, organomercurials are extensively bound by renal tissue, particularly the proximal tubular epithelium (Wedeen and Goldstein, 1963). Natriuresis ensues within about $\frac{1}{2}$ hour, in association with a fall in GFR in most cases. Potassium excretion usually rises too but may fall if it was initially high. Reabsorption of calcium and magnesium is depressed as much or more than that of sodium (Walser and Trounce, 1961; Wesson, 1962); acidification is little affected (Hilton, 1951; Weston *et al.*, 1951). Free water clearance (during water diuresis) may fail to raise in association with the increase in osmolar clearance (Goldstein *et al.*, 1961), suggest a predominantly distal action. However, the evidence on this point is conflicting (Heinemann *et al.*, 1959). During hydropenia, negative free water clearance also fails to rise (Porush and Abramson, 1965) or may fall (Seldin *et al.*, 1966). Stop-flow experiments have been variously interpreted as indicating a predominantly proximal (Vander *et al.*, 1958; McEvoy, 1968) or distal (R. W. Schmidt and Sullivan, 1966) site of action. Like other potent diuretics, organomercurials fail to alter fractional reabsorption of salt and water in the proximal tubule, when measured by the conventional recollection micropuncture technique (Dirks *et al.*, 1966), and lead to an increase in distal tubular fluid osmolality in the dog (Clapp and Robinson, 1968). Whether these observations reveal the site of action is conjectural.

A possible model of mercurial action is found in the frog skin (Linderholm, 1952) and in the toad bladder, where sodium transport is inhibited by chlormerodrin (Jamison, 1961; Pendleton *et al.*, 1968a). Mucosal-to-serosal sodium flux is inhibited and serosal-to-mucosal is increased. However, there are several differences between the response in toad bladder and in the kidney: the response in the former is not reversed by dimercaprol, while the renal response is reversed; an effect on short-circuit current is also seen following *p*-chloromercuribenzoate, which is a nondiuretic compound.

4. Thiazides

Several benzothiadiazines containing sulfonamide groups are clinically useful diuretics. The prototypes of this class were synthesized as analogs of acetazolamide, but it was soon found that their chloruretic action varied independently of carbonic anhydrase inhibition (Novello and Sprague, 1957). Chlorothiazide, the first clinically useful drug, has been the most widely studied. Others in common use include hydrochlorothiazide, trichlormethiazide, methylclothiazide, flumethiazide, and benzhydroflumethiazide. A detailed review of the pharmacology of these compounds has recently appeared (Peters and Roch-Ramel, 1969a). All have some carbonic anhydrase-inhibiting activity.

Little is known of their mechanism of action, other than that it involves inhibition of tubular reabsorption of sodium and chloride (as well as a small and variable degree of carbonic-anhydrase inhibition). Filtration rate is not greatly affected. Chlorothiazide is effective after adrenalectomy and, hence, does not act by inhibiting aldosterone (Kahn, 1962). From the observation that thiazides do not alter the ratio of sodium absorption to oxygen consumption, Peters and Roch-Ramel (1969a) infer that these drugs reduce sodium efflux from the lumen rather than augmenting passive influx.

Stop-flow experiments indicate a distal site of action (Sullivan and Pirch, 1966; McEvoy, 1968) when precautions are taken to prevent the fall in plasma sodium which usually occurs in such experiments (Fig. 13). Moreover, when these drugs are given during water diuresis, the rate of free water excretion either fails to rise in association with the ensuing increase in osmolar clearance (see Wesson, 1969) or more commonly falls (Earley *et al.*, 1961; Lant *et al.*, 1967). These results suggest inhibition of distal salt reabsorption, increase in distal water permeability, or both. Negative free water formation is unimpaired when these drugs are given during hydropenia (Earley *et al.*, 1961), perhaps indicating that sodium reabsorption in earlier portions of the ascending limb is less affected.

The proximal tubule apparently does not contribute to the natriuresis, as indicated by unchanging or increasing TF/P_{In} (Dirks *et al.*,

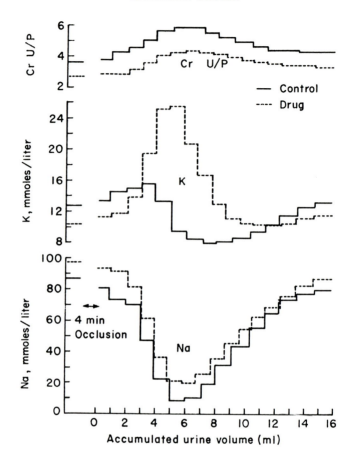

Fig. 13. Effect of a thiazide diuretic (bendroflumethiazide) on the stop-flow pattern in dogs. The distal dip in sodium excretion is considerably blunted, indicating inhibition of reabsorption at this site. Potassium secretion at the same site is augmented. Reprinted by permission from Sullivan and Pirch (1966).

1966). Furthermore, the limiting sodium gradient against which sodium reabsorption can proceed is unaffected (Holzgreve and Loeschke, 1967). Nevertheless, the shrinking drop technique reveals an inhibition of salt reabsorption in this segment (Holzgreve, 1968). The interpretation is discussed above (Section VIII, A).

GFR often falls. This circumstance further obscures the interpretation of micropuncture data in which single nephron filtration rates have not been recorded. The cause of the fall in GFR is evidently the diuresis itself, leading to increased intratubular pressure. Glomerular capillary pressure is little affected (Krause et al., 1967), and renal interstitial pressure falls (Martino and Earley, 1968).

Pendleton *et al.* (1968b) have recently shown that one drug in this class (bendroflumethiazide) will inhibit sodium transport in the toad bladder when it is applied to the serosal surface. Curiously, the opposite response is seen when it is applied to the mucosal surface. Further study of this *in vitro* system may shed light on biochemical mechanism of action.

5. OTHER SULFONAMIDES

a. *Acetazolamide*
This agent and a number of related compounds (Maren, 1969) exert their natriuretic action by inhibiting carbonic anhydrase. The mechanism of inhibition of bicarbonate reabsorption and the ensuing changes in tubular transport are discussed in Chapter 4. The localization of the site of action in the nephron is predominantly proximal, as would be anticipated from the distribution of the enzyme along the luminal membrane of the tubule. Thus, fractional reabsorption in the proximal segment is more unequivocally reduced by this agent than by most other diuretics (Dirks *et al.*, 1966; Holzgreve and Loeschke, 1967; Holzgreve, 1968). Furthermore, both positive and negative free water excretion increase when measured in appropriate circumstances, presumably owing to increased delivery of sodium to the diluting site (Porush and Abramson, 1965); furthermore, distal fluid sodium concentration increases (Clapp and Robinson, 1968).

b. *Furosemide*
This potent agent was introduced in 1965 (see Bank, 1968; Peters and Roch-Ramel, 1969b) and has already come into widespread use. It is similar in structure to the thiazides but lacks the thiadiazine ring. Its predominant site of action is apparently in the ascending limb, since it produces a profound reduction in either positive or negative free water excretion (Buchborn and Anastasakis, 1964; Suki *et al.*, 1965; Lant *et al.*, 1967), provided these values are initially high (Fig. 14). When free water clearance is initially low, the result may be little change despite the large increase in osmolar clearance (Le Zotte *et al.*, 1966). Its effect in reducing free water excretion appears to be diminished when it is given orally (Stříbrná and Schück, 1968). Like other diuretics, it inhibits proximal reabsorption as measured by the split oil drop technique (Ullrich *et al.*, 1966; Holzgreve, 1968; Knox *et al.*, 1969) but has little effect on fractional reabsorption in the proximal tubule (Dirks *et al.*, 1966; Rector *et al.*, 1967; Bennett *et al.*, 1968; Brenner *et al.*, 1969a). When precautions are taken to prevent any reduction of extracellular fluid volume or retrograde flow of tubular fluid into the collecting pipette, proximal fractional reabsorption is unaffected as GFR falls, or

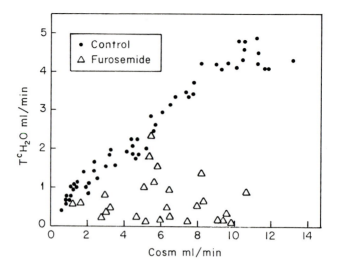

FIG. 14. Inhibition by furosemide of the concentrating mechanism in the dog. Negative free water formation (T^cH_2O) rises with solute excretion (Cosm) in controls receiving saline but not after furosemide. Reprinted by permission from Suki *et al.* (1965).

may be demonstrably reduced if GFR remains constant (Clapp *et al.*, 1969; Knox *et al.*, 1969). The limiting gradient against which the proximal nephron can reabsorb salt is reduced (Holzgreve and Loeschke, 1967). Oral glucose markedly reduces furosemide diuresis, suggesting a specific effect of the drug on glycolysis which can be overcome by increasing glucose concentration (Levin *et al.*, 1969).

An unusual feature of the action of this drug is an increase in glomerular capillary pressure, apparently by a direct vascular action, which may limit or prevent a fall in GFR (Krause *et al.*, 1967).

c. *Chlorthalidone and Chlorexolone*

These sulfonamides share many of the properties of the thiazides: they appear to act in the ascending limb as well as the distal tubule (Baba *et al.*, 1966; Lant *et al.*, 1967; McEvoy, 1968).

6. ETHACRYNIC ACID

An α, β-unsaturated ketone, this potent drug introduced in 1962 (Schultz *et al.*, 1962) does not resemble any of the other diuretics chemically. Pharmacologically, it closely resembles furosemide in its apparent lack of proximal effect in the intact kidney (Dirks *et al.*, 1966; Levine *et al.*, 1968) except when GFR is maintained (Clapp *et al.*, 1969), its principal action in the ascending limb (Earley and Friedler, 1964a; Lant *et al.*, 1967), and its effectiveness in either acidosis or alkalosis (Beyer *et al.*, 1965). It reduces free water excretion even more dramatically than does furosemide (Le Zotte *et al.*, 1966), but its actions are not additive with this drug. In the chicken, which has only rudimentary loops of Henle, ethacrynic acid is a powerful natriuretic, supporting the view that its actions are more generalized in the tubule (Nechay, 1967). Its pharmacology has recently been reviewed by Peters and Roch-Ramel (1969c).

7. SPIRONOLACTONE

An analog of aldosterone, this drug and its congeners induce diuresis exclusively by inhibiting the action of this hormone, and the magnitude of the resulting natriuresis, therefore, varies with the basal level of circulating aldosterone (Liddle, 1966; Herken, 1969a). In contrast to most other diuretics, it promotes potassium retention as a result of this action. Its action can be overcome by administering mineralocorticoids.

8. PTERIDINES

Triamterene and several related compounds resemble spironolactone in their effects, but possess an entirely unrelated chemical structure and do not act by inhibiting aldosterone (Herken, 1969b). This is clearly shown by the efficacy of triamterene in adrenalectomized subjects and by the additivity of the natriuretic effects of this drug with spironolactone (Wiebelhaus *et al.*, 1965; Liddle, 1966). Another compound, unrelated chemically, which exerts similar effects is amiloride (Bull and Laragh, 1968).

D. Other Compounds which Modify Sodium Transport

1. CARDIAC GLYCOSIDES

Injection into the renal artery of ouabain or strophanthidin exerts profound effects on sodium excretion. At the smallest doses, sodium reabsorption is facilitated (Palmer and Nechay, 1964; Nahmod and Walser, 1966); at larger doses it is markedly inhibited (Orloff and Burg, 1960; Cade *et al.*, 1961; Kupfer and Kosovsky, 1965; Nahmod and Walser, 1966). Further administration induces renal vasoconstriction. Studies by the stop-flow method indicate that distal tubular transport of sodium is inhibited (Wilde and Howard, 1960), but proximal reabsorption is also reduced in microperfused or isolated tubules (Schatzman *et al.*, 1958; Burg and Orloff, 1968). Transtubular potential in isolated collecting ducts is reduced (Burg *et al.*, 1968). The presence of adreno-cortical hormones is not a prerequisite for natriuresis (Cade *et al.*, 1961), but the presence of potassium in the renal perfusion medium is (Vogel and Tervooren, 1965). Clearly alterations in renal hemody-namics are not responsible for the natriuresis; furthermore, the drug is effective when administered into the renal portal system of the chicken (Orloff and Burg, 1960). Cortical and medullary ATP concentrations rise, suggesting reduced utilization (Kessler, 1969). Negative free water formation is almost completely eliminated, implying that sodium trans-port is particularly affected in the ascending limb; the amount of tissue-bound glycosides is likewise highest in outer medulla (Hendler *et al.*, 1969).

All of the available evidence is consistent with the hypothesis that the mechanism of natriuresis in response to cardiac glycosides administra-tion into the renal artery is inhibition of Na-K-ATPase. The role of this mechanism in the diuretic properties of digitalis in heart failure is cer-tainly minor, since the action of the drug upon the heart far outweighs its direct effect upon the kidney.

2. β-Diethylaminoethyldiphenylpropyl Acetate

Commonly known as SKF-525A, this compound has been widely employed experimentally as an inhibitor of microsomal drug-metabo-lizing enzymes. It also promotes natriuresis, evidently by inhibiting both proximal and distal sodium reabsorption (Marshall and William-son, 1964; Hook and Williamson, 1965c). Its action is additive with that of common diuretics (Hook and Williamson, 1964).

3. Catecholamines and Other Vasoactive Agents

The predominant effects of catecholamines and serotonin on sodium excretion are exerted by their vascular effects, (e.g., Blackmore, 1958; Langston *et al.*, 1962), and they have little or no direct action on tu-bular transport of sodium, as measured by the occlusion time method (Leyssac, 1965) or the shrinking drop technique (Fülgraff *et al.*, 1968b). Prostaglandin E inhibits sodium transport independently of any effect on GFR, but renal vasodilatation may be responsible (Johnston *et al.*, 1967).

IX. Nervous Influences

It has been known for years that renal denervation is followed by diuresis and natriuresis in the anesthetized, but not in the unanesthetized and unstressed dog (Berne, 1952; Surtshin *et al.*, 1952). The difference between the denervated and intact kidney of the anesthetized dog was attributed to tubular factors by Blake (1962), but Kamm and Levinsky (1965b) found unchanged sodium excretion when the increased GFR of the denervated kidney was prevented by an arterial clamp.

In man, impaired sympathetic function has little or no effect on sodium excretion in the resting state but leads to an exaggerated diuretic response to saline loading and an impairment of sodium conservation in response to sodium restriction (Gill, 1969). Anesthesia also augments saline diuresis (Gilmore and Michaelis, 1969). These and other results indicate that sympathetic impulses play an important role in the response of the kidney to alterations in effective blood volume, extracellular fluid volume, or intrathoracic pressure (Sieker *et al.*, 1954).

The efferent arc of this regulatory mechanism has not been clearly identified. Several factors appear to be involved. Increased sympathetic tone can reduce sodium excretion by reducing GFR, by promoting renin secretion and aldosterone production, by altering peritubular capillary hydrostatic or oncotic pressure, by redistributing renal blood flow, or conceivably by a direct effect on the tubular transport mechanisms independent of any vascular action. It is clear that at least under certain conditions, neither altered GFR nor altered mineralocorticoid activity is responsible for the observed changes in sodium excretion (Gill *et al.*, 1967; Gill, 1969).

There is also to be considered the possible role of autonomic supply to organs other than the kidney in modifying sodium excretion. Thus, chronic cardiac denervation diminishes the diuretic response to saline infusion, even though it does not alter the effect of saline on proximal tubular reabsorption (Knox *et al.*, 1967). Section of the vagi or their cervical cardiac branches does not alter the response (Keeler and Schnieden, 1958), but lesions in the paraventricular nuclei of the hypothalamus tend to increase sodium excretion (Keeler, 1959). The role of cardiac nerves in these phenomena has recently been reviewed by Gilmore (1968). Whether a natriuretic hormone is also involved in some of these effects remains to be established.

Hypertonic salt solution injected into the third ventricle of unanesthetized goats leads to a five- to tenfold increase in sodium excretion (Andersson *et al.*, 1966). Further study of intracranial sites responsive to alterations in the volume or tonicity of the extracelluar fluid is clearly indicated.

X. Glomerulotubular Balance

A. Proximal Sodium Reabsorption in Relation to GFR

A central problem in the renal regulation of sodium excretion is the interdependence which exists between tubular reabsorption and glomerular filtration. Under a variety of circumstances, the fraction of the glomerular filtrate reabsorbed in this segment is constant in the face of varying rate of filtration, a state often referred to as "perfect" glomerulotubular balance, though "proportionate" might be a better term. Equal changes in filtration and in the absolute rate of reabsorption may also occur in some situations. Under very few circumstances, by contrast, is the absolute rate of proximal transport constant despite varying filtration, i.e., nonexistent glomerulotubular balance. All gradations between these extremes have been observed in response to various experimental maneuvers, and rather widely discrepant results have been obtained from different laboratories. All agree, however, that glomerulotubular balance, even though it is often less than proportionate, is a characteristic feature of the intact kidney. Most of the experimental work has been summarized in Section IV. The principle hypotheses as to the mechanism of glomerulotubular balance are as follows:

1. Velocity-Dependent Reabsorption

The assumption that velocity must affect reabsorption is based upon a misconception, which has been discussed in Section IV, G and Section VIII, A. Nevertheless, velocity dependence by some unknown mechanism may exist. The only experimental evidence to refute it has been obtained in isolated tubules, in which glomerulotubular balance is nonexistent. One mechanism by which velocity could directly influence reabsorption is by affecting radial concentration gradients within the tubular lumen. At high flow, such gradients should be dissipated, and reabsorption might, therefore, increase. Although radial concentration gradients within the lumen for sodium or osmolality seem unlikely on theoretical grounds, this conclusion is not final (see Section IV) and the possibility exists that gradients within smaller channels, such as between microvilli, could be important *in situ* but not in the isolated nephron.

2. Reabsorption Dependent on Tubular Diameter

An increase in filtration rate, if it were not associated with a change in proximal reabsorption or downstream resistance, would necessarily lead to increased proximal fluid pressure. Unless interstitial pressure

rose *pari passu*, the tubules would dilate. If dilatation promotes proximal reabsorption, the change in reabsorption might be proportionate
to the change in filtration, and thus proportionate also to the change in
proximal tubule outflow. The more detailed hypothesis of Gertz and
the evidence for and against it has been presented (Section IV, F). At
least one group of investigators who championed this hypothesis have
abandoned it (Rodicio *et al.*, 1969), and it is now clear that luminal
diameter need not change appreciably even when glomerulotubular
balance is nearly proportionate (e.g., see Arrizureta-Muchnik *et al.*,
1969; Bojesen and Leyssac, 1969). Nevertheless, it is possible that tubular dilatation does promote reabsorption and that this mechanism
can produce some degree of glomerulotubular balance. Clearly, other
mechanisms must be invoked in those instances in which diameter is
unaltered.

The apparent constancy of reabsorption per unit tubular volume in
some experiments and the simple mathematical relationships which
follow from this form of interdependence have obscured the possibility
that some other form of dependence might exist between diameter and
reabsorption. For example, the electrical conductance of the tubule
might be a critical factor: the relationship between tubular diameter
and conductance has not been examined. It is unlikely to be proportional to the square of diameter: for a uniform cylinder composed of
homogeneous elastic material, conductance increases curvilinearly.
This function approaches the square of diameter for certain relative
values of inner and outer diameter (Fig. 15). The experimental data
are not yet sufficiently uniform to define the relationship between reabsorption rate and tubular diameter, under those circumstances when
diameter varies.

3. REABSORPTION DEPENDENT ON INTERSTITIAL PRESSURE OR VOLUME

Earley and Daugharty (1969) have suggested that a change in volume
or pressure of the renal interstitium, brought about by changes in
blood flow or in the balance of Starling forces across the postglomerular capillary, may in some unknown manner affect proximal sodium
reabsorption. Lewy and Windhager (1968) have proposed that this may
be the explanation of glomerulotubular balance. Rodicio *et al.* (1969)
have pointed out that the effects of aortic constriction, ureteral occlusion, and venous occlusion upon hydrostatic and oncotic pressure in
the postglomerular capillaries differ considerably, although all three
maneuvers may lead to reduced reabsorption. These authors suggest
that the transmural pressure gradient may be the critical factor. However, Brenner *et al.* (1969b) have established by direct measurement

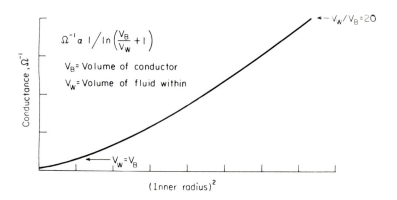

Fig. 15.   Theoretical model of the effect of tubular dilatation on its electrical conductance. The resistance of an elastic hollow cylinder of homogeneous material filled and surrounded with conducting fluid is (by Ohm's law) dependent on the inner and outer surface area and the wall thickness. Dilatation increases conductance, and this relationship becomes an approximately linear function of the square of radius as the ratio of the volume of the conductor to the volume of fluid within decreases.

that peritubular plasma concentration, during albumin infusion, varies with the rate of sodium reabsorption in the proximal tubule.

4. Intrarenal Hormones

Leyssac (1965) proposed that changes in the rate of flow of tubular fluid past the *macula densa*, subsequent to a change in GFR, might promote the release of renin and angiotensin (or other hormones) which would modify proximal reabsorption appropriately. As noted in Vol. IV, Chapter 2, angiotensin is clearly not the hormone responsible. But Thurau and Schnermann (1965) and Thurau *et al.* (1967) have shown that changes in sodium concentration in the fluid passing the *macula densa* induce profound changes in GFR, as indicated by collapse of the proximal tubule. Thus, glomerulotubular balance might be attributable to a mechanism which attunes glomerular filtration to the rate of tubular reabsorption, rather than the reverse. Indeed, the cause of the large "spontaneous" variations in GFR which are seen between individual rats has never been adequately explained. In such situations, where the initiating stimulus to altered renal function is unknown, this hypothesis is most plausible.

Recently Gottschalk and Leyssac (1968) have reexamined this hypothesis and have concluded that the proximal collapse observed after distal microinjection is an artifact, caused by leakage of fluid from the puncture site, an interpretation which Thurau rejects (Thurau, personal communication, cited by Gottschalk and Leyssac, 1968). Further study will be required to resolve this important question.

B. Distal Sodium Reabsorption in Relation to Inflow of Water and Sodium

Attempts to predict changes in sodium excretion from micropuncture observations on the proximal tubule have repeatedly failed, evidently because distal tubular activity may either fail to respond in the same direction, or may change in the opposite direction. This is the inference drawn from many studies in which a decrease in proximal reabsorption brought about by some experimental maneuver is not reflected in a corresponding increase in urinary excretion of sodium (e.g., Howards *et al.*, 1968). An alternative explanation of such data might be that the superficial proximal nephrons accessible to micropuncture are rejecting different fractions of filtered salt and water than are the remainder.

Another approach is to compare free-flow proximal with distal micropuncture observations during partial constriction of the renal artery (Landwehr *et al.*, 1968). Such data suggest a proportionality between loop transport of sodium and inflow, but it is not possible from such data to determine how much of this transport is attributable to the inaccessible portion of the proximal nephron as opposed to the thin limb or the thick ascending limb. Similar observations made during saline loading (Landwehr *et al.*, 1967) may reflect a response peculiar to this experimental stimulus, as noted below. Comparison of loop of Henle fluid with samples from surface convolutions in *Psammomys* indicates net influx of sodium in the descending limb and a large variable efflux in the ascending limb, which is apparently concentration-dependent (de Rouffignac and Morel, 1969).

A more definitive approach to this problem consists of perfusing individual loops of Henle at varying rates and measuring the composition and flow rate of the emerging distal fluid. Cortney *et al.* (1966) observed that distal fluid sodium concentration approached that of plasma as perfusion rate was increased. Schnermann (1968) observed variable changes in tubular fluid sodium concentration with perfusion rate, but a consistent increase in the absolute rate of sodium reabsorption. Morgan and Berliner (1969c) observed increased distal sodium concentration when the perfusion rate was either increased or decreased from a value of about 20 nl/minute (Fig. 16). The response to higher perfusion rate indicated decreased fractional but increased absolute reabsorption of sodium; the response to low perfusion rates was attributed to a greater degree of osmotic equilibration as well as in-

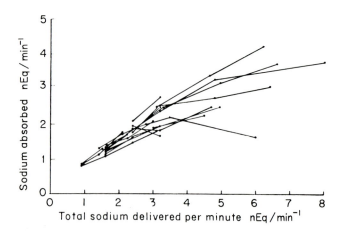

FIG. 16.   Sodium reabsorption by the loop of Henle as a function of perfusion rate of a saline solution in the rat. Although absolute rate of sodium reabsorption rises, fractional reabsorption falls. Reprinted by permission from Morgan and Berliner (1969c).

creased fractional sodium reabsorption. Further study of this important problem is needed.

Measurement of changes in free water excretion (during water diuresis) in response to induced alterations in proximal reabsorption has also been employed as an index of sodium transport in the thick ascending limb. This inference is valid only if no further water reabsorption occurs subsequently, during the conditions of the experiments, an assumption which may be open to question (Walser and Mudge, 1960; Aukland and Kjekshus, 1966). The use of negative free water excretion during hydropenia for the same purpose is even less supportable, since many factors other than distal sodium reabsorption could influence the results.

Apart from these uncertain changes in distal transport which may follow alterations in proximal outflow, the loop of Henle also plays a major role in determining proximal pressure (Gottschalk and Mylle, 1956). If luminal pressure or diameter is indeed an important determinant of salt reabsorption proximally, the relation between inflow and resistance of the loop becomes an important factor in autoregulation. Kruhoffer (1960) has considered these relationships in detail, and Bossert and Schwartz (1967) have evolved an interesting theoretical model of glomerulotubular balance based upon this concept. From measurements of proximal and distal pressures and flow rates, the resistance of the loop can be calculated. Schnermann (1968) and Brandis (1969) have in this way demonstrated that loop resistance does vary with flow.

XI. The Mechanism of Saline Diuresis

One of the most common and distressing disorders of electrolyte metabolism, edema, is also one of the easiest to reproduce experimentally. Administration of isotonic saline or similar solutions to experimental subjects produces a natriuretic response which eventually restores extracellular fluid volume to normal. This saline diuresis has been studied in great detail because its impairment in patients with edema accounts for their persistently overexpanded extracellular space. The fundamental mechanism remains elusive despite a wealth of investigation of almost every conceivable experimental variable. A number of factors have been identified which play a role in the response, and are listed below. Most workers agree, however, that the mechanisms clearly identified to date are less important than those as yet ill defined.

A. Glomerular Filtration Rate

Acute or chronic saline loading usually augments GFR, and for many years this was believed to be the mechanism of the ensuing natriuresis. Although increased arterial pressure and decreased plasma oncotic pressure are in part responsible for the rise in GFR, other unidentified factors also play a role (Hayslett *et al.*, 1967; Wesson, 1969). An intact adrenergic nervous system is not necessary for the response (Schrier *et al.*, 1967). As noted in preceding sections, glomerulotubular balance is usually fairly well maintained, so that the increment in salt excretion, on this basis alone, should not be much greater in relative terms than the increase in GFR. The earlier view that an undetectably small increment in GFR, if unassociated with a change in tubular reabsorption, could cause a great increase in sodium excretion is logically correct but practically irrelevant: situations in which glomerulotubular balance is nonexistent are rare indeed. Furthermore, as noted in Section IV, A, salt excretion may not change at all when GFR is increased in the absence of altered extracellular fluid volume. It is, therefore, open to question whether renal hemodynamics play any role in saline diuresis, even though the response to *reduction* of extracellular fluid volume may be largely dependent thereon.

B. Adrenocortical Hormones

When it became apparent that changes in tubular reabsorption must also contribute to saline diuresis, a hormone related to the known adrenocortical steroids with selective action on tubular reabsorption of sodium was postulated, and eventually identified as aldosterone. The effects of this substance on tubular transport of sodium are summarized in Section VII, C. Its role in the diuretic response to saline can be no greater than the magnitude of its sodium-retaining effect in normal subjects under control conditions. As noted above, a defect in sodium reabsorption in adrenalectomized subjects with normal extracellular fluid volume is difficult to demonstrate. Furthermore, competitive inhibition of aldosterone in normal subjects causes only a very modest natriuresis (Section VIII, C).

That neither filtration rate nor mineralocorticoid activity can account for the diuretic response to saline loading was suggested by a number of early clinical studies (e.g., Burnett *et al.*, 1953; Rosenbaum *et al.*, 1955) but more clearly brought into focus by the dog experiments of de Wardener *et al.* (1961), Levinsky and Lalone (1963), and Rector *et al.* (1964), in which these factors were carefully controlled or excluded. Chronic salt loading may, however, induce changes in proximal salt reabsorption which are prevented by simultaneous administration of aldosterone (Stumpe and Ochwadt, 1968). Thus, adrenocortical control may be an important factor normally, but other regulatory mechanisms become apparent in its absence.

C. Compositional Changes

Saline infusion reduces the hematocrit, lowers plasma oncotic pressure, lowers plasma potassium concentration, and increases chloride concentration. All of these changes, as noted in Section V, tend to promote natriuresis. However, various studies have eliminated all of these individually, or collectively, as major determinants (e.g., Bahlmann *et al.*, 1967b). The possibility that dilution of some unknown component, such as a metabolizable substrate (Waugh and Kubo, 1968), might be an important factor is more difficult to exclude with certainty. Nevertheless, it appears that these compositional changes can contribute to saline diuresis but are not essential to the response.

D. Redistribution of Renal Blood Flow

The experiments of Levinsky and Lalone (1963) in which saline infusion was combined with aortic clamping so as to achieve the same filtered load of sodium in the entire kidney could have increased the rate of filtration in some nephrons and decreased it in others. If the degree of glomerulotubular balance varied between these groups of nephrons, sodium excretion might rise. Earley and Friedler (1964b, 1965b) suggested that saline infusion might augment medullary blood flow and in this way impair distal sodium transport. Shuster *et al.* (1966) confirmed that noncortical blood flow rose with rapid saline infusion but showed that slower infusion had little effect even though it induced natriuresis; furthermore, aortic clamping did not prevent natriuresis despite reduced noncortical flow. Nissen (1968) estimated from measurement of oncotic pressure of superficial and deep renal venous drainage that fluid loading may induce shunts from afferent to efferent arterioles in the juxtamedullary glomeruli. Horster and Thurau (1968) have recently studied this problem in detail by measuring filtration rates of superficial and juxtamedullary glomeruli in salt-depleted and salt-loaded rats. The latter exhibited reduced filtration in juxtamedullary glomeruli but increased filtration in superficial nephrons, in support of Nissen's observations; overall GFR was essentially unchanged. Until glomerulotubular balance can be assessed in juxtamedullary nephrons, the possible role of this redistribution of filtration in determining sodium excretion remains conjectural.

E. Nervous Influences

These are considered in Section IX.

F. Arterial Pressure

In isolated kidneys perfused from saline-loaded dogs (S. J. McDonald and de Wardener, 1965), as well as in intact animals on desoxycorticosterone and vasopressin (Schrier *et al.*, 1967), the natriuretic response to volume expansion is correlated with the increment in mean arterial pressure. Metaraminol pretreatment augments the diuretic effect of saline in man (Vaamonde *et al.*, 1964). The effect of arterial pressure alone on sodium reabsorption is unequivocal (Section IV, B), and it is, therefore, probable that this factor contributes to the response to saline infusion.

G. Venous Pressure

As noted in Section IV, D, elevation of renal venous pressure may increase sodium excretion in oliguric animals but tends to inhibit the diuretic response to saline (Levinsky and Lalone, 1965; Friedler *et al.*, 1967; Wathen and Selkurt, 1969), though not invariably (Stamler *et al.*, 1958). In the latter circumstance filtration rate usually falls and fractional reabsorption in the proximal tubule increases (Cirksena *et al.*, 1966).

H. Natriuretic Hormone

Homer Smith suggested in 1957 that a humoral mechanism attuned to the volume of the body fluids might be responsible for the renal response to saline loading (H. W. Smith, 1957). Cross-circulation experiments by de Wardener and associates (1961) and by others (e.g., Pearce, 1968) supported this possibility and led them to postulate that the natriuretic hormone decays rapidly from the blood. As to the afferent mechanism of this response, they found that it was not inhibited by vagotomy, carotid denervation, or removal of the upper four thoracic sympathetic ganglia (Mills *et al.*, 1961). Cort and Lichardus (1963b), studying a closely related phenomenon – the natriuretic response to carotid occlusion – found that it could be inhibited by lesions in the posterior nucleus of the hypothalamus, even though the hypertensive response persisted. It was not inhibited by phenoxybenzamine or angiotensin (Cort and Lichardus, 1963c). From studies of oxytocin antagonists (Cort *et al.*, 1966), they concluded that natriuretic hormone is similar to but not identical with oxytocin. It is apparently a polypeptide of molecular weight 800–1000 which arises from the neurohypophysis and which disappears from plasma within 20 minutes on incubation at 34°C (Cort, 1968; Cort and Lichardus, 1968; Cort *et al.*, 1968). Whether this substance plays a role in the response to saline infusion as well as to carotid occlusion is uncertain.

According to Lockett (1966), dual hormones, one from the posterior hypothalamus and one from the hypophysis, are required for the diuretic response to saline. In addition to these data implicating the brain, there are observations pointing to a role of the liver: saline infusion into the portal vein is much more effective than systemic venous infusion in leading to inhibition of tubular sodium reabsorption (Daly *et al.*, 1967).

Rector *et al.* (1968) reported that plasma of saline-expanded animals contained an unidentified substance which inhibited proximal tubular salt transport – although it did not regularly lead to natriuresis. Bricker *et al.* (1969) have isolated from the plasma of saline-expanded dogs or uremic patients a substance which inhibits uptake of *p*-aminohippurate by kidney slices and also reduces sodium transport by frog skin. Sealy *et al.* (1969) have found a low molecular weight protein in the plasma and urine of salt-loaded subjects which promotes sodium excretion in rats. Many other reports of similar substances have appeared.

Despite these encouraging results, the status of natriuretic hormone remains in doubt. Not all workers have found natriuresis in cross-circulated animals (M. McDonald *et al.*, 1967), and a cooperative study from three laboratories failed to confirm the presence in the plasma of saline-loaded animals of an inhibitor of tubular transport (Wrigth *et al.*, 1969b). To further complicate the problem, a subsequent report from one of these same three laboratories indicates positive results in the plasma of blood-volume-expanded dogs (Clarkson *et al.*, 1969).

XII. Renal Role in Sodium Homeostasis

In normal subjects extracellular fluid volume and sodium balance vary through only a narrow range even in the face of substantial changes in intake or extrarenal losses of water and of salt. Although some degree of regulation of extrarenal losses and of salt appetite exists in man, by far the major role in achieving this homeostasis is attributable to the kidney. In this section, attention is directed towards the mechanisms by which renal regulation is achieved, other than those within the kidney itself.

As noted in preceding sections, blood pressure, venous pressure, and glomerular filtration rate each affect sodium excretion, more or less independently of each other. All three tend to be positively correlated with extracellular fluid volume or effective circulating blood volume. The mechanism by which GFR varies with extracellular fluid volume is unknown. Wesson (1969) has reviewed the evidence in detail, and has suggested that an unidentified hormone may regulate GFR in response to volume. Progressive increments in dietary sodium cause variable increases in GFR: in some studies, transient (Ladd and Raisz, 1949) or undetectable (Reinhardt and Behrenbeck, 1967) changes are seen despite measurable increase in extracellular fluid volume; in other studies (Gertz and Graun, 1967; Wesson, 1969) a modest rise in GFR results. Within a narrower range of dietary salt, sodium balance may be unaffected by sodium intake (Veverbrants and Arky, 1969). Any statement as to the relative importance of these hemodynamic factors (including sympathetic influences exerted through vasomotor actions), as compared with hormonal regulation, must be based on speculation or prejudice in our present state of knowledge.

Aldosterone secretion by the zona glomerulosa of the adrenal cortex is certainly another major component of renal sodium homeostasis. Its elaboration is controlled by two main mechanisms: (1) the renin-angiotensin system; and (2) the hypothalamo-pituitary axis via adrenocorticotrophic hormone (ACTH) release. In addition, pronounced hyponatremia (or hyperkalemia), may act directly on the gland to promote hormone secretion. A fourth mechanism which does not involve renin,

ACTH, or plasma electrolyte concentrations may also exist (Palmore *et al.*, 1969). The ACTH mechanism becomes significant only when glucocorticoid secretion is being maximally stimulated or when salt intake is reduced (Ganong and van Brunt, 1968). The renin mechanism is of greater importance, even in mediating the response to low salt intake, and is discussed in Chapters 2 and 3 of Vol. IV.

All the available evidence, some of which has been cited above, supports the inference that some other hormonal mechanism plays an important role in sodium homeostasis by means of modifying the tubular transport of sodium. For example, subjects on a low sodium intake exhibit a reduced natriuretic response to hypertonic (Black *et al.*, 1950) or hypotonic (Behrenbeck *et al.*, 1968) saline loading which cannot be explained by a lowered filtered load of sodium. Furthermore, sodium depletion induces an increase in proximal sodium transport which cannot be reproduced by aldosterone (Weiner *et al.*, 1969). Bricker (1967) and others believe that these other hormonal mechanisms may be of major importance. The final identification of these hormones and the stimulus to their release is an exciting prospect for future research.

REFERENCES

Andersson, B., Jobin, M., and Olsson, K. (1966). Stimulation of urinary salt excretion following injections of hypertonic NaCl-solution into the third brain ventricle. *Acta Physiol. Scand.* **67**, 127–128.

Anslow, W. P., Jr., and Wesson, L. G., Jr. (1955). Some effects of pressor-antidiuretic and oxytocic fractions of posterior pituitary extract on sodium, chloride, potassium and ammonium excretion in the dog. *Am. J. Physiol.* **182**, 561–566.

Arcila, H., Saimyoji, H., and Kessler, R. H. (1968). Accentuation of cyanide natriuresis by hypoxia. *Am. J. Physiol.* **214**, 1063–1067.

Ardill, B. L., Halliday, J. A., Morrison, J. D., Mulholland H. C., and Womersley, R. A. (1962). Interrelations of magnesium, phosphate and calcium metabolism. *Clin. Sci.* **23**, 67–75.

Arrizurieta-Muchnik, E. E., Lassiter, W. E., Lipham, E. M., and Gottschalk, C. W. (1969). Micropuncture study of glomerulotubular balance in the rat kidney. *Nephron* **6**, 418–436.

August, J. T., and Nelson, D. H. (1959). Adjustment to aldosterone or desoxycorticosterone acetate-induced sodium retention in patients with Addison's disease. *J. Clin. Invest.* **38**, 1964–1971.

August, J. T., Nelson, D. H., and Thorn, G. W. (1958). Response of normal subjects to large amounts of aldosterone. *J. Clin. Invest.* **37**, 1549–1555.

Aukland, K., and Kjeskshus, J. (1966). Tubular salt and water transport in hydrated dogs studied with push-flow technique. *Am. J. Physiol.* **210**, 971–979.

Aukland, K., and Krog, J. (1961). Influence of various factors on urine oxygen tension in dog. *Acta Physiol. Scand.* **52**, 350–365.

Baba, W. I., Lant, A. F., and Wilson, G. M. (1966). Studies on the mechanism and characteristics of action of a new phthalimidine diuretic, clorexolone. *Clin. Pharmacol. Therap.* **7**, 212–223.

Bahlmann, J. O., McDonald, S. J., Dunningham, J. G., and de Wardener, H. E. (1967a). The effect on urinary sodium excretion of altering the packed cell volume with albumin solutions without changing the blood volume in the dog. *Clin. Sci.* **32**, 395–402.

Bahlmann, J. O., McDonald, S. J., Ventom, M. G., and de Wardener, H. E. (1967b). The effect on urinary sodium excretion of blood volume expansion without changing the composition of the blood in the dog. *Clin. Sci.* **32**, 403–413.

Baines, A. D., and de Rouffignac, C. (1969). Functional heterogeneity of nephrons. II. Filtration rates, intraluminal flow velocities and fractional water reabsorption. *Arch. Ges. Physiol.* **308**, 260–276.

Baines, A. D., Gottschalk, C. W., and Leyssac, P. P. (1968). Proximal luminal volume and fluid reabsorption in the rat kidney. *Acta Physiol. Scand.* **74**, 440–452.

Baldwin, D. S., Kahana, E. M., and Clarke, R. W. (1950). Renal excretion of sodium and potassium in the dog. *Am. J. Physiol.* **162**, 655–664.

Bálint, P., and Forgács, I. (1966). Natriumreabsorption und Sauerstoffverbrauch der Niere bei osmotischer Belastung. *Arch. Ges. Physiol.* **288**, 332–341.

Bank, N. (1968). Physiological basis of diuretic action. *Ann. Rev. Med.* **19**, 103–118.

Barclay, J. A., Cooke, W. T., Kenney, R. A., and Nutt, M. E. (1947). The effect of water diuresis and exercise on the volume and composition of the urine. *Am. J. Physiol.* **148**, 327–337.

Barker, E. S., Elkinton, J. R., and Clark, J. K. (1959). Studies of the renal excretion of magnesium in man. *J. Clin. Invest.* **38**, 1733–1745.

Bartter, F. C., Liddle, G. W., Duncan, L. E., Jr., Barber, J. K., and Delea, C. (1956). The regulation of aldosterone secretion on man: The role of fluid volume. *J. Clin. Invest.* **35**, 1306–1315.

Beck, D., Levitin, H., and Epstein, F. H. (1959). Effect of intravenous infusions of calcium on renal concentrating ability. *Am. J. Physiol.* **197**, 118–1120.

Behrenbeck, D. W., and Reinhardt, H. W. (1967). Untersuchungen an wachen Hunden über die Einstellung der Natriumbilanz. II. Postprandiale Elektrolyt-und Wasserbilanz bei unterschiedlicher Kochsalzzufuhr. *Arch. Ges. Physiol.* **295**, 280–292.

Behrenbeck, D. W., Dörge, A., and Reinhardt, H. W. (1968). Untersuchungen an wachen Hunden über die Einstellung der Natriumbilanz. III. Electrolyt- bilanzen und Natriumrejektion nach akutem Natriumentzug durch Peritonealdialyse oder wiederholter Mannitolinfusion. *Arch. Ges. Physiol.* **300**, 226–243.

Bennett, C. M., Clapp, J. R., and Berliner, R. W. (1967). Micropuncture study of the proximal and distal tubule in the dog. *Am. J. Physiol.* **213**, 1254–1262.

Bennett, C. M., Brenner, B. M., and Berliner, R. W. (1968). Micropuncture study of nephron function in the rhesus monkey. *J. Clin. Invest.* **47**, 203–216.

Bentzel, C. J., Davies, M., Scott, W. N., Zatzman, M , and Solomon, A. K. (1968). Osmotic volume flow in the tubule of Necturus kidney. *J. Gen. Physiol.* **51**, 517–533.

Berne, R. M. (1952). Hemodynamics and sodium excretion of denervated kidney in anesthetized and unanesthetized dog. *Am. J. Physiol.* **171**, 148–158.

Beyer, K. H., Baer, J. E., Michaelson, J. K., and Russo, H. F. (1965). Renotropic characteristics of ethacrynic acid: A phenoxyacetic saluretic-diuretic agent. *J. Pharmacol. Exptl. Therap.* **147**, 1–22.

Black, D. A. K., Platt, R., and Stanbury, S. W. (1950). Regulation of sodium excretion in normal and salt-depleted subjects. *Clin. Sci.* **9**, 205–221.

Blackmore, W. P. (1958). Effect of serotonin on renal hemodynamics and sodium excretion in the dog. *Am. J. Physiol.* **193**, 639–643.

Blake, W. D. (1962). Relative roles of glomerular filtration and tubular reabsorption in denervation diuresis. *Am. J. Phyisol.* **202**, 777–780.

Blomhert, G. (1951). Thesis, University of Amsterdam, Scheltema and Holkema, Amsterdam.

Bloom, W. L. (1962). Inhibition of salt excretion by carbohydrate. *Arch. Internal. Med.* **109**, 80–86.

Blythe, W. B., and Welt, L. G. (1963). Dissociation between filtered load of sodium and its rate of excretion in the urine. *J. Clin. Invest.* **42**, 1491–1496.

Blythe, W. B., and Welt, L. G. (1965). Plasma sodium concentrations and urinary sodium excretion. *Trans. Assoc. Am. Physicians* **78**, 90–96.

Bojesen, E. (1954). The renal mechanism of "dilution diuresis" and salt excretion in dogs. *Acta Physiol. Scand.* **32**, 129–147.

Bojesen, E., and Leyssac, P. P. (1969). Proximal tubular reabsorption in the rat kidney as studied by the occlusion time and lissamine green transit time technique. *Acta Physiol. Scand.* **76**, 213–235.

Bossert, W. H., and Schwartz, W. B. (1967). Relation of pressure and flow to control of sodium reabsorption in the proximal tubule. *Am. J. Physiol.* **213**, 793–802.

Bott, P. A. (1943). Quantitative studies of composition of glomerular urine. XV. Concentration of sodium in glomerular urine of Necturi. *J. Biol. Chem.* **147**, 653–661.

Boulpaep, E. L. (1967). Ion permeability of the peritubular and luminal membrane of the renal tubular cell. *In* "Transport und Funktion Intracellulärer Elektrolyte" (F. Krück, ed.), pp. 98–105. Urban & Schwarzenberg, Munich.

Boylan, J. W., and Hong, S. K. (1966). Regulation of renal function in hypothermia. *Am. J. Physiol.* **211**, 1371–1378.

Brandis, M. (1969). About the flow resistance within the loop of Henle of the rat kidney after alteration of the extracellular volume. *Arch. Ges. Physiol.* **307**, R59.

Brandt, J. L., Zumoff, B., Castleman, L., Ruskin, H. D., Jones, A., and Zuckerman, S. (1956). Studies of the effects of large doses of bacterial pyrogen in the dog. I. The renal handling of salt and water. *J. Clin. Invest.* **35**, 1080–1088.

Brenner, B. M., Bennett, C. M., and Berliner, R. W. (1968). The relationship between glomerular filtration rate and sodium reabsorption by the proximal tubule of the rat nephron. *J. Clin. Invest.* **47**, 1358–1374.

Brenner, B. M., Keimowitz, R. I., Wright, F. S. and Berliner, R. W. (1969a). An inhibitory effect of furosemide on sodium reabsorption by the proximal tubule of the rat nephron. *J. Clin. Invest.* **48**, 290–300.

Brenner, B. M., Falchuk, K. H., Keimowitz, R. I., and Berliner, R. W. (1969b). The relationship between peritubular capillary protein concentration and fluid reabsorption by the renal proximal tubule. *J. Clin. Invest.* **48**, 1519–1531.

Bresler, E. H. (1960). Reabsorptive response of renal tubules to elevated sodium and chloride concentrations in plasma. *Am. J. Physiol.* **199**, 517–521.

Bricker, N. S. (1967). The control of sodium excretion with normal and reduced nephron populations. The pre-eminence of third factor. *Am. J. Med.* **43**, 313–321.

Bricker, N. S., Klahr, S., Bourgoignie, J., Miller, C. L., and Lubowitz, H. (1969). On a circulating inhibitor of sodium transport in uremia.*Symp. 4th Intern. Congr. Nephrol., Stockholm, 1969*, pp. 173–174.

Brooks, F. P., and Pickford, M. (1958). The effect of posterior pituitary hormones on the excretion of electrolytes in dogs. *J. Physiol. (London)* **142**, 468–493.

Brunner, E. P., Rector, F. C., Jr., and Seldin, D. W. (1966). Mechanism of glomerulotubular balance. II. Regulation of proximal tubular reabsorption by tubular volume, as studied by stopped-flow microperfusion. *J. Clin. Invest.* **45**, 603–611.

Buchborn, E., and Anastasakis, S. (1964). Angriffspunkt und Wirkungsmechanismus vom Furosemid am distalen Nephron des Menschen. *Klin. Wochschr.* **42**, 1127–1131.

Bull, M. B., and Laragh, J. H. (1968). Amiloride. A potassium-sparing natriuretic agent. *Circulation* **37**, 45-53.

Burg, M. B. (1969). Transport characteristics of isolated perfused proximal tubules. *In* "Renal Transport and Diuretics" (K. Thurau and H. Jahrmarker, eds.), pp. 109-122. Springer, Berlin.

Burg, M. B., and Orloff, J. (1968). Control of fluid absorption in the renal proximal tubule. *J. Clin. Invest.* **47**, 2016-2024.

Burg, M. B., Isaacson, L., Grantham, J., and Orloff, J. (1968). Electrical properties of isolated perfused rabbit renal tubules. *Am. J. Physiol.* **215**, 788-794.

Burnett, C. H., Seldin, D. W., and Walser, M. (1953). Observations on the electrolyte and water metabolism in Addison's disease during oral salt loading. *Trans. Assoc. Am. Physicians* **66**, 65-71.

Cade, J. R., Shalhoub, R. J., Canessa-Fischer, M., and Pitts, R. F. (1961). Effect of strophanthidin on renal tubules of dogs. *Am. J. Physiol.* **200**, 373-379.

Cafruny, E. J., Cho, K. C., and Gussin, R. Z. (1966). The pharmacology of mercurial diuretics. *Ann. N.Y. Acad. Sci.* **139**, 362-374.

Cannon, P. J., Dell, R. B., and Winters, R. W. (1968). Effect of diuretics on electrolyte and lactate gradients in dog kidney. *J. Lab. Clin. Med.* **72**, 192-203.

Castles, T. R., and Williamson, H. E. (1967). Mediation of aldosterone induced anti-natriuresis *via* RNA synthesis *de novo*. *Proc. Soc. Exptl. Biol. Med.* **124**, 717-719.

Chan, W. Y., and Sawyer, W. H. (1961). Saluretic actions of neurohypophysial peptides in conscious dogs. *Am. J. Physiol.* **201**, 799-803.

Chan, W. Y., and Sawyer, W. H. (1968). Intracranial action of oxytocin on sodium excretion by conscious dogs. *Proc. Soc. Exptl. Biol. Med.* **127**, 267-270.

Chertok, R. J., Hulet, W. H., and Epstein, B. (1966). Effects of cyanide, amytal, and DNP on renal sodium absorption. *Am. J. Physiol.* **211**, 1379-1382.

Chesley, L. C., and Tepper, I. (1958). Some effects of magnesium loading upon renal excretion of magnesium and certain other electrolytes. *J. Clin. Invest.* **37**, 1362-1372.

Chignell, C. F., and Titus, E. D. (1966). Effect of adrenal steroids on a Na^+- and K^+-requiring adenosine triphosphatase from rat kidney. *J. Biol. Chem.* **241**, 5083-5089.

Cirksena, W. J., Dirks, J. H., and Berliner, R. W. (1966). Effect of thoracic cava obstruction on response of proximal tubule sodium reabsorption to saline infusion. *J. Clin. Invest.* **45**, 179-186.

Clapp, J. R., and Robinson, R. R. (1966). Osmolality of distal tubular fluid in the dog. *J. Clin. Invest.* **45**, 1847-1853.

Clapp, J. R., and Robinson, R. R. (1968). Distal sites of action of diuretic drugs in the dog nephron. *Am. J. Physiol.* **215**, 228-235.

Clapp, J. R., Watson, J. F., and Berliner, R. W. (1963). Osmolality, bicarbonate concentration, and water reabsorption in proximal tubule of the dog nephron. *Am. J. Physiol.* **205**, 273-280.

Clapp, J. R., Nakajima, K., Nottebohm, G. A., and Robinson, R. R. (1969). Proximal site of action for furosemide and ethacrynic acid in the dog: Importance of GFR and ECF volume. *Free Commun., 4th Intern. Congr. Nephrol., Stockholm. 1969*, p. 71.

Clarkson, E. M., Talner, L. B., and de Wardener, H. E. (1969). The effect of plasma from blood volume expanded dogs on sodium, potassium and PAH transport of renal tubule fragments. *Free Commun., 4th Intern. Congr. Nephrol., Stockholm, 1969*, p. 370.

Clinton, M., and Thorn, G. W. (1943). Effect of desoxycorticosterone acetate administration on plasma volume and electrolyte balance of normal human subjects. *Bull. Johns Hopkins Hosp.* **72**, 255-264.

Cockett, A. T. K., Katz, Y. J., and Moore, R. S. (1968). Transport of sodium by the renal lymphatics during elevated central venous pressure. *Invest. Urol.* **5**, 483–491.

Cort, J. H. (1968). The source and chemical nature of the natriuretic activity of plasma evoked by saluretic "volume reflexes." *Can. J. Physiol. Pharmacol.* **46**, 325–333.

Cort, J. H., and Lichardus, B. (1963a). The effect of the carotid sinus pressor reflex on renal function and electrolyte excretion. *Physiol. Bohemoslov.* **12**, 291–299.

Cort, J. H., and Lichardus, B. (1963b). The role of the hypothalamus in the renal response to the carotid sinus pressor reflex. *Physiol. Bohemoslov.* **12**, 389–396.

Cort, J. H., and Lichardus, B. (1963c). The effect of dibenzyline and hypertensin on saluretic pressor and "volume" reflexes. *Physiol. Bohemoslov.* **12**, 304–309.

Cort, J. H., and Lichardus, B. (1968). Natriuretic hormone. *Nephron* **5**, 401–409.

Cort, J. H., Rudinger, J., Lichardus, B., and Hagemann, I. (1966). Effects of oxytocin antagonists on the saluresis accompanying carotid occlusion. *Am. J. Physiol.* **210**, 162–168.

Cort, J. H., Douša, T., Pliška, V., Lichardus, B., Sǎfǎřová, J., Vranešić, M., and Rudinger, J. (1968). Saluretic activity of blood during carotid occlusion in the cat. *Am. J. Physiol.* **215**, 921–927.

Cortney, M. A. (1969). Renal tubular transfer of water and electrolytes in adrenalectomized rats. *Am. J. Physiol.* **216**, 589–598.

Cortney, M. A., Mylle, M., Lassiter, W. E., and Gottschalk, C. W. (1965). Renal tubular transport of water, solute, and PAH in rats loaded with isotonic saline. *Am. J. Physiol.* **209**, 1199–1205.

Cortney, M. A., Nagel, W., and Thurau, K. (1966). A micropuncture study of the relationship between flow rate through the loop of Henle and sodium concentration in the early distal tubule. *Arch. Ges. Physiol.* **287**, 286–295.

Coxon, R. V., and Ramsay, D. J. (1967). The effect of water diuresis on electrolyte excretion in unanaesthetized dogs. *J. Physiol. (London)* **191**, 123–129.

Crutchfield, A. J., Jr., and Wood, J. E., Jr. (1948). Urine volume and renal sodium excretion during water diuresis. *Ann. Internal Med.* **28**, 28–40.

Daly, J. J., Roe, J. W., and Horrocks, P. (1967). A comparison of sodium excretion following the infusion of saline into systemic and portal veins in the dog: Evidence for a hepatic role in the control of sodium excretion. *Clin. Sci.* **33**, 481–487.

Daugharty, T. M., Belleau, L., Martino, J. A., and Earley, L. E. (1968). Interrelationship of physical factors affecting sodium reabsorption in the dog. *Am. J. Physiol.* **215**, 1442–1447.

Davis, B. B., Knox, F. G., and Berliner, R. W. (1967). Effect of vasopressin on proximal tubule sodium reabsorption in the dog. *Am. J. Physiol.* **212**, 1361–1364.

Davis, J. O., and Ball, W. C., Jr. (1958). Effects of a body cast on aldosterone and sodium excretion in dogs with experimental ascites. *Am. J. Physiol.* **192**, 538–542.

Davis, J. O., and Howell, D. S. (1953). Comparative effect of ACTH, cortisone, and DCA on renal function, electrolyte excretion and water exchange in normal dogs. *Endocrinology* **52**, 245–255.

de Rouffignac, C., and Morel, M. (1967). La perméabilité au sodium des différents segments du néphron étudiée chez le rat en diurèse saline à l'aide de microinjections intratubulaires de ^{22}Na. *Nephron* **4**, 92–118.

de Rouffignac, C., and Morel, F. (1969). Micropuncture study of water, electrolytes, and urea movements along the loops of Henle in Psammomys. *J. Clin. Invest.* **48**, 474–486.

de Wardener, H. E., Mills, I. H., Clapham, W. F., and Hayter, C. J. (1961). Studies on the efferent mechanism of the sodium diuresis which follows the administration of intravenous saline in the dog. *Clin. Sci.* **21**. 249–258.

Dicker, S. E. (1948). Renal excretion of sodium and potassium in rats. *J. Physiol. (London)* **107**, 8–13.

Dirks, J. H., and Seely, J. F. (1969). Micropuncture and diuretics. *Ann. Rev. Pharmacol.* **9**, 73–84.

Dirks, J. H., Cirksena, W. J., and Berliner, R. W. (1965). The effect of saline infusion on sodium reabsorption by the proximal tubule of the dog. *J. Clin. Invest.* **44**, 1160–1170.

Dirks, J. H., Cirksena, W. J., and Berliner, R. W. (1966). Micropuncture study of the effect of various diuretics on sodium reabsorption by the proximal tubules of the dog. *J. Clin. Invest.* **45**, 1875–1885.

Dubach, U. C., and Schmidt, U. (1969). Inhibition of (Na^+K^+)-stimulated adenosintriphosphatase in various structures of the rat nephron after furosemide. *Free Commun., 4th Intern. Congr. Nephrol., Stockholm, 1969*, p. 20.

Earley, L. E. (1966). Influence of hemodynamic factors on sodium reabsorption. *Ann. N.Y. Acad. Sci.* **139**, 312–327.

Earley, L. E., and Daugharty, T. M. (1969). Sodium metabolism. *New Engl. J. Med.* **281**, 72–86.

Earley, L. E., and Friedler, R. M. (1964a). Renal tubular effects of ethacrynic acid. *J. Clin. Invest.* **43**, 1495–1506.

Earley, L. E., and Friedler, R. M. (1964b). Observations on the mechanism of decreased tubular reabsorption of sodium and water during saline loading. *J. Clin. Invest.* **43**, 1928–1937.

Earley, L. E., and Friedler, R. M. (1965a). Studies on the mechanisms of natriuresis accompanying increased renal blood flow and its role in the renal response to extracellular volume expansion. *J. Clin. Invest.* **44**, 1857–1865.

Earley, L. E., and Friedler, R. M. (1965b). Changes in renal blood flow and possibly the intrarenal distribution of blood during the natriuresis accompanying saline loading in the dog. *J. Clin. Invest.* **44**, 929–941.

Earley, L. E., and Friedler, R. M. (1966). The effects of combined renal vasodilatation and pressor agents on renal hemodynamics and the tubular reabsorption of sodium. *J. Clin. Invest.* **45**, 542–551.

Earley, L. E., Kahn, M., and Orloff, J. (1961). The effects of infusions of chlorothiazide on urinary dilution and concentration in the dog. *J. Clin. Invest.* **40**, 857–866.

Earley, L. E., Martino, J. A., and Friedler, R. M. (1966). Factors affecting sodium reabsorption by the proximal tubule as determined during blockade of distal sodium reabsorption. *J. Clin. Invest.* **45**, 1668–1684.

Ebel, H., De Santo, N. G., and Hierholzer, K. (1968). Does a correlation exist between membrane-ATPase and steroid dependent sodium reabsorption in the rat kidney? *Arch. Ges. Physiol.* **300**, R28.

Ebel, H., Ehrich, J., and De Santo, N. G. (1969). The effect of diuretics on the ATPase activity of a plasma cell membrane enriched fraction of the rat kidney. *Arch. Ges. Physiol.* **307**, R77.

Elpers, M. J., and Selkurt, E. E. (1963). Effects of albumin infusion on the renal function in the dog. *Am. J. Physiol.* **205**, 153–161.

Feldman, D., Wende, C. V., and Kessler, E. (1961). The effect of aldosterone on oxidative enzymes of the rat kidney. *Biochim. Biophys. Acta* **51**, 401–403.

Fimognari, G. M., Fanestil, D. D., and Edelman, I. S. (1967). Induction of RNA and protein synthesis in the action of aldosterone in the rat. *Am. J. Physiol.* **213**, 954–962.

Finn, A. L., and Welt, L. G. (1963). Effect of aldosterone administration on electrolyte excretion and GFR in the rat. *Am. J. Physiol.* **204**, 243–244.

Foulkes, E. C., and Banks, R. O. (1968). Significance of urinary precession of sodium over simultaneously injected inulin. *Am. J. Physiol.* **215**, 574–581.

Freedman, P., Moulton, R., and Spencer, A. G. (1958). The effect of intravenous calcium gluconate on the renal excretion of water and electrolytes. *Clin. Sci.* **17**, 247–263.

Friedlander, S. K., and Walser, M. (1965). Some aspects of flow and diffusion in the proximal tubule of the kidney. *J. Theoret. Biol.* **8**, 87–96.

Friedler, R. M., and Earley, L. E. (1966). Reduced renal concentrating capacity during isotonic saline loading. *Proc. Soc. Exptl. Biol. Med.* **121**, 352–357.

Friedler, R. M., Belleau, L. J., Martino, J. A., and Earley, L. E. (1967). Hemodynamically induced natriuresis in the presence of sodium retention resulting from constriction of the thoracic inferior vena cava. *J. Lab. Clin. Med.* **69**, 565–583.

Frömter, E., and Hegel, U. (1966). Transtubuläre Potentialdifferenzen an proximalen and distalen Tubuli der Rattenniere. *Arch. Ges. Physiol.* **291**, 107–120.

Frömter, E., Wick, T., and Hegel, U. (1967). Untersuchungen über die Ausspritzmethode zur Lokalisation der Mikroelektrodenspitze bei Potentialmessungen am proximalen Konvolut der Rattenniere. *Arch. Ges. Physiol.* **294**, 265–273.

Fujimoto, M., Nash, F. D., and Kessler, R. H. (1964). Effects of cyanide, Q_{o_2}, and dinitrophenol on renal sodium reabsorption and oxygen consumption. *Am. J. Physiol.* **206**, 1327–1332.

Fülgraff, G., and Heidenreich, O. (1967). Mikropunktionsuntersuchunger über die Wirkung von Calciumionen auf die Resorptionskapazität und auf die prozentuale Resorption im proximalen Konvolut von Ratten. *Arch. Exptl. Pathol. Pharmakol.* **258**, 440–451.

Fülgraff, G., Meiforth, A., Sparwald, E., and Heidenreich, O. (1968a). Resorptionskapazität, Passagezeit und prozentuale Resorption im proximalen Tubulus von Ratten bei erhohter Ca^{++}- Konzentration. *Arch. Ges. Physiol.* **259**, 167–168.

Fülgraff, G., Meiforth, A., Osswald, H., and Heidenreich, O. (1968b). Die Wirkung von α- und β- Sympathicommetica auf die lokale Transportkapazität im proximalen Konvolut von Rattenniere. *Arch. Exptl. Pathol. Pharmakol.* **260**, 116.

Ganong, W. F., and Mulrow, P. J. (1958). Rate of change in sodium and potassium excretion after injection of aldosterone into the aorta and renal artery of the dog. *Am. J. Physiol.* **195**, 337–342.

Ganong, W. F., and van Brunt, E. E. (1968). Control of aldosterone secretion. *Handbook Exptl. Pharmacol.* [N.S.] **14**, Part 3, 4–116.

Garrod, O., Davies, S. A., and Cahill, G., Jr. (1955). The action of cortisone and desoxycorticosterone acetate on glomerular filtration rate and sodium and water exchange in the adrenalectomized dog. *J. Clin. Invest.* **34**, 761–776.

Gertz, K. H. (1963). Transtubuläre Natriumchloridfüsse und Permeabilität für Nichtelektrolyte im proximalen und distalen Konvolut der Rattenniere. *Arch. Ges. Physiol.* **276**, 336–356.

Gertz, K. H., and Graun, G. (1967). Die Lokalisation des Stromungswiderstandes innerhalb der Henleschen Schleife der Rattenniere. *Arch. Ges. Physiol.* **294**, R18.

Gertz, K. H., Kennedy, G. C., and Ullrich, K. J. (1964). Mikropunktionsuntersuchungen über die Flüssigkeitsrückresorption aus den einzelnen Tubulusabschnitten bei Wasserdiurese (Diabetes Insipidus). *Arch. Ges. Physiol.* **278**, 513–519.

Gertz, K. H., Mangos, J. A., Braun, G., and Pagel, H. D. (1965). On the glomerular tubular balance in the rat kidney. *Arch. Ges. Physiol.* **285**, 360–372.

Giebisch, G. (1968). Some electrical properties of single renal tubule cells. *J. Gen. Physiol.* **51**, 315s–325s.

Giebisch, G., Klose, R. M., Malnic, G., Sullivan, W. J., and Windhager, E. E. (1964a). Sodium movement across single perfused proximal tubules of rat kidneys. *J. Gen. Physiol.* **47**, 1175-1194.

Giebisch, G., Klose, R. M., and Windhager, E. E. (1964b). Micropuncture study of hypertonic sodium chloride loading in the rat. *Am. J. Physiol.* **206**, 687-693.

Giebisch, G., Malnic, G., Klose, R. M., and Windhager, E. E. (1966). Effect of ionic substitutions on distal potential differences in rat kidney. *Am. J. Physiol.* **211**, 560-568.

Gilbert, C. A., Bricker, L. A., Springfield, W. T., Jr., Stevens, P. M., and Warren, B. H. (1966). Sodium and water excretion and renal hemodynamics during lower body negative pressure. *J. Appl. Physiol.* **21**, 1699-1704.

Gill, J. R., Jr. (1969). The role of sympathetic nervous system in the regulation of sodium excretion by the kidney. *In* "Frontiers in Neuroendocrinology" (W. F. Ganong and L. Martini, eds.), pp. 289-305. Oxford Univ. Press, London and New York.

Gill, J. R., Jr., Mason, D. T., and Bartter, F. C. (1964). Adrenergic nervous system in sodium metabolism: Effects of guanethidine and sodium-retaining steroids in normal man. *J. Clin. Invest.* **43**, 177-184.

Gill, J. R., Jr., Carr, A. A., Fleischmann, L. E., Casper, A. G. T., and Bartter, F. C. (1967). Effects of pentolinium on sodium excretion in dogs with constriction of the vena cava. *Am. J. Physiol.* **212**, 191-196.

Gilmore, J. P. (1968). Contribution of cardiac nerves to the control of body salt and water. *Federation Proc.* **27**, 1156-1159.

Gilmore, J. P., and Michaelis, L. L. (1969). Influence of anesthesia on renal responses of the foxhound to intravascular volume expansion. *Am. J. Physiol.* **216**, 1367-1369.

Glabman, S., Aynedjian, H. S., and Bank, N. (1965). Micropuncture study of the effect of acute reductions in glomerular filtration rate on sodium and water reabsorption by the proximal tubules of the rat. *J. Clin. Invest.* **44**, 1410-1416.

Goldberg, M., McCurdy, D. K., and Ramirez, M. A. (1965). Differences between saline and mannitol diuresis in hydropenic man. *J. Clin. Invest.* **44**, 182-192.

Goldsmith, C., Rector, F. C., Jr., and Seldin, D. W. (1962). Evidence for a direct effect of serum sodium concentration on sodium reabsorption. *J. Clin. Invest.* **41**, 850-859.

Goldstein, M. H., Levitt, M. F., Hauser, A. D., and Polimeros, D. (1961). Effect of meralluride on solute and water excretion in hydrated man: comments on site of action. *J. Clin. Invest.* **40**, 731-742.

Gottschalk, C. W. (1958). Hydrostatic pressures in individual tubules and capillaries of the rat kidney. *In* "Factors Regulating Blood Flow" (G. P. Fulton and B. Zweifach, eds.), pp. 65-72. Am. Physiol. Soc., Washington, D.C.

Gottschalk, C. W. (1961). Micropuncture studies of tubular function in the mammalian kidney. *Physiologist* **4**, 35-55.

Gottschalk, C. W., and Leyssac, P. P. (1968). Proximal tubular function in rats with low inulin clearance. *Acta Physiol. Scand.* **74**, 453-464.

Gottschalk, C. W., and Mylle, M. (1956). Micropuncture study of pressures in proximal tubules and peritubular capillaries of the rat kidney and their relation to ureteral and renal venous pressures. *Am. J. Physiol.* **185**, 430-439.

Gottschalk, C. W., and Mylle, M. (1959). Micropuncture study of the mammalian urinary concentrating mechanism. Evidence for the countercurrent hypothesis. *Am. J. Physiol* **196**, 927-936.

Greene, I., and Hiatt, E. P. (1955). Renal excretion of nitrate and its effect on excretion of sodium and chloride. *Am. J. Physiol.* **180**, 179-182.

Hakim, A. A., and Lifson, N. (1969). Effects of pressure on water and solute transport by dog intestinal mucosa *in vitro. Am. J. Physiol.* **216**, 276-284.

Harrop, G. A., Soffer, L. J., Ellsworth, R., and Trescher, J. H. (1933). Studies on the suprarenal cortex. III. Plasma electrolytes and electrolyte excretion during suprarenal insufficiency in the dog. *J. Exptl. Med.* **58**, 17–38.

Hayslett, J. P., Kashgarian, M., and Epstein, F. H. (1967). Changes in proximal and distal tubular reabsorption produced by rapid expansion of extracellular fluid. *J. Clin. Invest.* **46**, 1254–1263.

Hayslett, J. P., Kashgarian, M., and Epstein, F. H. (1968). Functional correlates of compensatory renal hypertrophy. *J. Clin. Invest.* **47**, 774–782.

Hegel, U., Frömter, E., and Wick, T. (1967). Der elektrische Wandwiderstand des proximalen Konvolutes der Rattenniere. *Arch. Ges. Physiol.* **294**, 274–290.

Heidenreich, O. (1969). Quecksilberhaltige diuretica. *Handbook Exptl. Pharmacol.* [N. S.] **24**, 62–194.

Heinemann, H. O., Demartini, F. E., and Laragh, J. H. (1959). The effect of chlorothiazide on renal excretion of electrolytes and free water. *Am. J. Med.* **26**, 853–861.

Hendler, E. K., Torretti, J., Weinstein, E., and Epstein, F. H. (1969). Functional significance of the distribution of Na-K-ATPase within the kidney. *Free Commun. 4th Intern. Congr. Nephrol., Stockholm, 1969*, p. 19.

Herken, H. (1969a). Aldosteron-antagonisten. *Handbook Exptl. Pharmacol.* [N. S.] **24**, 436–493.

Herken, H. (1969b). Pseudo-antialdosterone. *Handbook Exptl. Pharmacol.* [N. S.] **24**, 494–549.

Herms, W., and Malvin, R. L. (1963). Effect of metabolic inhibitors on urine osmolality and electrolyte excretion. *Am. J. Physiol.* **204**, 1065–1070.

Herrmann, G., and Decherd, G. M., Jr. (1937). Further studies on the mechanism of diuresis with special reference to the action of some newer diuretics. *J. Lab. Clin. Med.* **22**, 767–779.

Hierholzer, K., Wiederholt, M., Holzgreve, H., Giebisch, G., Klose, R. M., and Windhager, E. E. (1965). Micropuncture study of renal transtubular concentration gradients of sodium and potassium in adrenalectomized rats. *Arch. Ges. Physiol.* **285**, 193–210.

Hierholzer, K., Wiederholt, M., and Stolte, H. (1966). Hemmung der Natriumresorption im proximalen und distalen Konvolut adrenalektomierter Ratten. *Arch. Ges. Physiol.* **291**, 43–62.

Hilger, H. H., Klümper, J. D., and Ullrich, K. J. (1958). Wasserrückresorption und Ionentransport durch die Sammelrohrzellen der Säugetierniere. *Arch. Ges. Physiol.* **267**, 218–237.

Hilton, J. G. (1951). Potentiation of diuretic action of mercuhydrin by ammonium chloride. *J. Clin. Invest.* **30**, 1105–1110.

Holliday, M. A., and Egan, T. J. (1962). Renal function in man, dog, and rat. *Nature* **193**, 748–750.

Holzgreve, H. (1968). Hemmung der lokalen und prozentualen Resorption im proximalen Konvolut de Rattenniere nach Gabe von Diuretica. *Arch. Exptl. Pathol. Pharmakol.* **260**, 146–147.

Holzgreve, H., and Loeschke, K. (1967). Natrium-, Kalium- und Chlorid-gleichgewichtskonzentrationen im proximalen Konvolut der Rattenniere nach Gabe von Diuretica. *Arch. Ges. Physiol.* **294**, R22.

Hook, J. B., and Williamson, H. E. (1964). Addition of the natriuretic action of SKF 525-A to the action of certain other natriuretic agents. *J. Pharmacol. Exptl. Therap.* **146**, 265–269.

Hook, J. B., and Williamson, H. E. (1965a). Lack of correlation between natriuretic activity and inhibition of renal Na-K-activated ATPase. *Proc. Soc. Exptl. Biol. Med.* **120**, 358–360.

Hook, J. B., and Williamson, H. E. (1965b). Addition of the saluretic action of furosemide to the saluretic action of certain other agents. *J. Pharmacol. Exptl. Thera.* **148**, 88–93.

Hook, J. B., and Williamson, H. E. (1965c). Localization of the site of the natriuretic action of SKF 525-A. *J. Pharmacol. Exptl. Therap.* **150**, 270–274.

Horster, M., and Thurau, K. (1968). Micropuncture studies on the filtration rate of single superficial and juxtamedullary glomeruli in the rat kidney. *Arch. Ges. Physiol.* **301**, 162–181.

Howards, S. S., Davis, B. B., Knox, F. G., Wright, F. S., and Berliner, R. W. (1968). Depression of fractional sodium reabsorption by the proximal tubule of the dog without sodium diuresis. *J. Clin. Invest.* **47**, 1561–1572.

Jamison, R. L. (1961). The action of a mercurial diuretic on active sodium transport, electrical potential and permeability to chloride of the isolated toad bladder. *J. Pharmacol. Exptl. Therap.* **133**, 1–6.

Jamison, R. L. (1968). Micropuncture study of segments of thin loop of Henle in the rat. *Am. J. Physiol.* **215**, 236–242.

Jick, H., Snyder, J. G., Moore, E. W., and Morrison, R. S. (1965). The effects of aldosterone and glucocorticoid on free water reabsorption. *Clin. Sci.* **29**, 25–32.

Johnston, H. H., Herzog, J. P., and Lauler, D. P. (1967). Effect of prostaglandin E_1 on renal hemodynamics, sodium and water excretion. *Am. J. Physiol.* **213**, 939–946.

Jorgensen, P. L. (1968). The effect of aldosterone and corticosterone on the $(Na^+ + K^+)$-activated ATP hydrolyzing enzyme system in kidneys of adrenalectomized rats. *Acta Physiol. Scand.* **73**, 21A–22A.

Kahn, M. (1962). Effect of chlorothiazide on electrolyte excretion in intact and adrenalectomized rats. *Am. J. Physiol.* **202**, 1141–1143.

Kamm, D. E., and Levinsky, N. G. (1964). Effect of plasma sodium elevation on renal sodium reabsorption. *Am. J. Physiol.* **206**, 1131–1136.

Kamm, D. E., and Levinsky, N. G. (1965a). Inhibition of renal tubular sodium reabsorption by hypernatremia. *J. Clin. Invest.* **44**, 1144–1150.

Kamm, D. E., and Levinsky, N. G. (1965b). The mechanism of denervation natriuresis. *J. Clin. Invest.* **44**, 93–102.

Kashgarian, M., Stoeckle, H., Gottschalk, C. W., and Ullrich, K. J. (1963). Transtubular electrochemical potential of sodium in proximal and distal tubules of rats during antidiuresis and water diuresis (diabetes insipidus). *Arch. Ges. Physiol.* **277**, 86–106.

Kashgarian, M., Warren, Y., and Levitin, H. (1965). Micropuncture study of proximal renal tubular chloride transport during hypercapnea in the rat. *Am. J. Physiol.* **209**, 655–658.

Katz, A. I., and Epstein, F. H. (1967). The physiological role of sodium-potassium activated adenosine triphosphatase in the active transport of cations across biological membranes. *Israel J. Med. Sci.* **3**, 155–166.

Katz, A. I., and Epstein, F. H. (1968). Physiologic role of sodium-potassium-activated adenosine triphosphatase in the transport of cations across biologic membranes. *New Engl. J. Med.* **278**, 253–261.

Katz, A. I., Hollingsworth, D. R., and Epstein, F. H. (1968). Influence of carbohydrate and protein on sodium excretion during fasting and refeeding. *J. Lab. Clin. Med.* **72**, 93–104.

Keck, W., Joppich, R., von Restorff, W., and Kramer, K. (1969). Renal hemodynamics, transtubular oncotic pressure gradient and sodium excretion after isotonic and isoncotic saline infusions and injections of hyperoncotic albumin. *Arch. Ges. Physiol.* **307**, R58.

Keeler, R. (1959). Effect of hypothalamic lesions on renal excretion of sodium. *Am. J. Physiol.* **197**, 847–849.

Keeler, R., and Schnieden, H. (1958). Investigation of mechanism of diuresis produced in the rat by an intravenous infusion of isotonic solution of sodium chloride. *Am. J. Physiol.* **195**, 137–141.

Kellogg, R. H., and Burack, W. R. (1954). Effect of adrenalectomy upon the diuresis produced by isotonic saline solutions in rats. *Am. J. Physiol.* **177**, 38–43.

Kelly, H. G., Cross, H. C., Turlon, M. R., and Hatcher, J. D. (1960). Renal and cardiovascular effects induced by intravenous infusion of magnesium sulfate. *Can. Med. Assoc. J.* **82**, 866–871.

Kelman, R. B. (1962). A theoretical note on exponential flow in the proximal part of the mammalian nephron. *Bull. Math. Biophys.* **24**, 303–317.

Kelman, R. B. (1965). Mathematical analysis of sodium reabsorption in proximal part of nephron in presence of nonreabsorbed solute. *J. Theoret. Biol.* **8**, 22–26.

Kessler, R. H. (1969). Adenine nucleotide concentration in renal cortex and medulla. *Symp. 4th Intern. Congr. Nephrol., Stockholm, 1969*, pp. 20–21.

Kessler, R. H., Landwehr, D., Quintanilla, A., Weseley, S. A., Kaufmann, W., Arcila, H., and Urbaitis, B. K. (1968). Effects of certain inhibitors on renal sodium reabsorption and ATP specific activity. *Nephron* **5**, 474–488.

Khuri, R. N., Goldstein, D. A., Maude, D. L., Edmonds, C., and Solomon, A. K. (1963). Single proximal tubules of necturus kidney. VIII. Na and K determination by glass electrodes. *Am. J. Physiol.* **204**, 743–748.

Kiil, F., Aukland, K., and Refsum, H. E. (1961). Renal sodium transport and oxygen consumption. *Am. J. Physiol.* **201**, 511–516.

Kinne, R., and Kirsten, R. (1968). Der Einfluss von Aldosteron auf die Aktivität mitochondrialer und cytoplasmatischer Enzyme in der Rattenniere. *Arch. Ges. Physiol.* **30**, 244–254.

Knippers, R., and Hchl, U. (1965). Die renale Ausscheidung von Magnesium, Calcium und Kalium nach Erhöhung der Magnesium-Konzentration im Plasma des Hundes. *Z. Ges. Exptl. Med.* **139**, 154–165.

Knox, F. G., Fleming, J. S., and Rennie, D. W. (1966). Effects of osmotic diuresis on sodium reabsorption and oxygen consumption of kidney. *Am. J. Physiol.* **210**, 751–759.

Knox, F. G., Davis, B. B., and Berliner, R. W. (1967). Effect of chronic cardiac denervation on renal response to saline infusion. *Am. J. Physiol.* **213**, 174–178.

Knox, F. G., Howards, S. S., Wright, F. S., Davis, B. B., and Berliner, R. W. (1968). Effect of dilution and expansion of blood volume on proximal sodium reabsorption. *Am. J. Physiol.* **215**, 1041–1048.

Knox, F. G., Wright, F. S., Howards, S. S., and Berliner, R. W. (1969). Effect of furosemide on sodium reabsorption by proximal tubule of the dog. *Am. J. Physiol.* **217**, 192–198.

Koch, K. M., Dume, T., Krause, H. H., and Ochwadt, B. (1967). Intratubulärer Druck, glomerulärer Capillardruck und Glomerulumfiltrat während Mannit-Diurese. *Arch. Ges. Physiol.* **295**, 72–79.

Koch, K. M., Aynedjian, H. S., and Bank, N. (1968). Effect of acute hypertension on sodium reabsorption by the proximal tubule. *J. Clin. Invest.* **47**, 1969–1709.

Kramer, K., and Deetjen, P. (1960). Beziehungen des O_2-Verbrauchs der Niere zu Durchblutung und Glomerulusfiltrat bei Anderung des arteriellen Druckes. *Arch. Ges. Physiol.* **271**, 782–796.

Krause, H. H., Dume, T., Koch, K. M., and Ochwadt, B. (1967). Intratubulärer Druck, glomerulärer Capillardruck und Glomerulumfiltrat nach Furosemid und Hydrochlorothiazid. *Arch. Ges. Physiol.* **295**, 80–89.

Kruhoffer, P. (1950). Studies on water-electrolyte excretion and glomerular activity in the mammalian kidney. Thesis, University of Copenhagen.

Kruhoffer, P. (1960). Handling of alkali metal ions by the kidney. *In* "The Alkali Metal Ions in Biology" (P. Kruhoffer, J. H. Thaysen, and N. A. Thorn, eds.), pp. 233–423. Handbuch Experimentellen Pharmakologie XIII, Springer, Berlin.

Kupfer, S., and Kosovsky, J. D. (1965). Effects of cardiac glycosides on renal tubular transport of calcium, magnesium, inorganic phosphate, and glucose in the dog. *J. Clin. Invest.* **44**, 1132–1143.

Ladd, M., and Raisz, L. G. (1949). Response of the normal dog to dietary sodium chloride. *Am. J. Physiol.* **159**, 149–152.

Landon, E. J., Jazab, N., and Forte, L. (1966). Aldosterone and sodium-potassium-dependent ATPase activity of rat kidney membranes. *Am. J. Physiol.* **211**, 1050–1056.

Landwehr, D. M., Klose, R. M., and Giebisch, G. (1967). Renal tubular sodium and water reabsorption in the isotonic sodium chloride-loaded rat. *Am. J. Physiol.* **212**, 1327–1333.

Landwehr, D. M., Schnermann, J., Klose, R. M., and Giebisch, G. (1968). Effect of reduction in filtration rate on renal tubular sodium and water reabsorption. *Am. J. Physiol.* **215**, 687–695.

Langston, J. B., Guyton, A. C., De Poyster, J. H., and Armstrong, G. G., Jr. (1962). Changes in renal function resulting from norepinephrine infusion. *Am. J. Physiol.* **202**, 893–896.

Lant, A. F., Baba, W. I., and Wilson, G. M. (1967). Localization of the site of action of oral diuretics in the human kidney. *Clin. Sci.* **33**, 11–27.

Lassen, N. A., Munck, O., and Thaysen, J. H. (1961). Oxygen consumption and sodium reabsorption in the kidney. *Acta Physiol. Scand.* **51**, 371–384.

Lassiter, W. E., Mylle, M., and Gottschalk, C. W. (1964). Net transtubular movement of water and urea in saline diuresis. *Am. J. Physiol.* **206**, 669–673.

Lauson, H. D., and Thompson, D. D. (1958). Effects in dogs of decrease in glomerular filtration rate on cation excretion during intravenous administration of unreabsorbable anions. *Am. J. Physiol.* **192**, 198–208.

Leaf, A., Bartter, F. C., Santos, R. F., and Wrong, O. (1953). Evidence in man that urinary electrolyte loss induced by Pitressin is a function of water retention. *J. Clin. Invest.* **32**, 868–878.

Leaf, A., Anderson, J., and Page, L. B. (1958). Active sodium transport by the isolated toad bladder. *J. Gen. Physiol.* **41**, 657–668.

Levin, N. W., Cortes, P., Colwell, J. A., and Herrera, E. (1969). Effect of furosemide on glucose and palmitate metabolism in the kidney. *Free Commun., 4th Intern. Congr. Nephrol., Stockholm, 1969* p. 203.

Levine, D. Z., Liebau, G., Fischbach, H., and Thurau, K. (1968). Micropuncture studies on the dog kidney. II. Reabsorptive characteristics of the proximal tubule during spontaneous and experimental variations in GFR and during drug induced natriuresis. *Arch. Ges. Physiol.* **304**, 365–375.

Levinsky, N. G., and Lalone, R. C. (1963). The mechanism of sodium diuresis after saline infusions in the dog. *J. Clin. Invest.* **42**, 1261–1276.

Levinsky, N. G., and Lalone, R. (1965). Sodium excretion during acute saline loading in dogs with vena cava constriction. *J. Clin. Invest.* **44**, 565–573.

Levitt, M. F., Halpern, M. H., Sweet, A. Y., and Gribetz, D. (1956). The effect of intravenous calcium infusion on electrolyte excretion in man. *J. Clin. Invest.* **35**, 720–721.

Levy, M. N., and Ankeney, J. L. (1952). Influence of glomerular filtration rate upon the renal tubular reabsorption of sodium. *Proc. Soc. Exptl. Biol. Med.* **79**, 491–494.

Lewy, J. E., and Windhager, E. E. (1968). Peritubular control of proximal tubular fluid reabsorption in the rat kidney. *Am. J. Physiol.* **214**, 943–954.

Leyssac, P. P. (1963). Dependence of glomerular filtration rate on proximal tubular reabsorption of salt. *Acta Physiol. Scand.* **58**, 236–242.

Leyssac, P. P. (1964). The effect of partial clamping of the renal artery on pressures in the proximal and distal tubules and peritubular capillaries in the rat kidney. *Acta Physiol. Scand.* **62**, 449–456.

Leyssac, P. P. (1965). The *in vivo* effect of angiotensin and noradrenaline on the proximal tubular reabsorption of salt in mammalian kidneys. *Acta Physiol. Scand.* **64**, 167–175.

Le Zotte, L. A., MacGaffey, K. M., Moore, E. W., and Jick, H. (1966). The effects of frusemide on renal concentration and dilution. *Clin. Sci.* **31**, 371–382.

Liddle, G. W. (1966). Aldosterone antagonists and triamterene. *Ann. N. Y. Acad. Sci.* **139**, 466–470.

Liebau, G., Levine, D. Z., and Thurau, K. (1968). Micropuncture studies on the dog kidney. I. The response of the proximal tubule to changes in systemic blood pressure within and below the autoregulatory range. *Arch. Ges. Physiol.* **304**, 57–68.

Linderholm, H. (1952). Active transport of ions through frog skin with special reference to the action of certain diuretics. *Acta Physiol. Scand.* **27**, Suppl. 97, 1–139.

Lindheimer, M. D., Lalone, R. C., and Levinsky, N. G. (1967). Evidence that an acute increase in glomerular filtration has little effect on sodium excretion in the dog unless extracellular volume is expanded. *J. Clin. Invest.* **46**, 256–265.

Lockett, M. F. (1966). Effects of saline loading on the perfused cat kidney. *J. Physiol. (London)* **187**, 489–500.

Lockett, M. F., and Roberts, C. N. (1963). Hormonal factors affecting sodium excretion in the rat. *J. Physiol. (London)* **167**, 581–590.

Loeb, R. F., Atchely, D., Benedict, E., and Leland, J. (1933). Electrolyte balance studies in adrenalectomized dogs with particular reference to the excretion of sodium. *J. Exptl. Med.* **57**, 775–792.

Ludens, J. H., Hook, J. B., and Williamson, H. E. (1967). Lack of effect of Actinomycin D on aldosterone induced antinatriuresis when administered after the hormone. *Proc. Soc. Exptl. Biol. Med.* **124**, 539–541.

McDonald, M., Schrier, R. W., and Lauler, D. P. (1967). Effect of acute extracellular volume expansion on cross-circulated dogs. *Nephron* **4**, 1–12.

McDonald, S. J., and de Wardener, H. E. (1965). The relationship between the renal arterial perfusion pressure and the increase in sodium excretion which occurs during an infusion of saline. *Nephron* **2**, 1–14.

McEvoy, J. (1968). Localization of the site of action of mersalyl, chlorothiazide and chlorthalidone in the renal tubule using the ischaemic stop flow technique. *Arch. Exptl. Pathol. Pharmakol.* **259**, 314–318.

Macey, R. I. (1963). Pressure flow pattern in a cylinder with reabsorbing walls. *Bull. Math. Biophys.* **25**, 1–9.

Macey, R. I. (1965). Hydrodynamics in the renal tubule. *Bull. Math. Biophys.* **27**, 117–124.

Macfarlane, W. V., Kinne, R., Walmsley, C. M., Siebert, B. D., and Peter, D. (1967). Vasopressins and the increase of water and electrolyte excretion by sheep, cattle and camels. *Nature* **214**, 979–981.

Malnic, G., Klose, R. M., and Giebisch, G. (1966a). Micropuncture study of distal tubular potassium and sodium transfer in rat nephron. *Am. J. Physiol.* **211**, 529–547.

Malnic, G., Klose, R. M., and Giebisch, G. (1966b). Microperfusion study of distal tubular potassium and sodium transfer in rat kidney. *Am. J. Physiol.* **211**, 548–559.

Malvin, R. L., Wilde, W. S., Vander, A. J., and Sullivan, L. P. (1958). Localization and characterization of sodium transport along the renal tubule. *Am. J. Physiol.* **195**, 549–557.

Manitius, A., Bensch, K., and Epstein, F. H. (1968). $(Na^+ - K^+)$-activated ATPase in kidney cell membranes of normal and methylprednisolone-treated rats. *Biochim. Biophys. Acta* **150**, 563–571.

Maren, T. H. (1969). Renal carbonic anhydrase and the pharmacology of sulfonamide inhibitors. *Handbook Exptl. Pharmacol.* [N. S.] **24**, 195–256.

Marsh, D. J., and Solomon, S. (1965). Analysis of electrolyte movement in thin Henle's loops of hamster papilla. *Am. J. Physiol.* **208**, 1119–1128.

Marshall, F. N., and Williamson, H. E. (1964). Natriuretic response during infusion of β-diethylaminoethyldiphenylpropyl acetate hydrochloride (SKF 525-A) into the renal artery. *J. Pharmacol. Exptl. Therap.* **143**, 395–400.

Martinez-Maldonado, M., Eknoyan, G., and Suki, W. (1969). Evidence for contribution of oxidative metabolism and anaerobic glycolysis to medullary sodium transport *in vivo*. *Free Commun., 4th Intern. Congr. Nephrol., Stockholm, 1969*, p. 22.

Martino, J. A., and Earley, L. E. (1967a). Demonstration of a role of physical factors as determinants of the natriuretic response to volume expansion. *J. Clin. Invest.* **46**, 1963–1978.

Martino, J. A., and Earley, L. E. (1967b). The effects of infusion of water on renal hemodynamics and the tubular reabsorption of sodium. *J. Clin. Invest.* **46**, 1229–1238.

Martino, J. A., and Earley, L. E. (1968). Relationship between intrarenal hydrostatic pressure and hemodynamically induced changes in sodium excretion. *Circulation Res.* **23**, 371–386.

Massry, S. G., Katz, A. I., Agmon, J., and Toor, M. (1968). Effect of water diuresis on electrolyte and hydrogen ion excretion in hot climate. *Nephron* **5**, 124–133.

Maude, D. L. (1968). Stop-flow microperfusion of proximal tubules in rat kidney cortex slices. *Am. J. Physiol.* **214**, 1315–1321.

Maude, D. L. (1969). Effects of K and ouabain on fluid transport and cell Na in proximal tubule *in vitro*. *Am. J. Physiol.* **216**, 1199–1206.

Maude, D. L., Shehadeh, I., and Solomon, A. K. (1966). Sodium and water transport in single perfused distal tubules of Necturus kidney. *Am. J. Physiol.* **211**, 1043–1049.

May, D. G., and Carter, M. K. (1967). Unilateral diuresis by infusing arecoline into renal portal system of hens. *Am. J. Physiol.* **212**, 1351–1354.

Mills, I. H. (1968). The cardiovascular system and renal control of sodium excretion. *Can. J. Physiol. Pharmacol.* **46**, 297–303.

Mills, I. H., de Wardener, H. E., Hayter, C. J., and Clapham, W. F. (1961). Studies on the afferent mechanism of the sodium chloride diuresis which follows intravenous saline in the dog. *Clin. Sci.* **21**, 259–264.

Morgan, T., and Berliner, R. W. (1968). Permeability of the loop of Henle, vasa recta, and collecting duct to water, urea, and sodium. *Am. J. Physiol.* **215**, 108–115.

Morgan, T., and Berliner, R. W. (1969a). An *in vivo* microperfusion study of factors affecting sodium reabsorption in the proximal tubule of the rat kidney. *Free Communic., 4th Intern. Congr. Nephrol., Stockholm, 1969*, p. 232.

Morgan, T., and Berliner, R. W. (1969b). Sodium and potassium transport in the distal tubule of the rat; studied by *in vivo* microperfusion. *Free Commun., 4th Intern. Congr. Nephrol., Stockholm*, p. 237.

Morgan, T., and Berliner, R. W. (1969c). A study by continuous microperfusion of water and electrolyte movements in the loop of Henle and distal tubule of the rat. *Nephron* **6**, 388–405.

Morgan, T., Sakai, F., and Berliner, R. W. (1968). *In vitro* permeability of medullary collecting ducts to water and urea. *Am. J. Physiol.* **214**, 574–581.

Mudge, G. H., and Weiner, I. M. (1957–1958). The mechanism of action of mercurial and xanthine diuretics. *Ann. N.Y. Acad. Sci.* **71**, 344–354.

Nagel, W., Horster, M., Wahl, M., Thurau, K., and Schnermann, J. (1966). Die tubuläre Resorptionskapazität für isotone NaCl-Lösung bei unterschiedlichen Glomerulumfiltraten und unter Angiotensineinwirkung. *Arch. Ges. Physiol.* **291**, R60.

Nahmod, V. E., and Walser, M. (1966). The effect of ouabain on renal tubular reabsorption and cortical concentration of several cations and on their association with subcellular particles. *Mol. Pharmacol.* **2**, 22–36.

Nechay, B. R. (1964). Potentiation of diuretic effects of methyl xanthines and pyrimidines by carbonic anhydrase inhibition. *J. Pharmacol. Exptl. Therap.* **144**, 276–283.

Nechay, B. R. (1967). Renal effect of ethacrynic acid in chickens, a species with a small countercurrent system. *J. Pharmacol. Exptl. Therap.* **158**, 471–474.

Nechay, B. R., Palmer, R. F., Chinoy, D. A., and Posey, V. A. (1967). The problem of $Na^+ + K^+$ adenosine triphosphatase as the receptor for diuretic action of mercurials and ethacrynic acid. *J. Pharmacol. Exptl. Therap.* **157**, 599–617.

Nissen, O. I. (1966). The filtration fractions of plasma supplying the superficial and deep venous drainage area of the cat kidney. *Acta Physiol. Scand.* **68**, 275–285.

Nissen, O. I. (1968). Changes in the filtration fractions in the superficial and deep venous drainage area of the cat kidney due to fluid loading. *Acta Physiol. Scand.* **73**, 320–328.

Nizet, A. (1967). Control by plasma potassium concentration of sodium excretion by isolated perfused dog kidney. *Arch. Ges. Physiol.* **297**, 162–165.

Nizet, A. (1968). Influence of serumalbumin and dextran on sodium and water excretion by the isolated dog kidney. *Arch. Ges. Physiol.* **301**, 7–15.

Novello, F. C., and Sprague, J. M. (1957). Benzothiadiazine dioxides as novel diuretics. *J. Am. Chem. Soc.* **79**, 2028–2030.

Nutbourne, D. M. (1968). The effect of small hydrostatic pressure gradients on the rate of active sodium transport across isolated living frog-skin membranes. *J. Physiol. (London)* **195**, 1–18.

Oken, D. E., Whittembury, G., Windhager, E. E., and Solomon, A. K. (1963). Single proximal tubules of Necturus kidney. V. Unidirectional sodium movement. *Am. J. Physiol.* **204**, 372–376.

Orloff, J., and Burg, M. (1960). Effect of strophanthidin on electrolyte excretion in chicken. *Am. J. Physiol.* **199**, 49–54.

Palmer, R. F., and Nechay, B. R. (1964). Biphasic renal effects of ouabain in the chicken: Correlation with a microsomal $Na^+ - K^+$ stimulated ATP-ase. *J. Pharmacol. Exptl. Therap.* **146**, 92–98.

Palmore, W. P., Marieb, N. J., and Mulrow, P. J. (1969). Stimulation of aldosterone secretion by sodium depletion in nephrectomized rats. *Endocrinology* **84**, 1342–1351.

Papper, S., Saxon, L., and Cohen, H. W. (1955). The effects of isotonic and hypertonic salt solutions on the renal excretion of sodium. *J. Clin. Invest.* **34**, 956.

Parmelee, M. L., and Carter, M. K. (1968). The diuretic effect of acetylcholine in the chicken. *Arch. Intern. Pharmacodyn.* **174**, 108–117.

Pearce, J. W. (1968). The renal response to volume expansion. *Can. J. Physiol. Pharmacol.* **46**, 305–313.

Pendleton, R. G., Sullivan, L. P., and Tucker, J. M. (1968a). The effect of chlormerodrin on the isolated toad bladder. *J. Pharmacol. Exptl. Therap.* **164**, 362–370.

Pendleton, R. G., Sullivan. L. P., Tucker, J. M., and Stephenson, R. E., III. (1968b). The effect of a benzothiadiazide on the isolated toad bladder. *J. Pharmacol. Exptl. Therap.* **164**, 348–361.

Peters, G., and Roch-Ramel, F. (1969a). Thiazide diuretics and related drugs. *Handbook Exptl. Pharmacol.* [N. S.] **24**, 257–385.

Peters, G., and Roch-Ramel, F. (1969b). Furosemide. *Handbook Exptl. Pharmacol.* [N. S.] **24**, 386–405.

Peters, G., and Roch-Ramel, F. (1969c). Ethacrynic acid and related drugs. *Handbook Exptl. Pharmacol.* [N. S.] **24**, 406–435.

Pinter, G. G., O'Morchoe, C. C. C., and Sikand, R. S. (1964). Effect of acetylcholine on urinary electrolyte excretion. *Am. J. Physiol.* **207**, 979–982.

Porter, G. A., Bogoroch, R., and Edelman, I. S. (1964). On the mechanism of action of aldosterone on sodium transport: The role of protein synthesis. *Proc. Natl. Acad. Sci. U.S.* **52**, 1326–1333.

Porush, J. G., and Abramson, R. G. (1965). The effect of hypertonic mannitol on renal sodium excretion in hydropenic man. *Clin. Sci.* **29**, 475–487.

Porush, J. G., Goldstein, M. H., Eisner, G. M., and Levitt, M. F. (1961). Effect of organomercurials on the renal concentrating operation in hydropenic man: comments on site of action. *J. Clin. Invest.* **40**, 1475–1485.

Pritchard, J. A. (1955). The use of the magnesium ion in the management of eclamptogenic toxemias. *Surg., Gynecol. Obstet.* **100**, 131–140.

Rapoport, S., and West, C. D. (1950). Ionic antagonism: effect of various anions on chloride excretion during osmotic diuresis in the dog. *Am. J. Physiol.* **162**, 668–676.

Rector, F. C., Jr., and Clapp, J. R. (1962). Evidence for active chloride reabsorption in the distal renal tubule of the rat. *J. Clin. Invest.* **41**, 101–107.

Rector, F. C., Jr., Van Giesen, G., Kiil, F., and Seldin, D. W. (1964). Influence of expansion of extracellular volume on tubular reabsorption of sodium independent of changes in glomerular filtration rate and aldosterone activity. *J. Clin. Invest.* **43**, 341–348.

Rector, F. C., Jr., Martinez-Maldonado, M., Brunner, F. P., and Seldin, D. W. (1966a). Evidence for passive reabsorption of NaCl in proximal tubule of rat kidney. *J. Clin. Invest.* **45**, 1060.

Rector, F. C., Jr., Brunner, F. P., and Seldin, D. W. (1966b). Mechanism of glomerulotubular balance. I. Effect of aortic constriction and elevated ureteropelvic pressure on glomerular filtration rate, fractional reabsorption, transit time, and tubular size in the proximal tubule of the rat. *J. Clin. Invest.* **45**, 590–602.

Rector, F. C., Jr., Brunner, F. P., Sellman, J. C., and Seldin, D. W. (1966c). Pitfalls in the use of micropuncture for the localization of diuretic action. *Ann. N.Y. Acad. Sci.* **139**, 400–407.

Rector, F. C., Jr., Sellman, J. C., Martinez-Maldonado, M., and Seldin, D. W. (1967). The mechanism of suppression of proximal tubular reabsorption by saline infusions. *J. Clin. Invest.* **46**, 47–56.

Rector, F. C., Jr., Martinez-Maldonado, M., Kurtzman, N. A., Sellman, J. C., Oerther, F., and Seldin, D. W. (1968). Demonstration of a hormonal inhibitor of proximal tubular reabsorption during expansion of extracellular volume with isotonic saline. *J. Clin. Invest.* **47**, 761–773.

Reinhardt, H. W., and Behrenbeck, D. W., (1967). Untersuchungen an wachen Hunden über die Einstellung der Natriumbilanz. I. Die Bedeutung des Extracellulärraumes für die Einstellung der Natrium-Tagesbilanz. *Arch. Ges. Physiol.* **295**, 266–279.

Renschler, H. E., Jaenkner, D., Kammerer, E. and Thoma, R. (1969). The influence of an intravenous glucose load on renal sodium excretion. *In* "Progress in Nephrology" (G. Peters and F. Roch-Ramel, eds.), pp. 385–389. Springer, Berlin.

Robb, C. A., Davis, J. O., Johnston, C. I., and Hartroft, P. M. (1968). Effects of cortisone on renal sodium excretion in rabbits. *Endocrinology* **82**, 1200–1208.

Robinson, J. R. (1954). "Reflections On Renal Function." Thomas, Springfield, Illinois.

Rodicio, J., Herrera-Acosta, J., Sellman, J. C., Rector, F. C., Jr., and Seldin, D. W. (1969). Studies on glomerulotubular balance during aortic constriction, ureteral obstruction, and venous occlusion in hydropenic and saline-loaded rats. *Nephron* **6**, 437–456.

Rosenbaum, J. D., Papper, S., and Ashley, M. M. (1955). Variations in renal excretion of sodium independent of change in adrenocortical hormone dosage in patients with Addison's disease. *J. Clin. Endocrinol.* **15**, 1459–1474.

Rosenfeld, S., Kraus, R., and McCullen, A. (1965). Effect of renin, ischemia, and plasma protein loading on the isolated perfused kidney. *Am. J. Physiol.* **209**, 835–843.

Samiy, A. H. E., Brown, J. L., and Globus, D. L. (1960). Effects of magnesium and calcium loading on renal excretion of electrolytes in dogs. *Am. J. Physiol.* **198**, 595–598.

Saugman, B. (1957). The excretion of easily diffusible anions in mammals. Thesis, University of Copenhagen.

Schatzmann, H. J., Windhager, E. E., and Solomon, A. K. (1958). Single proximal tubules of the Necturus kidney. II. Effect of 2,4-dinitrophenol and ouabain on water reabsorption. *Am. J. Physiol.* **195**, 570–574.

Schmidt, R. W., and Sullivan, L. P. (1966). Effect of meralluride on distal nephron transport of sodium, potassium, and chloride. *J. Pharmacol. Exptl. Therap.* **151**, 180–188.

Schmidt, U., and Dubach, U. C. (1969). Activity of (Na^+ K^+)-stimulated adenosintriphosphatase in the rat nephron. *Arch. Ges. Physiol.* **306**, 219–226.

Schnermann, J. (1968). Microperfusion study of single short loops of Henle in rat kidney. *Arch. Ges. Physiol.* **300**, 255–282.

Schnermann, J., Nagel, W., and Thurau, K. (1966). Die frühdistale Natriumkonzentration in Rattennieren nach renaler Ischämie und haemorrhagischer Hypotension. Ein Beitrag zur Pathogenese der postischämischen und post-haemorrhagischen Filtraterniedrigung. *Arch. Ges. Physiol.* **287**, 296–310.

Schnermann, J., Wahl, M., Liebau, G., and Fischbach, H. (1968). Balance between tubular flow rate and net fluid reabsorption in the proximal convolution of the rat kidney. I. Dependency of reabsorptive net fluid flux upon proximal tubular surface area at spontaneous variations of filtration rate. *Arch. Ges. Physiol.* **304**, 90–103.

Schnermann, J., Levine, D. Z., and Horster, M. (1969). A direct evaluation of the Gertz hypothesis on single rat proximal tubules *in vivo*; Failure of the tubular volume to be the sole determinant of the reabsorptive rate. *Arch. Ges. Physiol.* **308**, 149–165.

Schrier, R. W., McDonald, K. M., Jagger, P. I., and Lauler, D. P. (1967). The role of the adrenergic nervous system in the renal response to acute extracellular fluid volume expansion. *Proc. Soc. Exptl. Biol. Med.* **125**, 1157–1162.

Schrier, R. W., McDonald, K. M., Marshall, R. A., and Lauler, D. P. (1968). Absence of natriuretic response to acute hypotonic intravascular volume expansion in dogs. *Clin. Sci.* **34**, 57–72.

Schultz, E. M., Gragoe, E. J., Bicking, J. B., Bolhofer, W. A., and Sprague, J. M. (1962). α,β-unsaturated ketone derivatives of aryloxyacetic acids, a new class of diuretics. *J. Med. Pharm. Chem.* **5**, 660–662.

Sealy, J. E., Kirshman, J. D., and Laragh, J. H. (1969). Separation and characterization of a humoral natriuretic substance from plasma and urine of normal and hypertensive human subjects and sheep. *Free Commun., 4th Intern. Nephrol., Stockholm, 1969*, p. 371.

Segar, W. E., Riley, P. A., and Barila, T. G. (1956). Urinary composition during hypothermia. *Am. J. Physiol.* **185**, 528–532.

Seldin, D. W., Eknoyan, G., Siki, W. N., and Rector, F. C., Jr. (1966). Localization of diuretic action from the pattern of water and electrolyte excretion. *Ann. N.Y. Acad. Sci.* **139**, 328-343.

Selkurt, E. E. (1951). Effect of pulse pressure and mean arterial pressure modification on renal hemodynamics and electrolyte and water excretion. *Circulation* **4**, 541-551.

Selkurt, E. E., and Post, R. S., (1950). Renal clearance of sodium in the dog: effect of increasing sodium load on reabsorptive mechanism. *Am. J. Physiol.* **162**, 639-648.

Selkurt, E. E., Womack, I., and Dailey, W. N. (1965). Mechanism of natriuresis and diuresis during elevated renal arterial pressure. *Am. J. Physiol.* **209**, 95-99.

Shuster, A., Alexander, E., Lalone, R. C., and Levinsky, N. G. (1966). Renal blood flow, sodium excretion, and concentrating ability during saline infusion. *Am. J. Physiol.* **211**, 1181-1186.

Sieker, H. O., Gauer, O. H., and Henry, J. P. (1954). The effect of continuous negative pressure breathing on water and electrolyte excretion by the human kidney. *J. Clin. Invest.* **33**, 572-577.

Skou, J. C. (1957). The influence of some cations on an adenosine triphosphatase from peripheral nerves. *Biochim. Biophys. Acta* **23**, 394-401.

Skou, J. C. (1965). Enzymatic basis for active transport of Na$^+$ and K$^+$ across cell membrane. *Physiol. Rev.* **45**, 596-617.

Small, A., and Cafruny, E. J. (1967). Furosemide and hydrochlorothiazide do not have a common mode of action. *J. Pharmacol. Exptl. Therap.* **156**, 616-621.

Smith, H. W. (1951). "The Kidney: Structure and Function in Health and Disease." Oxford Univ. Press, London and New York.

Smith, H. W. (1957). Salt and water volume receptors. *Am. J. Med.* **23**, 623-652.

Stamler, J., Dreifus, L., Lichton, I. J., Marcus, E., Hasbrouck, E. E., and Wong, S. (1958). Effects of ascites formation on response to rapid water, sodium, and dextran loads in intact and diabetes insipidus Ringer's-infused dogs. *Am. J. Physiol.* **195**, 369-372.

Stein, R. M., Abramson, R. G., Bercovitch, D. D., and Levitt, M. F. (1965). Effects of unilateral renal arterial constriction on tubular reabsorption of sodium and water during an osmotic diuresis. *J. Clin. Invest.* **44**, 1720-1729.

Steinhausen, M. (1967a). Messungen des tubulären Harnstroms und der tubulären Reabsorption unter erhöhtem Ureterdruck. *Arch. Ges. Physiol.* **298**, 105-130.

Steinhausen, M. (1967b). Studies on the microcirculation of renal tubular flow under the special aspect of the glomerulotubular balance. *Bibliotheca Anat.* **9**, 135-140.

Steinhausen, M., Loreth, A., and Olson, S. (1965). Messungen des tubulären Harnstromes, seine Beziehungen zum Blutdruck und zur Inulin-Clearance. *Arch. Ges. Physiol.* **286**, 118-141.

Stříbrná, J., and Schück, O. (1968). A comparison of the site of action of intravenously and orally administered furosemide and ethacrynic acid in the human nephron. *Physiol. Bohemoslov.* **17**, 133-141.

Strickler, J. C., and Kessler, R. H. (1963). Effects of certain inhibitors on renal excretion of salt and water. *Am. J. Physiol.* **205**, 117-122.

Stumpe, K. O., and Ochwadt, B. (1968). Wirkung von Aldosteron auf die Natrium- und Wasserresorption im proximalen Tubulus bei chronischer Kochsalzbelastung. *Arch. Ges. Physiol.* **300**, 148-160.

Suki, W., Rector, F. C., Jr., and Seldin, D. W. (1965). The site of action of furosemide and other sulfonamide diuretics in the dog. *J. Clin. Invest.* **44**, 1458-1469.

Sullivan, L. P., and Pirch, J. H. (1966). Effect of bendroflumethiazide on distal nephron transport of sodium, potassium, and chloride. *J. Pharmacol. Exptl. Therap.* **151**, 168-179.

Surtshin, A., Mueller, C. B., and White, H. L. (1952). Effect of acute changes in glomerular filtration rate on water and electrolyte excretion: Mechanism of denervation diuresis. *Am. J. Physiol.* **169**, 159–173.

Taylor, C. B. (1963). The effect of mercurial diuretics on adenosinetriphosphatase of rabbit kidney *in vitro. Biochem. Pharmacol.* **12**, 539–550.

Thompson, D. D., and Pitts, R. F. (1952). Effects of alterations of renal arterial pressure on sodium and water excretion. *Am. J. Physiol.* **168**, 490–499.

Thurau, K., and Schnermann, J. (1965). Die Natriumkonzentration an den Macula densa Zellen als regulierender Faktor für das Glomerulumfiltrat (Mikropunktionsversuche). *Klin. Woschschr.* **43**, 410–413.

Thurau, K., and Wober, E. (1962). Zur Lokalisation der autoregulativen Widerstandsänderungen in der Niere: Mikropunktionsmessungen der Drucke in Tubuli und peritubulären Capillaren der Rattenniere bei Änderungen des arteriellen Druckes. *Arch. Ges. Physiol.* **274**, 553–566.

Thurau, K., Schnermann, J., Nagel, W., Horster, M., and Wahl, M. (1967). Composition of tubular fluid in the macula densa segment as a factor regulating the function of the juxtaglomerular apparatus. *Circulation Res.* **20–21**, Suppl. 2, 79–90.

Tobian, L., Coffee, K., Ferreira, D., and Meuli, J. (1964). The effect of renal perfusion pressure on the net transport of sodium out of distal tubular urine as studied with the stop-flow technique. *J. Clin. Invest.* **43**, 118–128.

Torelli, G., Milla, E., Faelli, A., and Costantini, S. (1966). Energy requirement for sodium reabsorption in the *in vivo* rabbit kidney. *Am. J. Physiol.* **211**, 576–580.

Uhlich, E., Baldamus, C. A., and Ullrich, K. J. (1969). The effect of aldosterone on sodium transport in the collecting ducts of the mammalian kidney. *Arch. Ges. Physiol.* **308**, 111–126.

Ullman, E. (1961). Acute anoxia and the excretion of water and electrolyte. *J. Physiol. (London)* **155**, 417–437.

Ullrich, K. J. (1967). Renal transport of sodium. *Proc. 3rd Intern. Congr. Nephrol., Washington, 1966*, pp. 48–61. Karger, Basel.

Ullrich, K. J., Schmidt-Nielsen, B., O'Dell, R., Pehling, G., Gottschalk, C. W., Lassiter, W. E., and Mylle, M. (1963). Micropuncture study of composition of proximal and distal tubular fluid in rat kidney. *Am. J. Physiol.* **204**, 527–531.

Ullrich, K. J., Rumrich, G., and Fuchs, G. (1964). Wasserpermeabilität und transtubulärer Wasserfluss corticaler Nephronabschnitte bei verschiedenen Diuresezuständen. *Arch. Ges. Physiol.* **280**, 99–119.

Ullrich, K. J., Baumann, K., Loeschke, K., Rumrich, G., and Stolte, H. (1966). Micropuncture experiments with saluretic sulfonamides. *Ann. N. Y. Acad. Sci.* **139**, 416–423.

Ussing, H. H., and Zerahn, K. (1951). Active transport of sodium as the source of electric current in the short-circuited isolated frog skin. *Acta Physiol. Scand.* **23**, 110–127.

Vaamonde, C. A., Sporn, I. N., Lancestremere, R. G., Belsky, J. L., and Papper, S. (1964). Augmented natriuretic response to acute sodium infusion after blood pressure elevation with metaraminol in normotensive subjects. *J. Clin. Invest.* **43**, 496–502.

Vander, A. J., Malvin, R. L., Wilder, W. S., and Sullivan, L. P. (1958). Localization of the site of action of mercurial diuretics by stop flow analysis. *Am. J. Physiol.* **195**, 558–562.

Vereerstraeten, P., and Toussaint, C. (1965). Réduction de la natriurèse par la perfusion d'albumine dans la veine porte rénale du coq. *Nephron* **2**, 355–366.

Vereerstraeten, P., and Toussaint, C. (1969). Effects of plasmapheresis on renal hemodynamics and sodium excretion in dogs. *Arch. Ges. Physiol.* **306**, 92–102.

Veverbrants, E., and Arky, R. A. (1969). Effects of fasting and refeeding. I. Studies on sodium, potassium and water excretion on a constant electrolyte and fluid intake. *J. Clin. Endocrinol.* **29**, 55–62.

Vogel, G., and Stoeckert, I. (1966). Die Bedeutung des Anions für die renal tubulären Transport von Na$^+$ und die Transporte von Glucose und PAH. *Arch. Ges. Physiol.* **292**, 309–315.

Vogel, G., and Tervooren, U. (1965). Die Bedeutung von Kalium für die renal tubulären *Arch. Ges. Physiol.* **284**, 103–107.

von Stackelberg, W. F. (1969). The effect of hydrostatic pressure difference on short circuit current and potential difference across the toad skin. *Arch. Ges. Physiol.* **307**, R55.

Vorburger, C. (1964). Die akute Wirkung des Diureticum Fursemid auf das Glomerulumfiltrat, die renale Hämodynamik, die Wasser-, Natrium-, Chlorid- und Kaliumausscheidung und auf den Sauerstoffverbrauch dei Nieren. *Klin. Woschschr.* **42**, 833–839.

Wahl, M., Nagel, W., Fischbach, H., and Thurau, K. (1967). On the application of the occlusion time method for measurements of lateral net fluxes in the proximal convolution of the rat kidney. *Arch. Ges. Physiol.* **298**, 141–153.

Wahl, M., Liebau, G., Fischbach, H., and Schnermann, J. (1968). Balance between tubular flow rate and net fluid reabsorption in the proximal convolution of the rat kidney. II. Reabsorptive characteristics during constriction of the renal artery. *Arch. Ges. Physiol.* **304**, 297–314.

Walker, A. M., Bott, P. A., Oliver, J., and MacDowell, M. C. (1941). Collection and analysis of fluid from single nephrons of mammalian kidney. *Am. J. Physiol.* **134**, 580–595.

Walser, M. (1966). Mathematical aspects of renal function: The dependence of solute reabsorption on water reabsorption, and the mechanism of osmotic natriuresis. *J. Theoret. Biol.* **10**, 307–326.

Walser, M. (1969). Reversible stimulation of sodium transport in the toad bladder by stretch. *J. Clin. Invest.* **48**, 1714–1723.

Walser, M., and Mudge, G. H. (1960). Renal excretory mechanisms. In "Mineral Metabolism" (C. L. Comar and F. Bronner, eds.), Vol. 1, Part 1A, pp. 288–337. Academic Press, New York.

Walser, M., and Rahill, W. J. (1963). Evidence for a single transport system for monovalent anions. *Physiologist* **6**, 292.

Walser, M., and Rahill, W. J. (1965a). Renal tubular reabsorption of iodide as compared with chloride. *J. Clin. Invest.* **44**, 1371–1381.

Walser, M., and Rahill, W. J. (1965b). Nitrate, thiocyanate, and perchlorate clearance in relation to chloride clearance. *Am. J. Physiol.* **208**, 1158–1164.

Walser, M., and Rahill, W. J. (1966a). Renal tubular reabsorption of bromide compared with chloride. *Clin. Sci.* **30**, 191–205.

Walser, M., and Rahill, W. J. (1966b). Renal tubular transport of fluoride compared with chloride. *Am. J. Physiol.* **210**, 1290–1292.

Walser, M., and Trounce, J. R. (1961). The effect of diuresis and diuretics upon the renal transport of alkaline earth cations. *Biochem. Pharmacol.* **8**, 157.

Washington, J. A., II, and Holland, J. M. (1966). Urine oxygen tension: Effects of osmotic and saline diuresis and of ethacrynic acid. *Am. J. Physiol.* **210**, 243–250.

Wathen, R. L., and Selkurt, E. E. (1969). Intrarenal regulatory factors of salt excretion during renal venous pressure elevation. *Am. J. Physiol.* **216**, 1517–1524.

Watson, J. F. (1966). Effect of saline loading on sodium reabsorption in the dog proximal tubule. *Am. J. Physiol.* **10**, 781–785.

Waugh, W. H., and Kubo, T. (1968). Antinatriuretic effect of exogenous metabolic substrates on the sodium diuresis of saline infusion. *Life Sci.* **7**, 325–335.

Webster, M. E., and Gilmore, J. P. (1964). Influence of kallidin-10 on renal function. *Am. J. Physiol.* **206**, 714–718.

Wedeen, R. P., and Goldstein, M. H. (1963). Renal tubular localization of chlormerodin labelled with mercury-203 by autoradiography. *Science* **141**, 438–440.

Weiner, M. W., Hayslett, J. P., Kashgarian, M., and Epstein, F. H. (1969). Accelerated reabsorption in the proximal tubule produced by sodium depletion. *Free Commun., 4th Intern. Congr. Nephrol., Stockholm, 1969*, p. 233.

Welt, L. G., and Orloff, J. (1951). The effects of an increase in plasma volume on the metabolism and excretion of water and electrolytes by normal subjects. *J. Clin. Invest.* **30**, 751–761.

Wesson, L. G., Jr. (1962). Organic mercurial effects on renal tubular reabsorption of calcium and magnesium and on phosphate excretion in the dog. *J. Lab. Clin. Med.* **59**, 630–637.

Wesson, L. G., Jr. (1969). "Physiology of the Human Kidney." Grune & Stratton, New York.

Weston, R. E., Grossman, J., and Leiter, L. (1951). The effect of mercurial diuretics on renal ammonia and titratable acidity production in acidotic human subjects with reference to site of diuretic action. *J. Clin. Invest.* **30**, 1262–1271.

Weston, R. E., Escher, D. J. W., Grossman, J., and Leiter, L. (1952). Mechanisms contributing to unresponsiveness to mercurial diuretics in congestive heart failure. *J. Clin. Invest.* **31**, 901–910.

Whittembury, G., and Fishman, J. (1969). Relation between cell Na extrusion and transtubular absorption in the perfused toad kidney: The effect of K, ouabain and ethacrynic acid. *Arch. Ges. Physiol.* **307**, 138–153.

Whittembury, G., Oken, D. E., Windhager, E. E., and Solomon, A. K. (1959). Single proximal tubules of Necturus kidney. IV. Dependence of H_2O movement on osmotic gradients. *Am. J. Physiol.* **197**, 1121–1127.

Wiebelhaus, V. D., Weinstock, J., Maass, A. R., Brennan, F. T., Sosnowski, C., and Larsen, T. (1965). The diuretic and natriuretic activity of triamterene and several related pteridines in the rat. *J. Pharmacol. Exptl. Therap.* **149**, 397–403.

Wiederholt, M. (1966). Mikropunktionsuntersuchungen am proximalen und distalen Konvolut der Rattennicre über Einfluss von Actinomycin D auf den mineralocorticoid-abhängigen Na-transport. *Arch. Ges. Physiol.* **292**, 334–342.

Wiederholt, M., and Wiederholt, B. (1968). Der Einfluss von Dexamethason auf die Wasser- und Elektrolytausscheidung adrenalektomierter Ratten. *Arch. Ges. Physiol.* **302**, 57–78.

Wiederholt, M., Hierholzer, K., Rumrich, G., and Holzgreve, H. (1964). Transtubuläre Na-Ströme im proximalen und distalen Tubulus adrenalektomierter Ratten. *Arch. Ges. Physiol.* **281**, R95.

Wiederholt, M., Stolte, H., Brecht, J. P., and Hierholzer, K. (1966). Mikropunktionsuntersuchungen über den Einfluss von Aldosteron, Cortison und Dexamethason auf die renale Natriumresoprtion adrenalektomierter Ratten. *Arch. Ges. Physiol.* **292**, 316–333.

Wiederholt, M., Hierholzer, K., Windhager, E. E., and Giebisch, G. (1967). Microperfusion study of fluid reabsorption in proximal tubules of rat kidneys. *Am. J. Physiol.* **213**, 809–818.

Wilde, W. S., and Howard, P. J. (1960). Renal tubular action of ouabain on Na and K transport during stop-flow and slow-flow technique. *J. Pharmacol. Exptl. Therap.* **130**, 232–238.

Wilkins, J. W., Jr., Green, J. A., Jr., and Weller, J. M. (1965). Effect of renal arterial pressure on the stop-flow sodium minimum. *Am. J. Physiol.* **209**, 1034–1038.

Williams, R. L., Pearson, J. E., Jr., and Carter, M. K. (1965). The saluretic effects of arecoline hydrochloride infused into the left renal artery of dogs. *J. Pharmacol. Exptl. Therap.* **147**, 32–39.

Williamson, H. E. (1963). Mechanism of the antinatriuretic action of aldosterone. *Biochem. Pharmacol.* **12**, 1449–1450.

Williamson, H. E., Skulan, T. W., and Shideman, F. E. (1961). Effects of adrenalectomy and desoxycorticosterone on stop-flow patterns of sodium and potassium in the rat. *J. Pharmacol. Exptl. Therap.* **131**, 49–55.

Willis, L. R., Ludens, J. H., and Williamson, H. E. (1968). Dependence of the natriuretic action of acetylcholine upon an increase in renal blood flow. *Proc. Soc. Exptl. Biol. Med.* **128**, 1069–1072.

Windhager, E. E. (1964). Electrophysiologic study of renal papilla of golden hamsters. *Am. J. Physiol.* **206**, 694–700.

Windhager, E. E. (1968). "Micropuncture Techniques and Nephron Function." Appleton, New York.

Windhager, E. E., and Giebisch, G. (1965). Electrophysiology of the nephron. *Physiol. Rev.* **45**, 214–244.

Windhager, E. E., Whittembury, G., Oken, D. E., Schatzmann, H. J., and Solomon, A. K. (1959). Single proximal tubules of the Necturus kidney. III. Dependence of H_2O movement on NaCl concentration. *Am. J. Physiol.* **197**, 313–318.

Windhager, E. E., Boulpaep, E. L., and Giebisch, G. (1967). Electrophysiological studies on single nephrons. *Proc. 3rd Intern. Congr. Nephrol., Washington, 1966.* Vol. 1, pp. 35–47. Karger, Basel.

Windhager, E. E., Lewy, J. E., and Spitzer, A. (1969). Intrarenal control of proximal tubular reabsorption of sodium and water. *Nephron* **6**, 247–259.

Winton, F. R. (1952). Intrarenal pressure and renal blood flow. *Trans. 3rd Conf. Renal Function, New York, 1951*, pp. 51–102. Josiah Macy Jr. Foundation, New York.

Wirz, H. (1956). Der osmotische Druck in der corticalen Tubuli der Rattenniere. *Helv. Physiol. Pharmacol. Acta* **14**, 353–362.

Wiswell, J. G. (1961). Some effects of magnesium loading in patients with thyroid disorders. *J. Clin. Endocrinol. Metab.* **21**, 31–38.

Wright, F. S., Knox, F. G., Howards, S. S., and Berliner, R. W. (1969a). Reduced sodium reabsorption by the proximal tubule of the Doca-escaped dogs. *Am. J. Physiol.* **216**, 869–875.

Wright, F. S., Brenner, B. M., Bennett, C. M., Keimowitz, R. I., Berliner, R. W., Schrier, R. W., Verroust, P. J., de Wardener, H. E., and Holzgreve, H. (1969b). Failure to demonstrate a hormonal inhibitor of proximal sodium reabsorption. *J. Clin. Invest.* **48**, 1107–1113.

Yunis, S. L., Bercovitch, D. D., Stein, R. M., Levitt, M. F., and Goldstein, M. H. (1964). Renal tubular effects of hydrocortisone and aldosterone in normal hydropenic man: Comments on sites of action. *J. Clin. Invest.* **43**, 1668–1676.

4 | RENAL SECRETION OF HYDROGEN

Floyd C. Rector, Jr.

I. Introduction

The fluids of the body contain a variety of constituents capable of buffering acids and alkali which serve to prevent wide fluctuations in pH. All of the buffer systems in a given compartment (intracellular, extracellular) are in equilibrium and a change in one buffer pair (conjugate acid and base) results in parallel changes in the other buffer systems. Although some of the buffer systems can be partially modified by alterations in metabolism, the homeostatic control of hydrogen ion

209

concentration in body fluids is focused primarily on the CO_2–bicarbonate buffer system. The pCO_2 in body fluids is regulated by ventilation, while the concentration of bicarbonate in extracellular fluids is controlled by the kidneys.

The regulation of plasma bicarbonate concentration by the kidneys involves two major processes. First, bicarbonate in glomerular filtrate is reabsorbed by the tubule. This is primarily a conservation process, preventing excessive loss of bicarbonate into the urine when plasma bicarbonate is below a certain critical or threshold level. When plasma bicarbonate rises above this level, tubular reabsorption does not increase proportionately to the quantity of bicarbonate in the filtrate, but remains relatively constant; the excess bicarbonate is excreted and the plasma concentration returns toward the threshold level. Second, the kidney regenerates that bicarbonate which is decomposed by the accession of metabolic acids (primarily H_2SO_4 and H_3PO_4) into the extracellular fluid. The regenerative process in some way involves the reclamation of filtered sodium, the production of new bicarbonate, and the excretion of the acid anions along with an equivalent amount of hydrogen. Since the ability of the renal tubule to reduce urine pH is limited, the hydrogen must, to a large extent, be excreted bound to buffer. The buffer may be either filtered and excreted with hydrogen as titratable acid or it may be produced in the tubule as NH_3 and excreted with hydrogen as ammonium ions.

Thus, the overall process of urine acidification involves reabsorption of filtered bicarbonate, generation of titratable acid, and production of ammonia. In terms of acid–base balance, however, the important value is net acid excretion, which is the sum of titratable acid and ammonium minus the bicarbonate excreted into the urine. The difference between total acidification and net acid excretion is equal to bicarbonate reabsorption. Since bicarbonate reabsorption exceeds net acid excretion by approximately 25-fold, net acid excretion represents only a small fraction (approximately 3 to 5%) of total acidification.

The acidification of the urine can be characterized in several ways. The capacity of the system may be evaluated from the maximal ability to reabsorb filtered bicarbonate. As plasma bicarbonate concentration is progressively raised, tubular reabsorption increases until a maximum is reached. The process thus exhibits some of the properties of a tubular maximum or Tm. However, at plasma concentrations far above that at which maximum reabsorption is achieved, reabsorption is a roughly linear function of glomerular filtration rate (GFR) (Pitts and Lotspeich, 1946). The system, therefore, does not exhibit a true Tm, but instead displays a constant value for reabsorption per unit glomerular filtrate.

Although this value does not represent a Tm in the true sense, the maximal value for reabsorption per unit GFR at high plasma bicarbonate concentrations by convention is termed the bicarbonate Tm. For man and dog the bicarbonate Tm is approximately 2.5 to 2.8 mEq/100 ml GFR (Pitts and Lotspeich, 1946; Pitts et al., 1949), whereas in the rat a value closer to 4.0 mEq/100 is observed (Guignard, 1966).

The mechanism of urine acidification can also be characterized by the ability to generate pH gradients between urine and blood. The maximum gradients are achieved when plasma bicarbonate concentration has been reduced by metabolic acidosis. The lowest achievable urine pH is 4 to 4.5, which represents a pH gradient between urine and blood of approximately 3 to 3.5 units. The formation of titratable acid and the excretion of ammonia are both related to the degree of reduction in urine pH. The lower the urine pH the greater the amount of hydrogen that reacts with the filtered buffers (phosphate, creatinine) to form titratable acid and the greater the quantity of ammonia trapped in the urine as ammonium.

II. Localization of Acidification in the Nephron

A. Bicarbonate Reabsorption

On the basis of early clearance studies in dogs (Pitts and Alexander, 1945) and micropuncture studies in Necturus (Montgomery and Pierce, 1937) it appeared that approximately 80% of filtered bicarbonate was reabsorbed in the proximal tubule by some isohydric process, while removal of the final 20% of filtered bicarbonate, lowering of urine pH, formation of titratable acid, and addition of ammonia all occurred in the distal tubule. More recent micropuncture studies, however, indicate that all of these processes occur more or less simultaneously in all portions of the nephron. In the normal rat 50 to 70% of the filtrate is reabsorbed in the proximal tubule. Associated with this reduction in volume there is a depression of tubular fluid pH to 6.8-7.0 and tubular fluid bicarbonate to 8 to 10 mEq/liter (Gottschalk et al., 1960; Giebisch et al., 1960; Rector, 1964). Thus, 80 to 90% of filtered bicarbonate is reabsorbed in the proximal tubule. Approximately 10% of the filtrate enters the distal convoluted tubule with a pH of approximately 6.3 and a bicarbonate concentration of 2 mEq/liter. Roughly 15% of filtered bicarbonate, therefore, is reabsorbed between the end of the proximal convolution and the beginning of the distal convolution. Presumably both the pars recta and the loop of Henle participate in the acidification process. Of the remaining 1% of filtered bicarbonate delivered distally most is reabsorbed in the distal convolution and only a negligible fraction enters the collecting ducts. The collecting ducts, although having very little capacity for acidification, appear to be the site for the final steep reduction in tubular fluid pH when buffer excretion is low (Ullrich et al., 1958; Hierholzer, 1961; Rector, 1964). However, when buffer excretion is high, the contribution of the collecting duct is trivial and the minimal pH is achieved by the end of the distal convolution (Rector, 1964). Qualitatively, a similar pattern of acidification is observed in the dog, although the concentration of bicarbonate in the proximal tubule is only slightly lower than the plasma level. During metabolic acidosis, however, proximal bicarbonate is reduced to approximately half the plasma concentration (Clapp, 1965; Clapp et al., 1965). The pattern of acidification in the Rhesus monkey appears to be similar to that observed in the rat (Bennett et al., 1968).

B. Titratable Acid Formation

The reduction of proximal pH results in the titration of the nonbicarbonate buffers in tubular fluid and suggests that the proximal tubule might participate in the formation of titratable acid. As far as the contribution to titratable acid in the final urine the role of the proximal tubule is questionable. If there were no further acidification beyond the proximal tubule, the reduction in volume of tubular fluid in a CO_2 permeable segment of the nephron would raise both the concentration of bicarbonate and the pH in the residual fluid (Gottschalk et al., 1960). The titratable acid would thus be dissipated by reaction with bicarbonate. Certainly, the titratable acid formed in the proximal tubule represents acid that can eventually appear in the urine, but this requires continued reabsorption of bicarbonate in the more distal portions of the nephron as tubular volume is progressively reduced.

C. Ammonia Secretion

From micropuncture studies it is apparent that ammonia is also secreted in both the proximal and distal portions of the nephron. In normal rat approximately 70% of excreted ammonia is present by the end of the proximal tubule (Glabman et al., 1963; Hayes et al., 1964). In normal dogs, ammonia is not detectable in proximal tubular fluid, but during metabolic acidosis approximately 50 to 70% of total urinary ammonia appears to be added in the proximal tubule (Clapp et al., 1965).

The significance of the ammonia added to proximal tubular fluid is not clear. Most likely ammonia is produced throughout the renal cortex and the rapidly diffusible NH_3 is in equilibrium throughout the cortex (Pitts, 1964). The total amount of ammonia in any tubular fluid compartment will be determined by tubular fluid pH, according to the reaction

$$NH_3 + H^+ \rightleftharpoons NH_4^+ \quad \text{(cell)}$$
$$\Updownarrow$$
$$NH_3 + H^+ \rightleftharpoons NH_4^+ \quad \text{(tubular fluid)}$$

Thus, the rate of ammonia excretion is determined by the pNH_3 of the renal cortex and the pH of the *final* tubular fluid, irrespective of whether or not ammonia is added to proximal tubular fluid. It is possible, however, that proximal tubular fluid might contribute ammonia directly to the terminal urine by means of changes occurring in the loop of Henle (Hayes *et al.*, 1966; Robinson and Owen, 1965; Sullivan, 1965). Ammonia-containing fluid leaving the proximal tubule is partially alkalinized by the process of water reabsorption in the descending limb of Henle's loop. At the same time fluid in the collecting duct is acidified. The pH gradient between the loop of Henle and the collecting duct favors the release of ammonia from loop fluid and trapping as ammonium in collecting duct fluid. Proximal fluid, therefore, may bypass the distal convolution and contribute its ammonia directly to the final urine. The advantage of this system is that, since ammonia is not formed in the medulla, the proximal tubular fluid serves as a source with which the terminal acidic tubular fluid can equilibrate. If this were not the case, the final pH drop occurring in the collecting duct would have little effect in augmenting ammonia excretion.

III. Mechanism of Urinary Acidification

A variety of possibilities have been suggested as mechanisms for acidifying urine. For many years it was recognized that acidification of the urine could be accomplished either by reabsorption of filtered alkali (e.g., $NaHCO_3$, Na_2HPO_4) leaving behind the filtered acids (H_2CO_3, NaH_2PO_4) or by secretion of acids into the tubular fluid. The experiments of Pitts and Alexander (1945) unequivocally demonstrated that the quantity of filtered H_2CO_3 and NaH_2PO_4 could not account for maximal rates of titratable acid excretion in acidotic dogs infused with sodium phosphate. They concluded that reabsorption of the alkaline portion of filtered buffers, while leaving the residual filtered acids in tubular fluid, could not account for maximal rates of acid excretion and that in some manner acid must be added to tubular fluid. These authors favored the view that cellular hydrogen was secreted in exchange for filtered sodium, although the secretion of molecular acids (HCl or H_3PO_4) or the generation of acid in the tubule [reabsorption of the hydroxyl of water thus liberating hydrogen; reabsorption of one carbonate from two bicarbonates generating one H_2CO_3 (Menaker, 1948); or sodium bicarbonate reabsorption coupled with the intratubular formation of H_2CO_3 from hydration of CO_2 as tubular bicarbonate concentration falls (Menaker, 1948)] could not be excluded. The secretion of molecular acids such as HCl, H_3PO_4, or H_2SO_4 was considered unlikely in view of the fact that no net secretion of chloride, phosphate, or sulfate can be demonstrated. The reabsorption of carbonate or hydroxyl ions did not appear likely because of the extremely low concentrations of these ions in biologic fluids, particularly in acid tubular fluid. Although certain of the proposed mechanisms of acidification can be excluded rather easily, it is much more difficult to choose between a mechanism involving hydrogen secretion and one involving $NaHCO_3$ reabsorption coupled with the hydration of CO_2 (diffusing into the lumen from plasma through CO_2-permeable tubular epithelium) to generate new H_2CO_3, which can then react with nonbicarbonate buffers to form titratable acid and ammonium ions.

Several lines of evidence have been adduced to favor the thesis that acidification in both proximal and distal tubules is mediated by a single process involving the secretion of cellular hydrogen, which is derived from the hydration of CO_2 under the catalytic influence of carbonic anhydrase. First, the high CO_2 tensions observed in alkaline urines have been interpreted by Pitts and Lotspeich (1946) as evidence of hydrogen secretion in the distal tubule. This finding, however, can also be explained by water abstraction in the collecting duct, thereby raising the concentration of bicarbonate and pH, and initiating a reaction between bicarbonate and the nonbicarbonate buffers (Reid and Hills, 1965). Second, inhibition of carbonic anhydrase with acetazolamide not only diminishes the excretion of ammonia and titratable acid, but can also promote the excretion of approximately 40% of the filtered bicarbonate. From this high rate of bicarbonate excretion Berliner (1952) concluded that acidification in both proximal and distal tubules is mediated by a carbonic anhydrase-dependent hydrogen secretory mechanism. Micropuncture studies have confirmed that acetazolamide inhibits acidification in the proximal tubule (Gottschalk *et al.*, 1960; Clapp *et al.*, 1963a), but as yet there is no direct demonstration of any role of carbonic anhydrase in the distal tubule. Moreover, carbonic anhydrase might facilitate acidification in a number of different ways [carrier-facilitated movement of bicarbonate either into the cell or from cell into blood; carrier-facilitated diffusion of CO_2 (Enns, 1967); intracellular catalysis of $CO_2 + H_2O$ or $CO_2 + OH^-$]; consequently, the demonstration of carbonic anhydrase-dependence does not prove hydrogen secretion. Third, the maximum rate of urinary acidification, as estimated from the bicarbonate Tm is augmented by raising and depressed by lowering CO_2 tension of plasma, presumably by an effect of CO_2 on intracellular pH (Brazeau and Gilman, 1953; Relman *et al.*, 1953; Dorman *et al.*, 1954). Although these observations *in toto* strongly suggest a hydrogen secretory mechanism, they do not conclusively establish that the mechanisms of acidification in proximal and distal tubules are identical nor do they exclude the possibility that direct reabsorption of bicarbonate ions participates to some extent in acidification of the urine.

The consequences of these two mechanisms, hydrogen secretion on the one hand and bicarbonate reabsorption on the other on intratubular pH_{tf} are entirely different and provide a theoretical basis for distinguishing between the two possibilities. As shown in Fig. 1, the secretion of hydrogen reacts with filtered bicarbonate to form H_2CO_3. The dehydration of H_2CO_3 to CO_2 is not instantaneous, consequently excess H_2CO_3 accumulates in the tubular fluid and lowers the pH below that predicted were H_2CO_3 and CO_2 in complete equilibrium (Walser and Mudge, 1960). The magnitude of the disequilibrium in the proximal tubule of the rat can be calculated as follows: Approximately 80% of

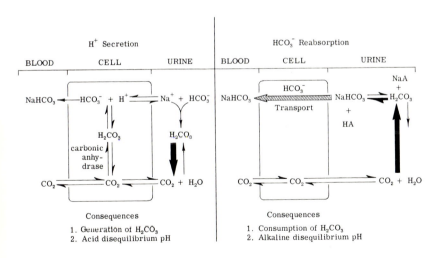

FIG. 1.   The theoretical portrayal of effects of hydrogen secretion versus bicarbonate reabsorption.

the filtered bicarbonate (20 mEq/liter filtrate) is reabsorbed in the proximal tubule. The transit time through the proximal tubule, estimated from the passage of lissamine green, is approximately 10 seconds (Rector et al., 1966). Thus, a given volume of filtrate is in contact with the proximal convoluted tubule only 10 seconds. The rate at which H_2CO_3 would be generated by proximal hydrogen secretion would be 2 mEq/liter/second. In a steady state the rate at which H_2CO_3 breaks down to CO_2 must also equal 2 mEq/liter/second. Assuming no diffusion of H_2CO_3 out of the tubule and the absence of carbonic anhydrase in the lumen, the luminal concentration of H_2CO_3, $[H_2CO_3]_L$, necessary to achieve this rate (R) of uncatalyzed breakdown can be calculated from the expression

$$R = K_{H_2CO_3}[H_2CO_3]_L - K_{CO_2}[CO_2]_L$$

where $K_{H_2CO_3} = 30$ sec^{-1}, $K_{CO_2} = 0.043$ sec^{-1} (Maren, 1967), and $[CO_2]_L =$ $[CO_2]_{plasma} = 1.2$ mmole/liter. The calculated $[H_2CO_3]_L$ is approximately 68 μmole/liter in contrast to the equilibrium concentration of 1.8 μmole/L. By substituting this value into the Henderson-Hasselbalch equation, assuming a true p$K_{H_2CO_3}$ of 3.57 and a tubular fluid bicarbonate concentration of 10 mEq/liter, an intratubular pH of 5.74 is obtained. In contrast, the calculated equilibrium pH (using the same bicarbonate concentration of 10 mEq/liter and an apparent p$K_{H_2CO_3}$ of 6.1) is 7.05. The difference between these two, which is termed the disequilibrium pH, is 1.3 units.

Direct reabsorption of bicarbonate ions, on the other hand, would not generate H_2CO_3 (Fig. 1). In fact, as the concentration of bicarbonate falls, the reaction of nonbicarbonate buffers with H_2CO_3 to form $NaHCO_3$ and titratable acid would lower the concentration of H_2CO_3 below its equilibrium concentration and generate an alkaline disequilibrium pH. This would result in the diffusion of CO_2 from plasma into the lumen, assuming the tubular epithelium were permeable to CO_2, and the generation of new H_2CO_3. However, the slow rate at which CO_2 is hydrated to H_2CO_3 would seriously limit the ability of this mechanism to form titratable acid. Berliner (1957) calculated that, if tubular fluid were not in contact with carbonic anhydrase, the uncatalyzed intratubular hydration of CO_2 is inadequate to account for the maximal rates of titratable acid excretion. A similar criticism can be raised against this as the mechanism of proximal acidification in either the rat or acidotic dog. The transformation of glomerular filtrate containing approximately 2.5 mmole/liter of phosphate to a fluid at pH 6.8 at the end of the proximal tubule generates approximately 0.7 mmole of titratable acid per liter of tubular fluid. The contact time per unit proximal tubular fluid is only 10 seconds, therefore the rate of titratable acid formation is 0.07 mmole/liter/second. This is the required rate at which H_2CO_3 must be formed from CO_2 in tubular fluid for this model to work. The maximum rate of H_2CO_3 formation (assuming luminal H_2CO_3 is reduced to such an exceedingly low concentration that the back reaction is negligible) is only

$$[CO_2]_{plasma} K_{CO_2} = (1.2 \text{ mmole/liter})$$
$$(0.043 \text{ sec}^{-1}) = 0.052 \text{ mmole/liter/second}$$

a value less than the required rate. For this mechanism to work, therefore, it would be essential that the tubular fluid be exposed to the catalytic effects of carbonic anhydrase.

It has been possible to distinguish between these two mechanisms by comparing the *in situ* intratubular pH and the pH of luminal fluid removed from the tubule and permitted to reach equilibrium (Rector *et al.*, 1965). The intratubular pH was measured directly with pH-sensitive glass microelectrodes inserted into the tubular lumina of rat kidney and the equilibrium pH was measured by aspirating tubular fluid into quinhydrone microelectrodes equilibrated with 5% CO_2. In the distal tubule of rats undergoing $NaHCO_3$ diuresis the intratubular pH was always lower than the equilibrium pH (Table I). The average difference (disequilibrium pH) was 0.85 pH units. This difference was obliterated by injecting carbonic anhydrase intravenously in amounts sufficient to

TABLE I

COMPARISON OF *in Vivo* INTRATUBULAR pH AND *in Vitro* EQUILIBRIUM pH OF PROXIMAL AND DISTAL TUBULAR FLUID[a]

Location	Treatment	*1* Intratubular pH	*2* Equilibrium pH	[1 − 2] Disequilibrium pH
Distal	$NaHCO_3$ infusion	6.85	7.73	−0.85
	$NaHCO_3$ infusion + carbonic anhydrase[b]	7.67	7.70	−0.03
Proximal	None	6.82	6.88	−0.06
	NaH_2PO_4 infusion	6.87	6.82	+0.05
	$NaHCO_3$ infusion	7.53	7.49	+0.04
	$NaHCO_3$ infusion + Cl-11,366[c]	6.71	7.56	−0.85

[a]Rector *et al.* (1965).

[b]Carbonic anhydrase infused intravenously to produce high levels of activity in the urine.

[c]CL-11,366—the potent carbonic anhydrase inhibitor, 2-benzenesulfonamido-1,3,4-thiadiazole-5 sulfonamide.

give high levels of activity in the urine. This effect of carbonic anhydrase proved that the disequilibrium pH was due to excess H_2CO_3 and that distal reabsorption of bicarbonate is mediated by secretion of hydrogen.

In contrast, in the proximal tubule the intratubular pH and the equilibrium pH were the same during both $NaHCO_3$ and Na_2HPO_4 diuresis (Table I). The absence of an acid disequilibrium during $NaHCO_3$ diuresis is clearly not compatible with the hydrogen secretory model, while the absence of an alkaline disequilibrium during Na_2HPO_4 is incompatible with the direct reabsorption of bicarbonate ions as shown in Fig. 1. This paradox necessitates that proximal tubular fluid be in contact with carbonic anhydrase, irrespective of which of the two basic mechanisms is operative.

Inhibition of carbonic anhydrase should clearly differentiate between these two mechanisms, giving an acid disequilibrium pH if hydrogen secretion were operative and a slight alkaline disequilibrium pH if bicarbonate reabsorption were involved. As shown in Table I, proximal intratubular pH was always significantly less than the equilibrium pH following inhibition of carbonic anhydrase. The average disequilibrium pH was 0.85 units. This clearly establishes that bicarbonate reabsorption in the proximal, as well as the distal tubule, is mediated by the secretion of hydrogen ions.

These results were recently confirmed by Vieira and Malnic (1968), who used micro-antimony electrodes for measuring intratubular pH. They found an acid disequilibrium pH normally present in the distal, but not in the proximal tubule. After inhibition of carbonic anhydrase with acetazolamide, an acid disequilibrium pH was also present in the proximal tubule.

IV. Localization of Carbonic Anhydrase

A. Functional Studies

The results of both Rector *et al.* (1965) and Vieira and Malnic (1968) clearly establish that hydrogen secretion is the major mechanism for acidification of tubular fluid in both proximal and distal tubules. The hydrogen secretory mechanisms in these two areas of the nephron, however, differ markedly with respect to the role of carbonic anhydrase (Fig. 2). Apart from its cellular action in maintaining intracellular concentration of hydrogen by catalyzing the hydration of CO_2, carbonic anhydrase subserves an additional function in the proximal tubule. Carbonic anhydrase appears to be in functional contact with proximal

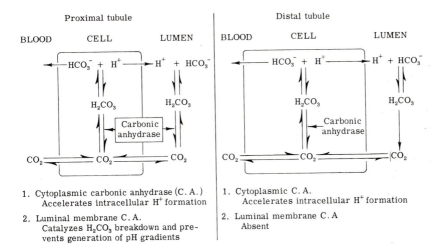

FIG. 2.   Role of carbonic anhydrase in facilitating hydrogen secretion in proximal and distal tubules.

tubular fluid so that H_2CO_3 formed by the reaction of secreted hydrogen with filtered bicarbonate is rapidly broken down to CO_2 and H_2O. Carbonic anhydrase, presumably located in the luminal membrane, prevents the accumulation of excess H_2CO_3. As a result of this action, the steady-state intratubular pH is approximately 1.0 to 1.5 units higher than it would be if carbonic anhydrase were not present in the luminal membrane. In the proximal tubule, therefore, carbonic anhydrase facilitates the transport of large quantities of hydrogen by both furnishing a supply of hydrogen and preventing the generation of steep pH gradients.

In contrast, the distal tubule does not contain carbonic anhydrase in its luminal membrane and must always secrete hydrogen against a concentration gradient even in the presence of high bicarbonate concentrations. As a consequence, pH in distal fluid is relatively constant despite wide variations in buffer and bicarbonate concentrations. What physiologic purpose is achieved by this omission of luminal carbonic anhydrase and the presence of a persistent pH gradient is not clear. If hydrogen gradients between distal tubule and blood were to contribute in any way to distal transtubular potential differences, then the absence of carbonic anhydrase in the luminal membrane would prevent wide variations in the potential difference as bicarbonate and buffer excretion fluctuates. This in turn might stabilize those distal functions, such as potassium excretion, which appear to be dependent in some way on distal potential differences (Giebisch et al., 1966).

B. Biochemical and Histochemical Studies

In view of the differences in the hydrogen secretory mechanism in the proximal and distal tubules, the localization of carbonic anhydrase within the kidneys becomes very important. Early biochemical studies were interpreted as showing that carbonic anhydrase was located only in the soluble fraction of the cell, with none in the particulate fractions (Datta and Shepard, 1959). However, studies by Karler and Woodbury (1960) and by Maren (1967) have demonstrated that roughly 10% of the total renal carbonic anhydrase activity is tightly bound to the endoplasmic reticulum. This finding therefore is consistent with the functional data indicating a fraction of carbonic anhydrase to be located in the luminal membrane of proximal tubular cells.

Carbonic anhydrase has been clearly demonstrated in both proximal and distal tubules by analysis of isolated tubules (Pollak *et al.*, 1965) and by histochemical stains for enzyme activity (Häusler, 1958). The histochemical staining technique (Häusler, 1958), which is dependent on the precipitation of $CoCO_3$ at sites of enzyme activity with subsequent conversion of $CoCO_3$ to CoS, gives different patterns in proximal and distal tubules. In the proximal tubule there is dense localization of enzyme along the peritubular membrane with less intense activity throughout the remainder of the cytoplasm; in addition there is precipitation of CoS in the tubular lumen, suggesting that the tubular fluid is exposed to enzymatic activity. In contrast, the distal tubule shows only diffuse activity throughout the cell cytoplasm without the dense localization along the peritubular surface, and, more importantly, without precipitate in the tubular lumen. These histochemical studies, while open to criticism concerning the specificity of the measurement, are consistent with the conclusion based on the measurements of intratubular pH that luminal fluid is exposed to carbonic anhydrase activity in the proximal but not in the distal tubule.

C. Consequences of Luminal Carbonic Anhydrase in the Proximal Tubule

1. Effect of Acetazolamide on Bicarbonate Titration Curves

In normal dogs, reabsorption of filtered bicarbonate is virtually complete at low plasma bicarbonate concentrations. As plasma bicarbonate concentration is progressively increased, reabsorption increases proportionately until a threshold is reached. Further increases in plasma bicarbonate increase reabsorption only modestly until a maximum reabsorptive capacity of Tm is achieved (Fig. 3). At the threshold level reabsorption is functioning at approximately 75% of its maximum ca-

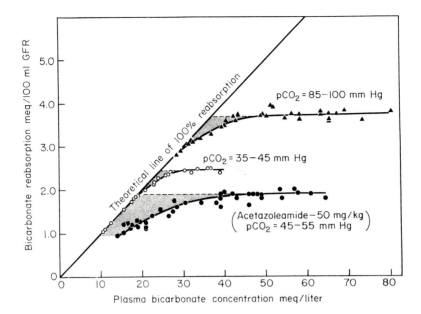

FIG. 3. Effect of plasma pCO_2 and acetazolamide on the relation between bicarbonate reabsorption and plasma bicarbonate concentration. The stippled area indicates bicarbonate excretion before the Tm was reached (Rector *et al.*, 1960).

pacity. A similar pattern is observed in respiratory acidosis (Fig. 3). It would appear that when the normal system is functioning close to Tm levels it cannot effect complete bicarbonate reabsorption, possibly because of sensitivity of the distal tubule to luminal pH when transporting at near-maximal rates. The splay of the normal titration curve, therefore, may be a function of the disequilibrium pH normally present in the distal tubule.

The shape of the bicarbonate titration curve is markedly different after administration of acetazolamide (Schwartz *et al.*, 1958; Rector *et al.*, 1960). It is evident from Figs. 3 and 4 that inhibition of carbonic anhydrase impairs the ability to generate a bicarbonate-free urine even at very low plasma bicarbonate concentrations. This inability to reabsorb bicarbonate completely is not the consequence of diminished intracellular hydrogen production, since raising arterial pCO_2 elevated the bicarbonate Tm but did not diminish the marked splaying of the bicarbonate titration curve (Fig. 4).

The most likely explanation of this phenomenon hinges about the role of carbonic anhydrase in the luminal membrane of the proximal tubule. Since luminal carbonic anhydrase prevents the accumulation of

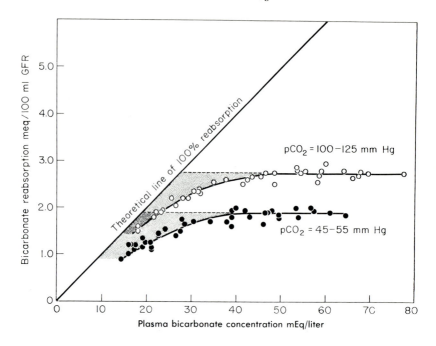

Fɪɢ. 4.   Failure of respiratory acidosis to eliminate the splay in the bicarbonate titration curve induced by acetazolamide (Rector *et al.*, 1960).

excess H_2CO_3, intratubular pH would not fall to limiting values until the reabsorption of bicarbonate was nearing completion. However, when carbonic anhydrase is inhibited, H_2CO_3 accumulates in the luminal fluid, lowering intratubular pH to a limiting value despite the presence of significant amounts of bicarbonate. As a result of the low intratubular pH, proximal hydrogen secretion would stop before bicarbonate concentration in the tubular fluid is significantly reduced. Consequently, the distal tubule is continually flooded with fluid containing a high bicarbonate concentration even during severe metabolic acidosis; the capacity of the distal tubule to reabsorb bicarbonate would be exceeded and bicarbonate would be excreted into the urine.

2. Effect of Acetazolamide on Urinary pCO_2

A second observation that may be explained by the luminal effects of carbonic anhydrase in the proximal tubule is the differing effects of $NaHCO_3$ and acetazolamide on urine CO_2 tensions. Guignard (1966) has recently observed that for a given level of bicarbonate and buffer excretion, the CO_2 tension gradient between urine and blood (urine pCO$_2$ — blood pCO$_2$) was greater following the administration of acetazolamide than during NaHCO$_3$ infusions. The most likely explanation for this finding is that, after inhibition of carbonic anhydrase, fluid leaving the proximal tubule and entering the loop of Henle contains excess H$_2$CO$_3$. In the loop of Henle H$_2$CO$_3$ would break down, tubular pH would rise, and acidic nonbicarbonate buffers would react with bicarbonate to form more H$_2$CO$_3$; this would generate a high medullary pCO$_2$ and raise the pCO$_2$ in collecting duct fluid.

3. EFFECT OF ACETAZOLAMIDE ON PROXIMAL AMMONIA

A third observation explained by the development of a proximal disequilibrium pH following inhibition of carbonic anhydrase is the differing effects of NaHCO$_3$ infusions and acetazolamide on proximal ammonia. Both NaHCO$_3$ infusions and acetazolamide raise the equilibrium pH (measured with quinhydrone electrodes) in the proximal tubule to approximately the same degree, yet NaHCO$_3$ obliterates proximal ammonia while acetazolamide has no effect on ammonia concentration (Hayes et al., 1966). Because of the disequilibrium pH in the proximal tubule acetazolamide has little effect on the actual intratubular pH despite the marked increase in bicarbonate concentration. Consequently, the pH-dependent trapping of ammonia as ammonium in proximal tubular fluid would be unaffected by acetazolamide. In contrast, NaHCO$_3$ infusions raise not only the equilibrium pH, but also the actual intratubular pH. Thus, the trapping of ammonium in proximal tubular fluid would be greatly diminished.

V. Source of Secreted Hydrogen

A. CO$_2$ and Water

The demonstration of an acid disequilibrium pH in the distal tubule normally and in the proximal tubule after inhibition of carbonic anhydrase, although establishing acid secretion as the primary mechanism involved in the acidification of tubular fluid, provides no insight into whether the acid is secreted into tubular fluid in molecular form (HCl, H$_3$PO$_4$, H$_2$SO$_4$) or by some direct or indirect exchange hydrogen for tubular sodium. The original argument of Pitts and Alexander (1945) against the molecular secretion of acid, namely that there is no good evidence for net secretion of any of the anions (not withstanding the probability of bidirectional flux across the tubule for both chloride and phosphate) still seems to be a relevant criticism, particularly when one considers the magnitude of the hydrogen secretion involved in the reabsorption of filtered bicarbonate.

The quantity of hydrogen involved in bicarbonate reabsorption far exceeds the supply of hydrogen arising from metabolism. The only means capable of supplying this demand is the diffusion of plasma CO_2 into the cell where it interacts with water or its products under the catalytic impact of carbonic anhydrase: (1) CO_2 may react with water to form H_2CO_3, which then contributes its hydrogen directly to the transport mechanism, or (2) hydroxyl ions produced when water is split in the process of pumping hydrogen out of the cell may react with CO_2 to form bicarbonate ions. Kinetic studies on the nature of the interaction between CO_2 and carbonic anhydrase suggest that bicarbonate rather than H_2CO_3 is the substrate bound to the enzyme (Maren, 1967). The reaction between CO_2 and hydroxyl ions to form bicarbonate, therefore, is the intracellular process most likely involved in the hydrogen secretory mechanism. Whichever of these two reactions are involved, however, it is clear that the rate of hydrogen secretion should be dependent on both the activity of carbonic anhydrase and the partial pressure of CO_2 in the renal tubular cell.

B. Role of pCO_2 and Carbonic Anhydrase Activity

Both carbonic anhydrase activity and plasma pCO_2 have been unequivocally shown to be determinants of the rate of hydrogen secretion. Inhibition of carbonic anhydrase prevents the elaboration of an acid urine, obliterates titratable acid formation, and promotes the excretion of a large fraction of filtered bicarbonate; although the rate of hydrogen secretion is seriously depressed, it is not completely abolished. The CO_2 tension of plasma also has a significant effect on the rate of hydrogen secretion with hypercapnea increasing and hypocapnea decreasing the bicarbonate Tm. Hypercapnea has been observed to exert some effect after complete inhibition of carbonic anhydrase, suggesting that these two factors may influence hydrogen secretion in a partially independent fashion.

The relative contributions of CO_2 tension and carbonic anhydrase activity to the maximum rate of hydrogen secretion, as well as the interdependence of their actions, have been extensively studied (Rector et al., 1960). The results of these studies are summarized below. The relation between the bicarbonate Tm and plasma pCO_2 is shown in Fig. 5. Normally the bicarbonate Tm is approximately 2.8 meq/100 ml GFR at a pCO_2 of 40 mm Hg. The bicarbonate Tm falls to 1.5 meq/100 ml

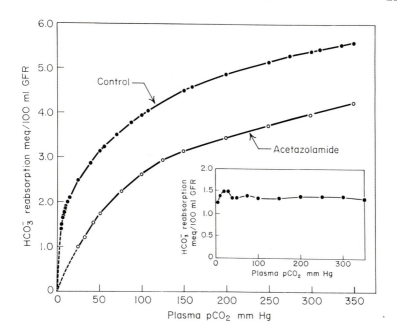

Fig. 5. Comparison of the relation between bicarbonate reabsorption and plasma pCO₂ with and without acetazolamide. The contribution of the carbonic anhydrase enzyme system at all levels of plasma pCO₂ is plotted in the inset as the difference between the upper and lower curves (Rector *et al.*, 1960).

GFR when pCO_2 is reduced to 10 mm Hg and increases progressively, although not in a linear fashion, when pCO_2 is elevated to very high levels. The failure of the bicarbonate Tm to increase proportionately as pCO_2 is raised may be due to partial saturation of the hydrogen transport system at higher CO_2 tensions. However, since the measurement of the bicarbonate Tm during severe hypercapnea requires very high plasma concentrations of bicarbonate, the curvilinear character of the curve in Fig. 5 may reflect in part the superimposed effects of ECF volume expansion rather than the intrinsic kinetics of the hydrogen secretory system.

Plasma pCO_2 is thought to influence bicarbonate reabsorption through its effects on the intracellular concentration of hydrogen ions, either by furnishing a plentiful supply of H_2CO_3 to the hydrogen transport system or by neutralizing hydroxyl ions generated by the pumping of hydrogen out of the cell. Both of these reactions are dependent on the enzyme carbonic anhydrase, thus it might be predicted that the sensitivity of the system to pCO_2 would be severely restricted following the inhibition of carbonic anhydrase. As shown by the lower curve in Fig. 5, this is clearly not the case; the hydrogen secretory mechanism is just as sensitive to pCO_2 folllowing the administration of a large dose of acetazolamide (20 mg/kg) as in the presence of an intact carbonic anhydrase enzyme system. It appears, therefore, that the regulatory effect of pCO_2 on the capacity to reabsorb bicarbonate is independent of carbonic anhydrase.

In contrast, the contribution of carbonic anhydrase activity to the bicarbonate Tm appears to be completely independent of pCO_2, at least over the range examined. A comparison of the relationship between the bicarbonate Tm and plasma pCO_2 in the presence and absence of carbonic anhydrase activity (upper and lower curves of Fig. 5) discloses that the difference between the two values (plotted in the insert of Fig. 5) is constant at all CO_2 tensions studied. The contribution of the carbonic anhydrase enzyme system to the bicarbonate Tm is approximately 1.4 meq/100 ml GFR and is completely independent of pCO_2.

On the basis of these studies it was suggested that bicarbonate reabsorption is mediated by two distinct hydrogen secretory mechanisms: one which is pCO_2-dependent, but carbonic anhydrase-independent, and a second which is carbonic anhydrase-dependent, pCO_2-independent. It was also suggested that these might represent spatially separate mechanisms located in different parts of the nephron. Recent micropuncture studies indicate, however, that carbonic anhydrase and pCO_2 exert their effects in the same area of the nephron, at least as far as the proximal tubule is concerned. Several different investigators (Gottschalk et al., 1960; Clapp et al., 1963a; Rector et al., 1965; Bennett et al., 1968) have found that acetazolamide inhibits bicarbonate reabsorption in the proximal convoluted tubule of the rat, dog, and squirrel monkey. The magnitude of the proximal inhibition, however, is not completely clear. Acetazolamide causes only a slight reduction in the proximal tubular fluid to plasma inulin ratio (Dirks et al., 1966), thus the fraction of filtered water reabsorbed in the proximal convoluted tubule is only slightly depressed. Clapp et al. (1963a) found that after acetazolamide proximal tubular bicarbonate concentrations, measured in CO_2-equilibrated quinhydrone microelectrodes, were almost double that of the plasma concentration. They calculated that proximal bicarbonate reabsorption was virtually abolished by inhibition of carbonic anhydrase. Other investigators (Frick, Kunau, Jr., Rector, Jr., and Seldin, unpublished data), however, have found that tubular fluid bicarbonate concentrations only occasionally exceed that of plasma following inhibition of carbonic anhydrase. If acetazolamide raised tubular fluid bicarbonate concentrations 10 to 20 mEq/liter above the plasma concentration, then the constraint of proximal isotonicity would necessitate a similar fall in the concentration of tubular fluid chloride below the level of the plasma chloride concentration; the tubular fluid to plasma chloride concentration ratio should fall significantly below 1.0, to a level between 0.8 and 0.9. Frick and associates found that the tubular fluid-to-plasma chloride ratios fell toward, but not below 1.0 following the administration of acetazolamide; the average TF/P chloride was 1.04. The failure of the TF/P chloride to fall below 1.0 was not the consequence of an induced metabolic acidosis, since similar results were obtained when plasma bicarbonate concentrations were raised to high levels by $NaHCO_3$ infusions. In part this discrepancy may be due to the considerable inaccuracies inherent in measuring bicarbonate concentrations in alkaline fluids with quinhydrone microelectrodes. In particular, slight losses of CO_2 from the electrode system can easily produce spuriously high values for bicarbonate concentration. The chloride method, on the other hand, is inherently much more accurate. The combined results of TF/P chloride, quinhydrone, and TF/P inulin measurements suggest that inhibition of carbonic anhydrase in the rat does not completely inhibit proximal bicarbonate reabsorption but does reduce it from a control level of 80% to a level of 40% of filtered bicarbonate reabsorbed.

The demonstration of a proximal action of pCO_2 has been much more difficult. In preliminary experiments both Clapp (1965) and Kunau and associates (1966) were unable to demonstrate any effect of pCO_2 on proximal bicarbonate reabsorption. The difficulty with such an experiment resides in the fact that in order to demonstrate an effect of pCO_2 it is necessary to induce metabolic alkalosis so that filtered bicarbonate is not rate-limiting. This in turn expands extracellular fluid (ECF) volume which may suppress proximal reabsorption and completely obscure the effects of hypercapnea. When these studies were repeated taking great care to control both the plasma concentration of bicarbonate and the degree of ECF volume expansion, hypercapnea could be clearly shown to stimulate proximal reabsorption of bicarbonate (Frick et al., unpublished observations). Under these conditions the concentration of bicarbonate at the end of the proximal convolution was 22 mEq/liter at a pCO_2 of 33 mm Hg and 13 mEq/liter at a pCO_2 of 90 mm Hg. These micropuncture studies, therefore, establish that pCO_2, as well as carbonic anhydrase activity, influences the rate of hydrogen secretion in the proximal tubule.

On the basis of the micropuncture studies, it can be concluded that the ability to characterize bicarbonate reabsorption into a pCO_2-dependent, carbonic anhydrase-independent and a carbonic anhydrase-dependent, pCO_2-independent system cannot be ascribed to two distinct hydrogen secretory mechanisms situated in different parts of the nephron. The apparent lack of interaction between the regulatory effects of carbonic anhydrase and CO_2 tension (Fig. 5) on a single hydrogen secretory mechanism might be explained as follows. The major contribution of carbonic anhydrase might be related to its location in the luminal membrane of the proximal tubule and its role in dissipating luminal H_2CO_3 generated by the process of hydrogen secretion. Inhibition of carbonic anhydrase blocks this process, resulting in the accumulation of excess H_2CO_3 and the generation of a rate-limiting disequilibrium pH. For this reason alone, independent of any intracellular effects of the enzyme, the rate of hydrogen secretion would diminish. Moreover, this process would be virtually independent of pCO_2, since as CO_2 tension is raised the intracellular concentration of H_2CO_3, the rate of luminal generation of H_2CO_3, and the luminal concentration of H_2CO_3 would all increase more or less proportionately; the limiting pH gradient imposed by the disequilibrium in the luminal fluid would be approximately the same at all CO_2 tensions. Thus, if the major contribution of carbonic anhydrase to the system were its luminal action, this fraction of the bicarbonate Tm would be pCO_2-independent.

The nature of the mechanism mediating bicarbonate reabsorption after inhibition of carbonic anhydrase has been the subject of considerable controversy. Maren (1967) has presented evidence that high doses of acetazolamide and other carbonic anhydrase inhibitors completely inhibit renal carbonic anhydrase (greater than 99.9% inhibition) and that the reaction between CO_2 and H_2O must be completely reduced to the uncatalyzed rate. Despite this extreme degree of inhibition, bicarbonate reabsorption proceeds at an appreciable rate following administration of the inhibitor. Maren (1967) has calculated that the uncatalyzed hydration of CO_2 can account for only 10 to 20% of the observed rate of bicarbonate reabsorption, and has suggested that the reabsorption of bicarbonate following inhibition of the enzyme is mediated by direct reabsorption of bicarbonate ions rather than hydrogen secretion.

Two lines of evidence, however, are against such an interpretation. First, bicarbonate reabsorption following administration of acetazolamide is almost completely CO_2-dependent, as shown by the lower curve in Fig. 5; at an extrapolated CO_2 tension of zero there appears to be little if any residual bicarbonate reabsorption. Second, the marked acid disequilibrium pH (0.8 units) observed in the proximal tubule after the administration of a potent carbonic anhydrase inhibitor

(Table I) indicates that most, if not all, of the bicarbonate was reabsorbed by a process involving hydrogen secretion. After inhibition of carbonic anhydrase in the rat approximately 40% of filtered bicarbonate is reabsorbed in the proximal tubule. This is approximately 12 mEq/liter of filtrate or 1.2 mEq/liter/second. From this rate the calculated intraluminal concentration of H_2CO_3 would be 18 μmole/liter and the intratubular pH would be 6.4, or 1.0 pH units below the calculated equilibrium value. The observed disequilibrium value of 0.85 was very close to this value. The slightly smaller observed disequilibrium value could have been due to errors in measurement, diffusion of some of the excess H_2CO_3 out of the lumen without breaking down to CO_2, or to the direct reabsorption of a small fraction of bicarbonate. The close agreement between the calculated and observed disequilibrium pH, however, is evidence that the major fraction of bicarbonate reabsorption is mediated by hydrogen secretion even after complete inhibition of carbonic anhydrase.

The sources of the hydrogen for the secretory process under these conditions is somewhat of a mystery. If Maren's estimate that with large doses of inhibitor carbonic anhydrase is 99.9% inhibited is correct, the rate of hydration of CO_2 is insufficient to account for the observed rates of hydrogen secretion. Moreover, the uncatalyzed rate of CO_2 hydration is capable of contributing such a small fraction to the total rate of hydrogen secretion that changing pCO_2 should have little effect on the system. These difficulties might be obviated in several ways. First, if the hydrogen pump generates hydroxyl ions by splitting water, the concentration of hydroxyl ions would rise after inhibition of carbonic anhydrase, but increased passive diffusion of hydroxyl out of the cell might prevent the cell from becoming sufficiently alkaline to stop hydrogen secretion. To the extent that hydroxyl can diffuse out of the cell, the need for reaction with CO_2 is circumvented. Although this process might be capable of sustaining a high rate of hydrogen secretion in the absence of carbonic anhydrase activity, it would also be independent of CO_2 tension and consequently would not exhibit the observed pCO_2 sensitivity of the carbonic anhydrase-independent system. A second possibility is that a hydrogen pump located at the peritubular surface of the cell might derive hydrogen from the buffers and H_2CO_3 in blood. A final possibility is that, due to structural orientation within the cell, carbonic anhydrase is much less completely inhibited than would be predicted from the *in vitro* kinetic constants and that there is sufficient residual enzyme activity to maintain the reactions $CO_2 + H_2O \rightleftharpoons H_2CO_3$ and $CO_2 + OH \rightleftharpoons HCO_3$ near equilibrium. If this latter possibility were in fact true, the intracellular phase of the hydrogen secretory process would be pCO_2-dependent, carbonic anhydrase-independent, while the luminal phase of hydrogen secretion would be carbonic anhydrase-dependent and pCO_2-independent.

One corollary of this model is that bicarbonate reabsorption in the proximal tubule would be both sensitive to pCO_2 and dependent on carbonic anhydrase, while distal reabsorption would be sensitive to pCO_2, but insensitive to carbonic anhydrase inhibition since it does not have luminal carbonic anhydrase. Suitable studies to determine whether distal hydrogen secretion is sensitive to pCO_2 have not been performed. The distal tubule, however, does appear to be relatively insensitive to the inhibitory effects of acetazolamide. Micropuncture studies utilizing the shrinking-drop technique of Gertz, in which the disappearance of a small droplet of isotonic $NaHCO_3$ was measured, failed to show any clear-cut inhibition of bicarbonate reabsorption by the administration of carbonic anhydrase inhibitors (Rector, 1964). Carbonic anhydrase has clearly been shown to reside in distal tubular cells (Pollak et al., 1965), but whether inhibition of its activity has any significant effect on the rate of distal hydrogen secretion cannot definitely be answered until the results from more precise studies are available.

VI. Mechanism of Hydrogen Secretion

Several investigators (Pitts, 1958; Bank, 1962) have suggested that hydrogen secretion, at least in the proximal tubule, might be a passive process driven by the transtubular potential difference. In support of this hypothesis, Bank (1962) found a correlation between the transtubular potential and the minimal pH established in the proximal tubule. However, following the inhibition of carbonic anhydrase during $NaHCO_3$ diuresis the generation of an acid disequilibrium pH results in rather steep transtubular pH gradients, averaging 0.7 pH units (Rector et al., 1965), which are difficult to attribute to electrical forces. According to the Nernst equation

$$[E_T = -61 \text{ mV} (pH_{blood} - pH_{TF})]$$

a transtubular potential difference (E_T) of -42 mV would be required to generate the 0.7 transtubular pH gradient, under equilibrium conditions of zero net hydrogen secretion. Since considerable hydrogen was being secreted under these experimental conditions, the potential would have to be much greater than -42 mV to account for hydrogen secretion during carbonic anhydrase inhibition. Malnic et al. (1964)

found potentials to be only -25 mV after inhibition of carbonic anhydrase, an electrical force insufficient to account for hydrogen secretion under these circumstances. Recent studies by Frömpter and Hegel (1966) make passive secretion of hydrogen even less likely. Frömpter and Hegel have presented convincing evidence that the proximal transtubular potential difference in the rat is zero and that previous measurements giving a value of -20 mV were due to electrode tip artifacts. If there is no significant potential difference across the normal proximal tubule, then the observed proximal acidification clearly cannot be attributed to passive processes and must be mediated by some mechanism involving active transport of hydrogen ions.

In the distal tubule, the transtubular potential differences are much higher and are sufficient to account for minimum pH values achieved under conditions where the rate of secretion is very small. During $NaHCO_3$ diuresis the average distal potential difference is approximately 55 mV, while the average distal transtubular pH gradient is 0.65 units (Rector et al., 1965). Thus, the potential is sufficient to generate the observed pH gradients, provided there was little or no net movement of hydrogen. However, whether the potential is also sufficient to drive distal hydrogen secretion at a near maximal rate, as it must have been under these conditions, is not clear. At the present time it is not possible to determine whether distal hydrogen secretion is also an active transport process or whether it is simply the passive consequence of the transtubular potential.

VII. Regulation of the Rate of Hydrogen Secretion

A. Relation between Hydrogen Secretion and Sodium and Chloride Reabsorption

Although the precise manner by which hydrogen is secreted into the tubular fluid is unknown, the process must be intimately interdigitated with the reabsorption of sodium and chloride. Since sodium, chloride, and bicarbonate account for the greatest fraction of all ions in the glomerular filtrate, the sum of chloride reabsorption and hydrogen secretion must be approximately equal to sodium reabsorption. This raises several important questions concerning the mechanisms for regulating hydrogen secretion. First, do changes in the absolute rate of sodium reabsorption produce proportionate changes only in chloride reabsorption, leaving hydrogen secretion relatively constant, or does hydrogen secretion change in parallel fashion? Second, to what extent can the rate of hydrogen secretion be regulated independently of sodium reabsorption? To the extent that hydrogen secretion can be altered independently of sodium reabsorption, there must be an obligatory inverse relation between chloride reabsorption and hydrogen secretion. In examining the homeostatic control of hydrogen secretion, therefore, it is necessary to consider all factors which might influence either the rate of sodium reabsorption or the proportions between hydrogen secretion and chloride reabsorption.

Pitts and Lotspeich (1946) observed that the maximum rate of bicarbonate reabsorption is not constant, but varies proportionately to either spontaneous or chronically induced changes in GFR. Under these conditions bicarbonate reabsorption expressed as meq/100 ml GFR is constant. This relationship between bicarbonate reabsorption and GFR is similar to that observed between sodium reabsorption and GFR and suggests a linkage between the two. Thompson and Barrett (1954), on the other hand, failed to obtain this relation when GFR was acutely reduced by inflating a balloon in the aorta above the renal arteries. In their experiments the maximum rate of bicarbonate reabsorption remained constant as GFR was reduced, and the value of reabsorption per 100 ml GFR rose. The extent to which sodium reabsorption paralleled the change in GFR in these studies, however, is not known. This problem has been reexamined in more detail recently (Frick *et al.*, unpublished observations) by investigating the effects of acutely lowering GFR on the relation between sodium, chloride, and bicarbonate reabsorption in the proximal convoluted tubule, an area of the nephron known to exhibit good glomerulotubular balance with respect to sodium and water. Constriction of the aorta above the renal arteries during saline diuresis reduced the GFR by approximately 40%, yet the tubular fluid-to-plasma ratios of inulin, sodium, chloride, and bicarbonate were all unchanged. In these experiments glomerulartubular balance was almost perfect and the fractional reabsorptions of water, sodium, chloride, and bicarbonate were all maintained constant. The absolute rates of reabsorption of sodium, chloride, and water and the secretion of hydrogen, therefore, were all changing proportionally to GFR. This indicates that the mechanism for maintaining glomerulotubular balance involves not only sodium reabsorption, but also the secretion of hydrogen ions. This participation of hydrogen secretion in glomerulotubular balance suggests that, at least in the proximal tubule, the absolute rate of hydrogen secretion is in some way geared to the absolute rate of sodium reabsorption.

Alterations in extracellular fluid volume have clearly been shown to influence the rate of sodium reabsorption, independently of GFR and aldosterone (DeWardener *et al.*, 1961; Levinsky and Lalone, 1963; Rector *et al.*, 1964b). This change in sodium reabsorption is mediated in part by release of a natriuretic hormone (Rector *et al.*, 1968) and in part by changes in intrarenal hemodynamics (Martino and Earley, 1967). These factors associated with variations in ECF volume appear to influence not only the reabsorption of sodium, but also the rate of hydrogen secretion. For example, infusions of hypertonic $NaCl$ have been observed to depress bicarbonate reabsorption in both normal (Pitts and Lotspeich, 1946) and hypercapneic dogs (Hilton *et al.*, 1956). Although this effect was attributed to competitive inhibition between chloride and bicarbonate for a common reabsorptive pathway, a more likely explanation is that expansion of ECF volume produced proportionate suppression of sodium reabsorption and hydrogen secretion. More direct evidence for an effect of ECF volume expansion on hydrogen secretion has been obtained by Kunau and associates (1966). In a series of micropuncture studies in rats they observed that isohydric expansion of ECF volume with Ringer's bicarbonate solution reduced the tubular fluid-to-plasma inulin ratio from 2.0 to 1.3, did not change the tubular fluid-to-plasma sodium ratio and increased the tubular fluid bicarbonate concentration from 8 to 12 meq/liter in the proximal convoluted tubule. Thus, expansion of ECF volume suppressed sodium reabsorption and hydrogen secretion in the proximal tubule more or less proportionately, again suggesting close linkage of the two processes.

The effect of ECF volume expansion on hydrogen secretion probably introduces a serious error in the measurement in the maximum bicarbonate reabsorptive capacity, since in a bicarbonate titration study the plasma bicarbonate concentration is raised experimentally by an infusion of $NaHCO_3$. In part, therefore, the apparent tubular maximum may be due to suppression of the system by ECF volume expansion, preventing further increase in hydrogen secretion in response to the elevated concentration of bicarbonate in the filtrate, rather than reflecting a true intrinsic limitation in the system.

A similar parallel increase in sodium reabsorption and hydrogen secretion in response to contraction in ECF volume is much more difficult to demonstrate because of the limitations imposed by the quantity of filtered sodium. Under certain circumstances, which will be discussed in detail below, the stimulus for complete sodium reabsorption in response to contracted ECF volume may drive hydrogen secretion at a high rate if the availability of reabsorbable anion (chloride) in the glomerular filtrate is reduced by substitution with either bicarbonate or poorly reabsorbable anions (phosphate, sulfate, nitrate).

B. Rate of Hydrogen Secretion Relative to Chloride Reabsorption

The linkage between the rate of sodium reabsorption and the rate of hydrogen secretion results in the proportionate variation of bicarbonate reabsorption with variations in GFR, the suppression of bicarbonate reabsorption by expansion of ECF volume, and, under some circumstances, the stimulation of bicarbonate reabsorption by contraction of ECF volume. The level at which the concentration of bicarbonate in plasma is maintained, however, will be determined, not by the absolute rate of hydrogen secretion, but rather by those factors which regulate the proportions between hydrogen secretion and chloride reabsorption. This point is the key to an understanding of the manner in which the regulation of acid–base balance is dissociated from the regulation of ECF volume. As ECF volume is altered a variety of factors (GFR, aldosterone, intrarenal hemodynamics) will exert their action, changing the absolute rate of sodium reabsorption and secondarily the absolute rates of both chloride reabsorption and hydrogen secretion. At whatever absolute rate the system may be operating, however, acid–base balance can be independently regulated by varying the ratio between hydrogen secretion and chloride reabsorption.

The ratio of bicarbonate to chloride in the reabsorbate normally is approximately 25:100 and is relatively fixed. The bicarbonate:chloride ratio in plasma, therefore, will normally be maintained at this value. If the concentration of bicarbonate in plasma is elevated by administration of $NaHCO_3$, bicarbonate and chloride will still be reabsorbed in approximately the same ratio of 25:100 and the excess bicarbonate in the filtrate will be excreted. The renal threshold for bicarbonate, and consequently the plasma concentration of bicarbonate, therefore, is set by the ratio of hydrogen secretion to chloride reabsorption. The concentration of bicarbonate in plasma can be maintained at a higher than normal level only if the renal threshold for bicarbonate is raised. This requires that the secretion of hydrogen be increased relative to the reabsorption of chloride. There appear to be two major mechanisms for inducing such a relative change. The first mechanism involves the stimulation of sodium reabsorption under conditions where chloride reabsorption cannot be increased; this discrepancy, presumably by altering transmembrane electromotive forces, may secondarily accelerate hydrogen secretion. This mechanism, on occasion, operates in complete disregard of the acid–base status of the animal and may result in a chronic metabolic alkalosis. The second mechanism, on the other hand, involves a direct stimulation of hydrogen secretion and appears to operate in a fashion more closely oriented toward the homeostatic control of acid–base balance.

1. EFFECT OF A DISCREPANCY BETWEEN SODIUM AND CHLORIDE REABSORPTION

The first mechanism, involving a discrepancy between sodium and chloride reabsorption, may be activated in two ways: (1) by an infusion of sodium salts of poorly reabsorbable anions, and (2) by chloride depletion. The infusion of Na_2SO_4 or other sodium salts of poorly reabsorbable anions, particularly in salt-depleted animals, has been observed to increase the transtubular potential in the distal tubule (Clapp et al., 1962) and consequently would be predicted to enhance hydrogen secretion in the distal tubule. In accord with their effects on distal transtubular potential, the infusion of these sodium salts of poorly reabsorbable anions effects more complete bicarbonate reabsorption as the bicarbonate Tm is approached (Rector and Seldin, 1962), lowers urine pH (Schwartz et al., 1955), and increases the excretion of hydrogen in the form of titratable acid (Bank and Schwartz, 1960). If these salts are administered chronically to salt-depleted animals, a mild metabolic alkalosis may supervene.

A physiologically more important means of generating a discrepancy between sodium and chloride reabsorption is by selective depletion of chloride. Schwartz and his associates (Schwartz et al., 1961; Gulyassy et al., 1962; Atkins and Schwartz, 1962; Needle et al., 1964; Kassirer et al., 1965; Kassirer and Schwartz, 1966b) have shown that a variety of maneuvers (exposure to and then removal from high CO_2 tensions; administration of sodium nitrate; gastric aspiration) in dogs and man maintained on a rigidly chloride-free diet will sustain a chronic metabolic alkalosis with plasma bicarbonate concentrations in the range of 30 to 32 mEq/liter. There appear to be two essential factors operative in all of the various circumstances studied: (1) contraction of ECF volume (secondary to the low NaCl diet) with subsequent stimulation of sodium reabsorption, and (2) elevation of the bicarbonate:chloride concentration ratio in glomerular filtrate by prerenal or preexistent factors. The reabsorption of sodium must be stimulated to such an intense degree that the urine is virtually sodium-free. Under these circumstances the tubule no longer has the ability to regulate the ratio at which bicarbonate and chloride are returned to the blood along with the reabsorbed sodium. This alone is insufficient to stimulate increased hydrogen secretion; severe uncomplicated ECF volume depletion does not by itself generate a metabolic alkalosis. On the other hand, if the salt-depleted animal is administered a sodium salt of a poorly reabsorbable anion (Na_2SO_4, Na_2HPO_4, $NaNO_3$) the sodium will be retained along with newly generated bicarbonate and the anion will be excreted with hydrogen. Alternatively, if the ratio of bicarbonate to chloride in plasma is increased above normal by prerenal factors (prior exposure to hypercapnea, gastric aspiration), the alkalosis will persist since the reabsorption of chloride cannot be selectively increased because of the limited quantity of chloride in the filtrate and the reabsorption of bicarbonate cannot be selectively depressed because of the overriding demands of sodium reabsorption. The peculiar role of chloride in this process is related entirely to the fact that NaCl and $NaHCO_3$ are the only two important physiologically reabsorbable sodium salts; consequently only with access to chloride can the ECF volume be reexpanded without generating or maintaining a metabolic alkalosis. Most importantly it is not the reduction in plasma chloride concentration *per se*, but rather the ECF volume contraction and stimulation of sodium reabsorption that is important in maintaining the relatively high rate of hydrogen secretion. This has been clearly demonstrated by Cohen (1967), who gave chloride-depleted alkalotic dogs an isotonic infusion containing chloride and bicarbonate in the same ratio as existed in the animals' plasma. In response to this infusion, ECF volume was reexpanded, the stimulus to sodium reabsorption was diminished, the ratio between hydrogen secretion and chloride reabsorption was restored to normal, the excess bicarbonate in the filtrate was excreted, and the metabolic alkalosis was corrected.

2. ROLE OF INTRACELLULAR pH

In the salt-depleted state the overriding demands imposed by the intense stimulation of sodium reabsorption may determine the ratio at which chloride and bicarbonate are added to renal venous blood irrespective of the acid–base status of the animal. However, when dietary intake of salt and ECF volume are normal, the bicarbonate:chloride concentration ratio will be determined by those factors which act primarily on hydrogen secretion. Under these conditions the system responds more appropriately to changes in acid–base equilibrium. One hypothesis is that factors which influence hydrogen secretion do so by their effects on cell pH.

Experiments by Brazeau and Gilman (1953), Relman *et al.* (1953), and Dorman *et al.* (1954) showed that the bicarbonate Tm was elevated by raising plasma CO_2 tension and was depressed by lowering plasma pCO_2, completely independent of blood pH. On the basis of these studies it was concluded that intracellular pH was of signal importance in controlling the rate of hydrogen secretion, while the extracellular pH played little if any role. It is difficult to exclude an effect of extracellular pH from this type of study, however, for several reasons. First, to assure a maximum rate of hydrogen secretion it is necessary to have an excess of bicarbonate in the glomerular filtrate. If pCO_2 is kept constant, it is not possible to lower blood pH without imposing a limit on the rate of hydrogen secretion by reducing the level of bicarbonate in the filtrate. Second, raising plasma bicarbonate concentration sufficiently to achieve the maximum rate of reabsorption requires the infusion of $NaHCO_3$ and the concomitant expansion of ECF volume. The expansion of ECF volume may suppress both the reabsorption of sodium and the secretion of hydrogen and thereby obscure important effects of other factors such as pH and bicarbonate concentration.

Despite these objections the striking regulatory effect exerted by pCO_2 in the absence of any clearly demonstrable effect of extracellular pH suggests that the hydrogen secretory system is controlled primarily by intracellular pH and that the system responds in such a fashion as to return cell pH towards normal. According to this model, the homeostatic function of the hydrogen secretory system is primarily oriented towards control of renal intracellular pH, and only incidentally towards control of blood pH.

The pH of intracellular fluid is determined, not only by pCO_2, but also by the concentration of bicarbonate in the cell, consequently any factor altering the intracellular concentration of bicarbonate will influence hydrogen secretion. In the steady state the rate at which bicarbonate is removed from the cell must equal the rate of hydrogen secretion (Fig. 6). It is generally accepted that bicarbonate ions generated by the process of hydrogen secretion are removed from the cell by passive diffusion down an electrochemical gradient. (The alternative possibility that the cellular bicarbonate is decomposed by reacting with hydrogen

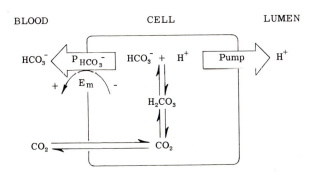

FIG. 6.   Factors controlling pH of the renal tubular cell. In steady state, HCO_3 removal $= H^+$ secretion. HCO_3 removal: (a) Permeability (P_{HCO_3-}); (b) $[HCO_3^-]_{cell} - [HCO_3^-]_{plasma}$; (c) membrane potential. H^+ secretion: (a) Pump activity; (b) $[H^+]_{cell}$, pCO_2 and $[HCO_3^-]_{cell}$.

ions passively diffusing across the peritubular membrane into the cell along electrochemical gradients would be equally consistent with the discussion that follows.) The rate of removal, therefore, is dependent upon the permeability coefficient for bicarbonate (or hydrogen), the concentration gradient for bicarbonate (or hydrogen), and the electrical potential across the peritubular membrane. Alteration of any of these factors will change the rate of bicarbonate removal and secondarily influence hydrogen secretion. Conversely, if the rate of hydrogen secretion is abruptly changed, the intracellular concentration of bicarbonate will change to a new steady-state value, provided permeability and the peritubular transmembrane potential are unaltered. Thus, any factor which might affect the rate of hydrogen secretion independently of intracellular pH, such as the availability of bicarbonate and buffers in the glomerular filtrate, will secondarily alter the rate at which bicarbonate is generated in the cell and change intracellular pH.

a. *Effect of Acute and Chronic Respiratory Acidosis.* In acute respiratory acidosis cell pH is reduced and the hydrogen secretory mechanism is stimulated. Hydrogen secretion cannot rise proportionately, however, because of the limited supply of bicarbonate in the filtrate. To some extent, tissue buffers are titrated to form extracellular bicarbonate which can then be filtered and increase the quantity of hydrogen acceptor in tubular fluid. This permits hydrogen secretion to increase but to only a limited extent. In addition, even in the presence of an unlimited supply of filtered bicarbonate, hydrogen secretion does not increase linearly as pCO_2 is acutely elevated (Fig. 5). Consequently, the rate of hydrogen secretion is not sufficient either to raise cell bicarbonate high enough to correct cell pH or to maintain plasma bicarbonate at a level which will completely compensate the respiratory acidosis. As a result of the intracellular acidosis, the production of ammonia will increase, net acid will rise, and new bicarbonate will be generated and added to extracellular fluid (Carter *et al.*, 1959; Polak *et al.*, 1961).

Within the first 24 hours of hypercapnea (pCO_2 approximately 80 mm Hg) plasma bicarbonate concentration in the dog increases from 22 to 30 mEq/liter, primarily as a consequence of the titration of tissue buffers (Giebisch *et al.*, 1955a; Cohen *et al.*, 1964). Thereafter, as net acid is increased (primarily as ammonia) and new bicarbonate is added to extracellular fluid, plasma bicarbonate increases slowly, reaching a plateau of about 36 meq/liter on the 4th or 5th day. After 4 to 5 days in the rat (Carter *et al.*, 1959), and 8 to 10 days in the dog, net acid excretion returns to normal and a new steady state is achieved (Polak *et al.*, 1961; Schwartz *et al.*, 1965). The delay in reaching the new steady-state concentration of plasma bicarbonate is not entirely the consequence of the slow rate at which new bicarbonate can be generated by the kidney and added to the body fluids. A similar delay in reaching the steady state is also observed in dogs given large quantities of $NaHCO_3$ in their diet (Van Ypersele de Strihou *et al.*, 1962). This suggests that the gradual approach to a new steady state in respiratory acidosis is a consequence of adaptive changes in the hydrogen secretory mechanism.

Sullivan and Dorman (1955) have also observed adaptive changes in the hydrogen secretory mechanism in response to chronic hypercapnea. During acute respiratory acidosis (pCO_2 approximately 90 mm Hg) they found the bicarbonate Tm to be approximately 3.4 mEq/100 ml GFR, whereas after chronic exposure to the same degree of hypercapnea the Tm was approximately 4.5 mEq/100 ml GFR. Several possible factors might be responsible for this adaptive change. Stimulation of adrenal cortex with increased secretion of adrenal hormones has been suggested as a possible cause for the adaptive increase in bicarbonate reabsorption. With the exception of the study of Grollman and Gamble (1959), who noted slight metabolic alkalosis in normokalemic dogs given DOCA, ACTH, or cortisone, adrenal steroids have been shown to alter the maximum rate of hydrogen secretion only if potassium deficiency is permitted to occur. If potassium deficiency is prevented, adrenal steroids have no significant effect on the rate of hydrogen secretion (Seldin *et al.*, 1956; Giebisch *et al.*, 1955b). Although adrenal steroids alone are not a likely explanation for the adaptive changes, potassium depletion is a possible factor. Modest losses of potassium during chronic respiratory acidosis are noted in animals receiving dietary salt but not in those maintained on a salt-free diet, yet the adaptive change is similar in both groups of animals (Polak *et al.*, 1961). Moreover, the changes in acid excretion are different in potassium depletion and in chronic hypercapnea. In animals given DOCA and Na_2SO_4 to induce potassium depletion, ammonia excretion is persistently elevated, whereas ammonia increases only transiently during chronic respiratory acidosis, and has returned to normal levels at a time when the adaptive increase in the maximum bicarbonate reabsorptive capacity is evident. It seems unlikely, therefore, that potassium deficiency plays any important role in the adaptive response to hypercapnea. Another possibility is that acutely elevating bicarbonate reabsorption by hypercapnea tends to expand ECF volume and that this serves to diminish the response to the elevated pCO_2. With time, chloride is lost from the body, permitting an elevation of plasma bicarbonate concentration without a concomitant overexpansion of ECF volume. This possibility, however, has been virtually ruled out by the experiments of Polak *et al.* (1961) showing that dogs maintained on either a high salt diet or a salt-free diet exhibit the same delay in achieving a new steady state and attain exactly the same plasma bicarbonate concentration in response to prolonged respiratory acidosis. At the present time, therefore, there is no adequate explanation for the adaptive increase in the maximum rate of hydrogen secretion in response to chronic hypercapnea.

The exact manner in which the hydrogen secretory mechanism adapts during chronic hypercapnea also is not clear. The adaptive change might occur at either the peritubular bicarbonate removal step or the luminal hydrogen secretory step (Fig. 6). A primary change at the bicarbonate removal step, either by increasing permeability to bicarbonate (or hydrogen) or by increasing the peritubular transmembrane potential, is highly unlikely since this would tend to lower the intracellular concentration of bicarbonate and shift cell pH further from the normal value. A more likely possibility is that in some manner the activity of the hydrogen transport mechanism located in the luminal surface of the cell is enhanced. An adaptive change at this step would tend to raise the intracellular concentration of bicarbonate. The augmentation of pump activity would presumably increase until intracellular bicarbonate was generated at a rate sufficient to raise cell pH towards a normal value. The fact that ammonia excretion returns towards normal in the steady state supports the view that the adaptive change in the hydrogen secretory mechanism has corrected, rather than worsened, the intracellular acidosis. Since the rate of bicarbonate removal during chronic hypercapnea must be increased commensurate with the rate of hydrogen secretion, the concentration gradient for bicarbonate (or hydrogen) between cell and plasma must be increased. Consequently, the plasma concentration of bicarbonate will increase proportionately less than the intracellular concentration, so that during the steady state when intracellular pH has returned towards normal, the plasma bicarbonate is not elevated sufficiently to achieve complete compensation of the acidosis. This formulation is consistent with the observations of Carter *et al.* (1959), Polak *et al.* (1961), and Schwartz *et al.* (1965) that during chronic hypercapnea blood pH does not return to normal, but remains slightly acid.

b. Role of Potassium. A large number of observations suggest an intimate relation between the secretion of hydrogen and potassium. Stimulating hydrogen secretion by means of hypercapnea depresses potassium secretion (Denton *et al.*, 1952; Dorman *et al.*, 1954), whereas lowering the rate of hydrogen secretion by either acetazolamide (Berliner *et al.*, 1951) or respiratory alkalosis (Singer *et al.*, 1952; Stanbury and Thomson, 1952) accelerates potassium secretion. Conversely, the administration of potassium salts raises urine pH, lowers the excretion of ammonia and titratable acid, and blocks the reabsorption of bicarbonate (Loeb *et al.*, 1932; Winkler and Smith, 1942; Berliner *et al.*, 1950; Roberts *et al.*, 1953; Orloff and Davidson, 1959; Rector *et al.*, 1962). Potassium deficiency, on the other hand, enhances the reabsorption of bicarbonate and the excretion of ammonia and titratable acid (Kennedy *et al.*, 1949; Broch, 1950; Roberts *et al.*, 1955; Giebisch *et al.*, 1955b). These studies indicate that there is an apparent reciprocal relation between potassium and hydrogen secretion and suggest the possibility that these two ions compete for a common secretory pathway (Berliner *et al.*, 1951; Berliner, 1952).

The exact role of potassium in modulating hydrogen secretion has recently been subjected to extensive reappraisal by Schwartz and his associates (Atkins and Schwartz, 1962; Kassirer *et al.*, 1965; Kassirer and Schwartz, 1966a). These investigators have found that in both man and dog the metabolic alkalosis associated with moderate potassium deficiency (induced by either gastric aspiration or dietary means) can be completely corrected by the administration of NaCl, without repleting the potassium deficiency. In reviewing the literature they were able to find only 10 well-documented cases of hypokalemic alkalosis which were resistant to the administration of NaCl. Probably many more cases of saline-resistant alkalosis exist, but have not been reported. The difference between these cases of saline-resistant hypokalemic alkalosis, and the cases of the experimentally induced hypokalemia studied by Schwartz *et al.* is not known, but may be related to more severe depletion of potassium in the saline-resistant cases. These data suggest that, although severe potassium deficiency may augment hydrogen secretion, the effects observed with modest potassium depletion are primarily the consequence of ECF volume deficit rather than potassium deficiency per se.

In addition to cases of saline-resistant hypokalemic alkalosis (usually produced by vomiting, diarrhea, or diuretics) a large number of patients with either primary aldosteronism, Cushing's syndrome, or administration of exogenous mineralocorticoids develop hypokalemic metabolic alkalosis which is neither prevented nor corrected by the administration of large amounts of NaCl. In fact, in these circumstances the increased renal loss of potassium is dependent on the adequate intake of sodium; if all sodium salts are removed from the diet hypokalemic alkalosis does not develop, while the administration of any sodium salt, including NaCl, results in the prompt loss of potassium and the generation of a metabolic alkalosis (Seldin *et al.*, 1956). Prevention of potassium deficiency by the administration of large amounts of supplemental KCl prevents the alkalosis. The ease with which saline-resistant hypokalemic alkalosis can be induced by adrenal steroids, in contrast to the difficulty encountered where the potassium deficiency is induced by other means (gastrointestinal losses), suggests that stimulation of sodium–hydrogen exchange by the adrenal steroids, perhaps in the distal tubule, may play an important role in elevating bicarbonate reabsorption. It is equally apparent, however, that excess adrenal steroids alone are not sufficient to augment hydrogen secretion, and that there must be an associated potassium deficiency.

In addition to the difficulties arising from the effects of contracted ECF volume and the stimulatory action of adrenal steroids, evaluation of the role of hypokalemia on hydrogen secretion is complicated by species differences. In hypokalemic dogs expansion of ECF volume will completely correct the metabolic alkalosis in the absence of excess adrenal steroids. In man, administration of saline appears to correct the alkalosis associated with moderate potassium depletion, but not that associated with more severe deficiencies or with hyperadrenocorticism. In hypokalemic rats omission of excess mineralocorticoids and administration of NaCl will not completely correct the metabolic alkalosis (Seldin *et al.*, 1956; Luke and Levitin, 1967), clearly indicating an effect of potassium deficiency per se.

The mechanism by which potassium influences hydrogen secretion has not been clearly elucidated. On the basis of the reciprocal relation between hydrogen and potassium secretion it has been suggested that hydrogen and potassium compete for a common secretory pathway (Berliner *et al.*, 1951; Berliner, 1952). Since potassium is reabsorbed throughout most of the nephron and is secreted only in the latter half of the distal convoluted tubule and collecting duct (Bloomer *et al.*, 1963; Marsh *et al.*, 1963; Malnic *et al.*, 1964; Watson *et al.*, 1964) competitive inhibition of hydrogen secretion by potassium should be limited to these more distal portions of the nephron.

Micropuncture studies, however, do not support this view and suggest that variations in potassium exert a major effect on hydrogen secretion in the proximal tubule. Rector *et al.* (1964a) found that bicarbonate concentration at the end of the proximal convoluted tubule was significantly lower in hypokalemic alkalotic rats than in animals made equally alkalotic by the infusion of $NaHCO_3$. Conversely, Clapp and Bernstein (1968) observed that the acute administration of KCl produced a rise in proximal bicarbonate concentration. Although these experiments suggest that potassium may influence hydrogen secretion in the proximal tubule, ECF volume was not sufficiently controlled to permit such a conclusion. In the studies of Rector *et al.* (1964a), the control animals were made alkalotic by the infusion of $NaHCO_3$. Thus the higher proximal bicarbonate concentrations in these animals than in the noninfused hypokalemic rats may have been the suppressive effects of ECF volume expansion in the control rats, rather than the enhancing effects of hypokalemia in the potassium of deficient rats. Similarly, the acute elevation of proximal bicarbonate concentration following the infusion of KCl (Clapp and Bernstein, 1968) may have been due to overexpansion of ECF volume rather than any direct effect of potassium on the rate of hydrogen secretion.

Kunau *et al.* (1968) have reexamined the effect of hypokalemia on proximal bicarbonate reabsorption in rats, taking great care to control the expansion of ECF volume. The control rats were made alkalotic by an infusion of 0.15 M $NaHCO_3$, while the hypokalemic rats were given an equal volume of fluid containing 37 mEq/liter of $NaHCO_3$ and 88 mEq/liter of NaCl. Bicarbonate concentration at the end of the proximal tubule was 8 mEq/liter in the hypokalemic and 22 mEq/liter in the control rats. When the hypokalemic rats were given an even greater volume of fluid, proximal bicarbonate concentration was still lower than in the control rats.

These results establish that hypokalemia per se in some manner stimulates hydrogen secretion in the proximal convoluted tubule. Whether there is also an effect in the distal tubule cannot be determined by the studies of Kunau *et al.* (1968), but in the absence of contrary evidence it is reasonable to assume that potassium exerts its effect along the entire nephron. Since potassium is secreted only in the distal tubule, the acceleration of hydrogen secretion in the proximal tubule of potassium-deficient rats indicates that potassium must be influencing hydrogen secretion by some mechanism other than competition for a common secretory pathway.

The most reasonable hypothesis is that potassium influences hydrogen secretion by modifying cell pH. In the face of a constant pCO_2 potassium could influence cell pH only by altering the steady state intracellular concentration of bicarbonate. This could occur in one of two ways: (1) potassium could modify the permeability of the peritubular membrane to bicarbonate (or hydrogen), or (2) potassium could change the peritubular transmembrane potential (Fig. 6). In rats the normal transmembrane potential of skeletal muscle is −89 mV; this is increased to 95–100 mV by hypokalemia and depressed to 60–70 mV by hyperkalemia. If hypokalemia produced similar changes in the electrical force across the peritubular surface of renal tubular cells, bicarbonate removal would be accelerated and intracellular bicarbonate would be maintained at a lower than normal concentration. The resulting intracellular acidosis would augment both hydrogen secretion and ammonia production. Hyperkalemia, on the other hand, would have the reverse effects.

C. Effect of Composition of Glomerular Filtrate on Hydrogen Secretion

1. Effect of Metabolic Acids

The absolute rate of hydrogen secretion is influenced not only by those factors which affect the maximum capacity of the system (hydrogen pump activity, stimulus to sodium reabsorption, intracellular pH), but also by the availability of hydrogen receptors in glomerular filtrate and tubular fluid. In addition, the buffer composition of the glomerular filtrate determines the ultimate fate of the secreted acid. If the concentration of bicarbonate in plasma and glomerular filtrate is very high, all of the secreted hydrogen will be consumed by reaction with bicarbonate; under these conditions the maximum rate of hydrogen secretion will be achieved. If, on the other hand, the concentration of bicarbonate in plasma and glomerular filtrate is very low, only a portion of the secreted hydrogen will be utilized in bicarbonate reabsorption, while the remainder will be diverted into nonbicarbonate buffers and excreted as titratable acid and ammonium; under these conditions net acid excretion ($TA + NH_4 - HCO_3^-$) will be maximal but total hydrogen secretion will be significantly less than the secretory capacity.

Hydrogen which reacts with filtered bicarbonate to form H_2CO_3, and eventually CO_2 and H_2O, is recycled back into the cell and does not contribute to the net elimination of acid (Fig. 7). Only the small percent of secreted hydrogen which is bound to urinary buffer, either as titratable acid or ammonium, serves to rid the body of metabolically produced or exogenously administered acids (Fig. 7). Therefore, the factors which govern the distribution of secreted hydrogen between filtered bicarbonate and nonbicarbonate buffers determine to what extent the available hydrogen will be used to conserve filtered bicarbonate and to what extent to generate new bicarbonate.

The diversion of secreted hydrogen into nonbicarbonate buffers requires that the pH of tubular fluid be lowered below that of glomerular filtrate. To the extent that sodium, chloride, bicarbonate, and water reabsorption (particularly in the proximal portions of the ne-

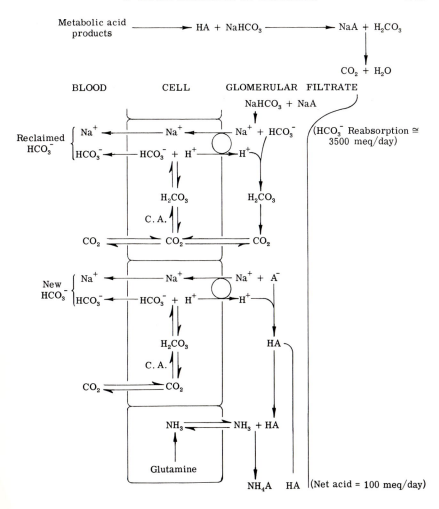

FIG. 7. Distribution of secreted hydrogen between bicarbonate reabsorption and net acid excretion.

phron) occur proportionately, bicarbonate concentration remains relatively constant; tubular fluid pH changes very little and secreted hydrogen is preferentially utilized in bicarbonate reabsorption. As bicarbonate reabsorption nears completion, however, the concentration of bicarbonate and the pH of tubular fluid fall; secreted hydrogen then begins to react with the nonbicarbonate buffers.

The most important physiologic factor influencing the point along the nephron at which the pH of tubular fluid begins to fall and the magnitude of the final pH gradient between urine and blood is the concentration of bicarbonate in the glomerular filtrate. When plasma bicarbonate concentration is raised the acidification of tubular fluid is reduced and the pH gradient between urine and blood is diminished. In contrast, when plasma bicarbonate is lowered, the acidification occurs much earlier (i.e., more proximal) in the tubule and the final pH gradient between urine and blood is enhanced (Gottschalk *et al.*, 1960; Giebisch *et al.*, 1960; Rector, 1964; Clapp *et al.*, 1965).

Metabolic acidosis by lowering plasma bicarbonate concentration reduces the quantity of secreted hydrogen consumed by bicarbonate reabsorption and increases the amount of hydrogen excreted as titratable acid and ammonium ions. If there is a plentiful supply of filtered buffers (phosphate, creatinine), titratable acid will be formed. If, on the other hand, there is a paucity of buffer in the glomerular filtrate, ammonia will be produced in the tubular cell from neutral precursors (primarily glutamine) and added to tubular fluid. Although the tubules are capable of generating pH gradients as great as 3.5 units, only approximately 30% of the metabolic acids can be excreted as titratable acid, while the remaining 70% are excreted as urinary ammonium.

According to current concepts ammonia produced in the tubular epithelium enters both blood and tubular fluid by diffusion of the nonionic NH_3. It is assumed that all compartments within the kidney are in equilibrium with NH_3, and that the total amount of ammonia $NH_3 + NH_4^+$) trapped in each phase (blood, cell, tubular fluid) will be determined by the relative pH of the various compartments, and to some by the flow rates of both blood and tubular fluid (Orloff and Berliner, 1956; Milne *et al.*, 1958; Pitts, 1964). The rapid diffusibility of free NH_3 with trapping as ammonium ions permits rapid changes in the excretion of ammonia without commensurate changes in production; the ammonia is simply redistributed between blood and urine.

In acute metabolic acidosis the quantity of bicarbonate in glomerular filtrate is reduced, the tubular fluid becomes acid earlier in the nephron, the urine becomes more acid, there is titration of nonbicarbonate filtered buffers to form titratable acid and there is diversion of ammonia from blood into urine with increased excretion of ammonium ions. However, due to the limited ability of the tubule to increase its production of ammonia acutely, as well as the limited supply of filtered buffer, the reduced amount of hydrogen consumed in bicarbonate reabsorption is not matched by a commensurate increase in the quantity of hydrogen excreted as ammonium and titratable acid. Consequently, the total amount of hydrogen secretion is reduced. As discussed previously, in the steady state the rate of bicarbonate removal across the peritubular surface of the cell must equal the rate of hydrogen transport across the luminal surface (Fig. 6). If, for any reason, the rate of hydrogen secretion is reduced, the rate at which bicarbonate is generated within and removed from the cell must also be reduced. Assuming that the permeability and transmembrane potential of the peritubular membrane are unchanged, then in the steady state the concentration of bicarbonate in the cell must be reduced, giving rise to an intracellular acidosis. The administration of a metabolic acid, therefore, by reducing the quantity of hydrogen receptor in the filtrate will limit the rate of hydrogen secretion and generate an intracellular acidosis. If sustained, the intracellular acidosis will produce an adaptive acceleration in ammonia production, which when added to tubular fluid will act as a hydrogen acceptor and permit total hydrogen secretion to return towards normal levels; in this new steady state, however, less of the secreted hydrogen will be involved in bicarbonate reabsorption and more will be excreted into the urine as ammonium.

REFERENCES

Atkins, E. L., and Schwartz, W. B. (1962). Factors governing correction of the alkalosis associated with potassium deficiency; the critical role of chloride in the recovery process. *J. Clin. Invest.* **41**, 218–229.
Bank, N. (1962). Relationship between electrical and hydrogen ion gradients across rat proximal tubule. *Am. J. Physiol.* **203**, 577–582.
Bank, N., and Schwartz, W. B. (1960). The influence of anion penetrating ability on urinary acidification and the excretion of titratable acid. *J. Clin. Invest.* **39**, 1516–1525.
Bennett, C. M., Brenner, B. M., and Berliner, R. W. (1968). Micropuncture study of nephron function in the rhesus monkey. *J. Clin. Invest.* **47**, 203–216.
Berliner, R. W. (1952). Renal secretion of potassium and hydrogen ions. *Federation Proc.* **11**, 695–700.
Berliner, R. W. (1957). Some aspects of ion exchange in electrolyte transport by the renal tubules. *In* "Metabolic Aspects of Transport Across Cell Membranes" (Q. R. Murphy, ed.), pp. 203–220. Univ. of Wisconsin Press, Madison, Wisconsin.
Berliner, R. W., Kennedy, T. J., Jr., and Hilton, J. G. (1950). Renal mechanisms for excretion of potassium. *Am. J. Physiol.* **162**, 348–367.
Berliner, R. W., Kennedy, T. J., Jr., and Orloff, J. (1951). Relationship between acidification of the urine and potassium metabolism. *Am. J. Med.* **11**, 274–282.
Bloomer, H. A., Rector, F. C., Jr., and Seldin, D. W. (1963). The mechanism of potassium reabsorption in the proximal tubule of the rat. *J. Clin. Invest.* **42**, 277–285.
Brazeau, P., and Gilman, A. (1953). Effect of plasma CO_2 tension on renal tubular reabsorption of bicarbonate. *Am. J. Physiol.* **175**, 33–38.
Broch, O. J. (1950). Low potassium alkalosis with acid urine in ulcerative colitis. *Scand. J. Clin. Lab. Invest.* **2**, 113–119.
Carter, N. W., Seldin, D. W., and Teng, H. C. (1959). Tissue and renal response to chronic respiratory acidosis. *J. Clin. Invest.* **38**, 949–960.
Clapp, J. R. (1965). The effect of alterations in acid-base balance on bicarbonate reabsorption by the dog proximal tubule. *Clin. Res.* **13**, 302.

248 FLOYD C. RECTOR, JR.

Clapp, J. R., and Bernstein, B. A. (1968). Bicarbonate reabsorption by the dog nephron during potassium depletion or acute hyperkalemia. *Clin. Res.* **16**, 60.

Clapp, J. R., Rector, F. C., Jr., and Seldin, D. W. (1962). Effects of unreabsorbed anions on proximal and distal transtubular potentials in rats. *Am. J. Physiol.* **202**, 781-786.

Clapp, J. R., Watson, J. F., and Berliner, R. W. (1963a). Effect of carbonic anhydrase inhibition on proximal tubular bicarbonate reabsorption. *Am. J. Physiol.* **205**, 693-696.

Clapp, J. R., Watson, J. F., and Berliner, R. W. (1963b). Osmolality, bicarbonate concentration and water reabsorption in proximal tubule of the dog nephron. *Am. J. Physiol.* **205**, 273-280.

Clapp, J. R., Owen, E. E., and Robinson, R. R. (1965). Contribution of the proximal tubule to urinary ammonia excretion by the dog. *Am. J. Physiol.* **209**, 269-272.

Cohen, J. J. (1967). On the mechanism of selective chloride retention during the correction of metabolic alkalosis. *Clin. Res.* **15**, 355.

Cohen, J. J., Brackett, N. W., and Schwartz, W. B. (1964). The nature of the carbon dioxide titration curve in the normal dog. *J. Clin. Invest.* **43**, 777-786.

Datta, P. K., and Shepard, T. H. (1959). Intracellular localization of carbonic anhydrase in rat liver and kidney tissues. *Arch. Biochem. Biophys.* **81**, 124-129.

Denton, D. A., Maxwell, M., McDonald, I. R., Munro, J., and Williams, W. (1952). Renal regulation of the extracellular fluid in acute respiratory acidaemia. *Australian J. Exptl. Biol. Med. Sci.* **30**, 489-510.

DeWardener, H. E., Mills, I. H., Clapham, W. F., and Hayter, C. J. (1961). Studies on the efferent mechanism of the sodium diuresis which follows the administration of intravenous saline in the dog. *Clin. Sci.* **21**, 249-258.

Dirks, J. H., Cirksena, W. J., and Berliner, R. W. (1966). Micropuncture study of the effect of various diuretics on sodium reabsorption by the proximal tubules of the dog. *J. Clin. Invest.* **45**, 1875-1885.

Dorman, P. J., Sullivan, W. J., and Pitts, R. F. (1954). The renal response to acute respiratory acidosis. *J. Clin. Invest.* **33**, 82-90.

Enns, T. (1967). Facilitation by carbonic anhydrase of carbon dioxide transport. *Science* **155**, 44-47.

Frömter, E., and Hegel, U. (1966). Transtubulare Potentialdifferenzen an proximalen und distalen Tubuli der Rattenniere. *Arch. Ges. Physiol.* **291**, 107-120.

Giebisch, G., Berger, L., and Pitts, R. F. (1955a). The extrarenal response to acute acid-base disturbances of respiratory origin. *J. Clin. Invest.* **34**, 231-245.

Giebisch, G., MacLeod, M. B., and Pitts, R. F. (1955b). Effect of adrenal steroids on renal tubular reabsorption of bicarbonate. *Am. J. Physiol.* **183**, 377-386.

Giebisch, G., Windhager, E. E., and Pitts, R. F. (1960). Mechanism of urinary acidification. *In* "Biology of Pyelonephritis" (E. L. Quinn and E. H. Cass, eds.), pp. 277-287. Little, Brown, Boston, Massachusetts.

Giebisch, G., Klose, R. M., and Malnic, G. (1966). Renal tubular potassium transport. *Proc. 3rd Intern. Congr. Nephrol., Washington, D.C.* **I**, 62-75.

Glabman, S., Klose, R. M., and Giebisch, G. (1963). Micropuncture study of ammonia excretion in the rat. *Am. J. Physiol.* **205**, 127-132.

Gottschalk, C. W., Lassiter, W. E., and Mylle, M. (1960). Localization of urine acidification in the mammalian kidney. *Am. J. Physiol.* **198**, 581-585.

Grollman, A. P., and Gamble, J. L., Jr. (1959). Metabolic alkalosis, a specific effect of adrenocortical hormones. *Am. J. Physiol.* **196**, 135-140.

Guignard, J. P. (1966). Mecanisme de la reabsorption renale des bicarbonates chez le rat. *Helv. Physiol. Pharmacol. Acta* **24**, 193-226.

Gulyassay, P. F., Van Ypersele de Strihou, C., and Schwartz, W. B. (1962). On the mechanism of nitrate-induced alkalosis. The possible role of selective chloride depletion in acid-base regulation. *J. Clin. Invest.* **41**, 1850–1862.

Häusler, G. (1958). Zur Technik und Spezifität des histochemischen Carbonanhydrasenachweises in Modellversuch und in Gewebsschnitten von Rattentieren. *Histochemie* **1**, 29–47.

Hayes, C. P., Jr., Mayson, J. S., Owen, E. E., and Robinson, R. R. (1964). A micropuncture evaluation of renal ammonia excretion in the rat. *Am. J. Physiol.* **207**, 77–83.

Hayes, C. P., Jr., Owen, E. E., and Robinson, R. R. (1966). Renal ammonia excretion during acetazolamide or sodium bicarbonate administration. *Am. J. Physiol.* **210**, 744–750.

Hierholzer, K. (1961). Secretion of potassium and acidification in collecting ducts of mammalian kidney. *Am. J. Physiol.* **201**, 318–324.

Hilton, J. G., Capeci, N. E., Kiss, G. T., Kruesi, O. R., Glaviano, V. V., and Wegria, R. (1956). The effect of acute elevation of the plasma chloride concentration on the renal excretion of bicarbonate during acute respiratory acidosis. *J. Clin. Invest.* **35**, 481–487.

Karler, R., and Woodbury, D. M. (1960). Intracellular distribution of carbonic anhydrase. *Biochem. J.* **75**, 538–543.

Kassirer, J. P., and Schwartz, W. B. (1966a). Correction of metabolic alkalosis in man without repair or potassium deficiency. A re-evaluation of the role of potassium. *Am. J. Med.* **40**, 19–26.

Kassirer, J. P., and Schwartz, W. B. (1966b). The response of normal man to selective depletion of hydrochloric acid. Factors in the genesis of persistent gastric alkalosis. *Am. J. Med.* **40**, 10–18.

Kassirer, J. P., Berkman, P. M., Lawrenz, D. R., and Schwartz, W. B. (1965). The critical role of chloride in the correction of hypokalemic alkalosis in man. *Am. J. Med.* **38**, 172–189.

Kennedy, T. J., Jr., Winkley, J. H., and Dunning, M. F. (1949). Gastric alkalosis with hypokalemia. *Am. J. Med.* **6**, 790–794.

Kunau, R. T., Jr., Frick, A., Rector, F. C., Jr., and Seldin, D. W. (1966). Effect of extracellular fluid volume expansion, potassium deficiency, and pCO_2 on bicarbonate reabsorption in the rat kidney. *Clin. Res.* **14**, 380.

Kunau, R. T., Jr., Frick, A., Rector, F. C., Jr., and Seldin, D. W. (1968). Micropuncture study of the proximal tubular factors responsible for the maintenance of alkalosis during potassium deficiency in the rat. *Clin. Sci.* **34**, 223–231.

Levinsky, N. G., and Lalone, R. C. (1963). The mechanism of sodium diuresis after saline infusion in the dog. *J. Clin. Invest.* **42**, 1261–1276.

Loeb, R. F., Atchley, D. W., Richards, D. W., Jr., Benedict, E. M., and Driscoll, M. E. (1932). On the mechanism of nephrotic edema. *J. Clin. Invest.* **11**, 621–639.

Luke, R. G., and Levitin, H. (1967). Impaired renal conservation of chloride and acid-base changes associated with potassium depletion. *Clin. Sci.* **32**, 511–526.

Malnic, G., Klose, R. M., and Giebisch, G. (1964). Micropuncture study of renal potassium excretion in the rat. *Am. J. Physiol.* **206**, 674–686.

Maren, T. H. (1967). Carbonic anhydrase: Chemistry, physiology, and inhibition. *Physiol. Rev.* **47**, 595–781.

Marsh, D. J., Ullrich, K. J., and Rumrich, G. (1963). Micropuncture analysis of the behavior of potassium ions in rat renal cortical tubules. *Arch. Ges. Physiol.* **277**, 107–119.

Martino, J. A., and Earley, L. E. (1967). Demonstration of a role of physical factors as determinants of the natriuretic response to volume expansion. *J. Clin. Invest.* **46**, 1963–1978.

Menaker, W. (1948). Buffer equilibria and reabsorption in the production of urinary acidity. *Am. J. Physiol.* **154**, 174–184.

Milne, M. D., Scribner, B. H., and Crawford, M. A. (1958). Non-ionic diffusion and the excretion of weak acids and bases. *Am. J. Med.* **24**, 709–729.

Montgomery, H., and Pierce, J. A. (1937). The site of acidification of the urine within the renal tubule in amphibia. *Am. J. Physiol.* **118**, 144–152.

Needle, M. A., Kaloyanides, G. J., and Schwartz, W. B. (1964). The effects of selective depletion of hydrochloric acid on acid-base and electrolyte equilibrium. *J. Clin. Invest.* **43**, 1836–1846.

Orloff, J., and Berliner, R. W. (1956). The mechanism of ammonia excretion in the dog. *J. Clin. Invest.* **35**, 223–235.

Orloff, J., and Davidson, D. G. (1959). The mechanism of potassium excretion in the chicken. *J. Clin. Invest.* **38**, 21–30.

Pitts, R. F. (1958). Some reflections on mechanisms of action of diuretics. *Am. J. Med.* **24**, 745–763.

Pitts, R. F. (1964). Renal production and excretion of ammonia. *Am. J. Med.* **36**, 720–742.

Pitts, R. F., and Alexander, R. S. (1945). The nature of the renal tubular mechanism for acidifying the urine. *Am. J. Physiol.* **144**, 239–254.

Pitts, R. F., and Lotspeich, W. D. (1946). Bicarbonate and the renal regulation of acid-base balance. *Am. J. Physiol.* **147**, 138–154.

Pitts, R. F., Ayer, J. L., and Schiess, W. A. (1949). The renal regulation of acid-base balance in man. III. The reabsorption and excretion of bicarbonate. *J. Clin. Invest.* **28**, 35–44.

Polak, A., Haynie, G. D., Hayes, R. M., and Schwartz, W. B. (1961). Effects of chronic hypercapnea on electrolyte and acid-base equilibrium. I. Adaptation. *J. Clin. Invest.* **40**, 1223–1237.

Pollak, V. E., Mattenheimer, H., DeBruin, H., and Weinman, K. (1965). Experimental metabolic acidosis: The enzymetic basis of ammonia production by the dog kidney. *J. Clin. Invest.* **44**, 169–181.

Rector, F. C., Jr. (1964). Micropuncture studies on the mechanism of urinary acidification. "Renal Metabolism and Epidemiology of Some Renal Diseases," pp. 9–31. Maple Press, York, Pennsylvania.

Rector, F. C., Jr., and Seldin, D. W. (1962). Influence of unreabsorbed anions on renal threshold and Tm for bicarbonate. *Am. J. Physiol.* **202**, 313–318.

Rector, F. C., Jr., Seldin, D. W., Roberts, A. D., Jr., and Smith, J. S. (1960). The role of plasma CO_2 tension and carbonic anhydrase activity in the renal reabsorption of bicarbonate. *J. Clin. Invest.* **39**, 1706–1721.

Rector, F. C., Jr., Buttram, H., and Seldin, D. W. (1962). An analysis of the mechanism of the inhibitory influence of K+ on renal H+ secretion. *J. Clin. Invest.* **41**, 611–617.

Rector, F. C., Jr., Bloomer, H. A., and Seldin, D. W. (1964a). Effect of potassium deficiency on the reabsorption of bicarbonate in the proximal convolution of the rat kidney. *J. Clin. Invest.* **43**, 1976–1982.

Rector, F. C., Jr., Van Giesen, G., Kiil, F., and Seldin, D. W. (1964b). Influence of expansion of extracellular volume on tubular reabsorption of sodium independent of changes in glomerular filtration rate and aldosterone activity. *J. Clin. Invest.* **43**, 341–348.

Rector, F. C., Jr., Carter, N. W., and Seldin, D. W. (1965). The mechanism of bicarbonate reabsorption in the proximal and distal tubules of the kidney. *J. Clin. Invest.* **44**, 278–290.

Rector, F. C., Jr., Brunner, F. P., and Seldin, D. W. (1966). Mechanism of glomerulotubular balance. I. Effect of aortic constriction and elevated ureteropelvic pressure on glomerular filtration rate, fractional reabsorption, transit time, and tubular size in the proximal tubule of the rat. *J. Clin. Invest.* **45**, 590–602.

Reid, E. L., and Hills, A. G. (1965). Diffusion of carbon dioxide out of the distal nephron in man during antidiuresis. *Clin. Sci.* **28**, 15–28.

Relman, A. S., Etsten, B., and Schwartz, W. B. (1953). The regulation of renal bicarbonate reabsorption by plasma carbon dioxide tension. *J. Clin. Invest.* **32**, 972–978.

Roberts, K. E., Magida, M. G., and Pitts, R. F. (1953). Relationship between potassium and bicarbonate in blood and urine. *Am. J. Physiol.* **172**, 47–54.

Roberts, K. E., Randall, H. T., Sanders, H. L., and Hood, M. (1955). Effects of potassium on renal tubular reabsorption of bicarbonate. *J. Clin. Invest.* **34**, 666–672.

Robinson, R. R., and Owen, E. E. (1965). Intrarenal distribution of ammonia during diuresis and antidiuresis. *Am. J. Physiol.* **208**, 1129–1134.

Schwartz, W. B., Jenson, R. L., and Relman, A. S. (1955). Acidification of the urine and increased ammonia excretion without change in acid-base equilibrium: sodium reabsorption as a stimulus to the acidifying process. *J. Clin. Invest.* **34**, 673–680.

Schwartz, W. B., Falbriard, A., and Relman, A. S. (1958). An analysis of bicarbonate reabsorption during partial inhibition of carbonic anhydrase. *J. Clin. Invest.* **37**, 744–751.

Schwartz, W. B., Hays, R. M., Polak, A., and Haynie, G. D. (1961). Effects of chronic hypercapnea on electrolyte and acid-base equilibrium. II. Recovery, with special reference to the influence of chloride intake. *J. Clin. Invest.* **40**, 1238–1249.

Schwartz, W. B., Brackett, N. C., and Cohen, J. J. (1965). The response of extracellular hydrogen ion concentration to graded degrees of chronic hypercapnea: The physiologic limits of the defense of pH. *J. Clin. Invest.* **44**, 291–301.

Seldin, D. W., Welt, L. G., and Cort, J. H. (1956). The role of sodium salts and adrenal steroids in the production of hypokalemic alkalosis. *Yale J. Biol. Med.* **29**, 229–247.

Singer, R. B., Clark, J. K., Barker, E. S., and Elkington, J. R. (1952). The effects of acute respiratory alkalosis on electrolyte excretion and renal hemodynamics in man. *J. Clin. Invest.* **31**, 663.

Stanbury, S. W., and Thomson, A. E. (1952). The renal response to respiratory alkalosis. *Clin. Sci.* **11**, 357–374.

Sullivan, L. P. (1965). Ammonium excretion during stopped flow: a hypothetical ammonium countercurrent system. *Am. J. Physiol.* **209**, 273–282.

Sullivan, W. J., and Dorman, P. J. (1955). The renal response to chronic respiratory acidosis. *J. Clin. Invest.* **34**, 268–276.

Thompson, D. D., and Barrett, M. J. (1954). Renal reabsorption of bicarbonate. *Am. J. Physiol.* **176**, 201–206.

Ullrich, K. J., Eigler, F. W., and Pehling, G. (1958). Sekretion von Wasserstoffionen in den Sammelrohren der Saugetieniere. *Arch. Ges. Physiol.* **267**, 491–496.

Van Ypersele de Strihou, C., Gulyassy, P. F., and Schwartz, W. B. (1962). Effects of chronic hypercapnea on electrolyte and acid-base equilibrium. III. Characteristics of the adaptive and recovery process as evaluated by provision of alkali. *J. Clin. Invest.* **41**, 2246–2252.

Vieira, F. L., and Malnic, G. (1968). Hydrogen ion secretion by rat renal cortical tubules as studied by an antimony microelectrode. *Am. J. Physiol.* **214**, 710–718.

Walser, M., and Mudge, G. H. (1960). Renal excretory mechanisms. *In* "Mineral Metabolism" (C. L. Comer and F. Bronner, eds.), pp. 287–336. Academic Press, New York.

Watson, J. F., Clapp, J. R., and Berliner, R. W. (1964). Micropuncture study of potassium concentration in proximal tubule of dog, rat and Necturus. *J. Clin. Invest.* **43**, 595–605.

Winkler, A. W., and Smith, P. K. (1942). Renal excretion of potassium salts. *Am. J. Physiol.* **138**, 94–103.

5 | RENAL METABOLISM AND TRANSFER OF AMMONIA

*Sulamita Balagura-Baruch**

*Established Investigator of the American Heart Association.

I. Perspectives

A. The Role of Ammonia in the Acid–Base Equilibrium of the Body

Ammonia* excretion is important for removal of excess acid from the body and hence, for preservation of acid–base equilibrium, due to the fortunate combination of the following characteristics (Pitts, 1968a): (1) Ammonia in solution exists as the readily permeant form, the free base (NH_3), and as the poorly permeant form, ammonium ion (NH_4^+). The degree of ionization depends on the pH of the solution. Acidification increases and alkanization decreases the proportion of ammonium ion to free base. (2) Ammonia, formed in renal tubular epithelium from precursor amino acids, diffuses from cells into urine and blood. In each phase, a fraction is converted to ammonium ion according to the hydrogen ion concentration. Thus, acid urines represent a "sink" for trapping of ammonia in its cationic form, favoring continued diffusion of ammonia from cells into urine. (3) Ammonia participates in sodium conservation by forming ammonium salts with anions that would otherwise obligate sodium excretion.

Excretion of strong acids is limited by the inability of renal epithelium to maintain concentration gradients of hydrogen ions between urine and blood greater than 800/1. In other words, the kidney does not form urine of pH below 4.4–4.8. Consequently, in states leading to depletion of body buffer stores, such as diabetes, starvation, loss of base, and ingestion of acid, a main mechanism for preservation of acid–base balance within limits compatible with life lies in enhancement of ammonia production by the kidney. In the process, no energy is expended by the body. Ammonia is a natural waste product of amino acid metabolism. Its production and release are, in metabolic terms, quite inexpensive.

---

*"Ammonia" is used here as a general term to include free base ammonia (NH_3) and ammonium ion (NH_4^+). For this latter purpose, some authors prefer the term "ammonium."

B. Historical Review

Although both urine acidity and the pernicious effects of acid loading had been recognized well before the beginning of this century (Walter, 1877), it was only in 1911 that the presence of ammonia in urine was correlated with acid excretion by Henderson. This author first identified ammonia output as part of the mechanisms for conservation of body neutrality. With Palmer, he observed that in normal man the excess acid produced by foodstuffs is excreted as ammonia and as titratable acidity, and that in advanced nephritis ammonia elimination is impaired. Strangely, they favored the view that urine ammonia varies in relation to nitrogen metabolism rather than in relation to blood pH (Henderson and Palmer, 1914, 1915).

Soon afterwards, Marriott and Howland (1918) observed in humans greater ammonia excretion following ingestion of a strong acid than after equimolar amounts of a weak acid, and Haldane and Kennaway (1920) observed enhanced ammonia output during CO_2 breathing and depressed output during hyperventilation or ingestion of sodium bicarbonate. The interpretation of these results invoked effects of blood pH on ammonia metabolism in the liver, accepted at the time as the source of blood and urine ammonia.

This role was transferred to the kidney a year later, when Nash and Benedict (1921) found in dogs that ammonia concentration in renal venous blood is twice as high as that in arterial blood and in blood from the cava. Although they considered the possibility that renal ammonia might derive from amino acids, they dismissed it in favor of the established view of urea as source of blood ammonia. Their alternate consideration was confirmed only 22 years later when Van Slyke and associates (1943) reported in a terse Letter to the Editor that most of the ammonia formed by the kidney derives from glutamine.

In the meantime, most of the experimentation revolved around verifying Nash and Benedict's discovery and establishing the relation between ammonia output and body neutrality. Results from studies *in vitro* strengthened the theory that the kidney produces ammonia. This was observed for the first time *in vitro* on kidney cultures from doe embryos by Holmes and Watchorn in 1927, and confirmed for chopped rat kidney by Patey and Holmes in 1929. It soon became evident that no other tissue incubated with glucose in aerobiosis produces ammonia (Dickens and Greville, 1933) and that acidification of the incubating media enhances ammonia synthesis (Holmes and Patey, 1930). In the light of our present knowledge, it is hard to understand why it was not postulated that amino acids are sources of ammonia *in vivo* when it was observed that addition of glycine, aspartate, and lysine greatly stimulate ammonia formation *in vitro* (Patey and Holmes, 1929; Holmes and Patey, 1930).

Work on the dog (Hendrix and Sanders, 1923) and man (Van Slyke *et al.*, 1926) firmly established that changes of ammonia excretion are part of the response of the body to acid stress, and that increments are associated with acidosis produced either by acid administration or by disease states such as diabetes. However, there was little agreement on whether the effects occur in response to acid–base factors in urine, blood, or tissues. Some had observed elevations of ammonia output without urine acidification (Gamble *et al.*, 1924). Others, like Briggs (1934), favored the latter as the stimulus for ammonia excretion. In fact, Briggs, by first advancing the thesis that ammonia excretion correlates better with acid–base factors of urine than with tissue acidity, introduced one of the issues most debated up to the present. It is generally conceded now that the opposite view is true.

Despite the large amount of information amassed during the first half of this century on ammonia excretion in health and disease, in man and in several other species, real insight into the relation and relevance of the process to acid–base homeostasis was lacking until Pitts elucidated the mechanisms of urine acidification, as follows. Hydrogen ion secretion from tubular cells into luminal fluid serves to titrate basic salts into acidic salts, to reabsorb bicarbonate, and to excrete acid combined with ammonia. In this manner, then, the kidney participates in replenishing base to body buffer stores, in continuous jeopardy of depletion by acid residues of normal metabolism (Pitts and Alexander, 1945; Pitts, 1948).

These views and additional studies in chronic acidosis were presented by Pitts during the Federation of American Societies for Experimental Biology Meetings in 1948. Besides explaining the nature of urine acidification, they shaped the concept of body adaptation to chronic acidosis by enhanced ammonia excretion. Most importantly, the work of Pitts outlined the trails of research on this and related subjects followed up to the present throughout the world.

At present there is no doubt that the nature of ammonia transfer across renal cells (Section II) is one of nonionic diffusion, as formulated in theoretical terms by Jacobs in 1940 from observations on plant cells, postulated for kidney by Pitts in 1948, suggested by Orloff and Berliner (1956), Owen and Robinson (1965), and several others (Section II), and conclusively proven by Stone and co-workers in 1967. Thus, preformed ammonia brought to the kidney in arterial blood and that synthesized within renal cells form a homogeneous pool. The free base attains diffusion equilibrium in all renal phases, i.e., it distributes rapidly and evenly among peritubular blood, interstitial fluid, and luminal fluid in all cortical and medullary segments of the nephron.

The metabolic pathways of renal ammonia metabolism (Section III) have been delineated in general terms by observing the effects of amino acids on rates of ammonia production by intact kidney and by slices or homogenates. Since renal epithelium is well supplied with enzymes involved in deamidation, deamination, and transamination reactions, several amino acids are potential ammonia precursors. However, it is generally conceded that glutamine is the main source of ammonia in mammalian kidney, due to the combined favorable characteristics of ample arterial supply, high permeability of tubular epithelium and mitochondria, abundant renal content of glutaminases, and fast intrarenal turnover rates. The precise origin of ammonia released by the kidney to urine and blood is known only in the chronically acidotic dog, from studies by Pitts and associates. About 50% of the ammonia released by the kidney derives from the amide nitrogen of glutamine, 16–25% from its amino group, 16–25% from preformed arterial ammonia, and 2–8% from the amino nitrogen of alanine. Whether the information can be safely extrapolated to include man and other animal forms in diverse states of acid–base equilibrium remains to be established.

During prolonged acid stress the rates of ammonia excretion, at any urine pH value, exceed those in acute acidosis (Section IV). This response is called adaptation. It occurs throughout the animal kingdom. Adaptation seems to depend on intracellular acid–base changes in renal cells rather than on extracellular fluid factors, such as blood pH and bicarbonate concentration. Thus, adaptation correlates well with decreases of potassium concentration and of pH inferred to occur in renal cells from observations of changes in muscle cells and plasma electrolytes in conditions leading to adaptation.

The nature of the control of ammonia production (Section V) represents an active field of investigation at present. So far, the causes for adaptation in acidosis remain obscure. In 1952, Davies and Yudkin demonstrated increased glutaminase activity in kidneys of chronically acidotic rats. This study prompted numerous experiments designed to confirm the findings in the rat and other species. At present, it is generally accepted that adaptation is not caused by enzyme induction. Rather, production seems to depend on feedback regulation by the end products of the ammonia-forming reactions, namely, glutamate, α-ketoglutarate, and ammonia. Little is known about the operation of these factors *in vivo* during alterations of acid–base equilibrium of the body.

There is no doubt that the topic of regulation of renal ammonia production will represent a challenging source of experimental inquiry for a long time.

II. Transfer of Ammonia

A. The Chemical Nature of Ammonia and Permeability Properties

Ammonia in solution exists as free base ammonia (NH_3) and as ammonium ion (NH_4^+), in relative proportions determined by the hydrogen ion concentration.

$$NH_3 \underset{-H^+}{\overset{+H^+}{\rightleftharpoons}} NH_4^+$$

Free base   Ammonium ion

The uncharged molecule (NH_3) is a base, for it binds protons to give the acid form (NH_4^+). The charged form (NH_4^+) is an acid, for it releases protons to give free base (NH_3). Hence, the system is a buffer.

In contrast to most other weak electrolytes, one of the constituents, the free base, is a gas. In this respect the ammonia system resembles the familiar bicarbonate/carbonic acid system; it also shares the advantage of fast diffusion of gases across cell membranes. Since dissolved free base is in equilibrium with gaseous ammonia, the concentration in solution ($[NH_3]$) and the partial pressure (pNH_3) are related by the solubility coefficient (α) as follows:

$$pNH_3 = \frac{[NH_3]}{\alpha} \times 22.09 \tag{1}$$

In normal human plasma at $37°C$, α has a value of 0.91 liter (STPD)/liter plasma $\times$ mm Hg of pNH_3 as determined by Jacquez et al. (1959).

The two forms of ammonia in solution differ substantially in their abilities to cross cell membranes. The free base is highly lipid-soluble, hence freely permeant. In contrast, ammonium ion is water-soluble and poorly permeant (Jacobs and Stewart, 1936). These are general properties of weak electrolytes (Jacobs, 1940), for un-ionized molecules cross cell membranes by dissolving in the abundant lipid components, whereas ionized molecules traverse membranes through a limited area of water-filled pores, representing a minimal fraction of total membrane area.

The relative proportions of free base and ammonium ion in solution are determined by the pK_{ab} of the system and by the hydrogen ion concentration of the solution, as indicated in the Henderson-Hasselbalch equation:

$$pH = pK_{ab} + \log \frac{[NH_3]}{[NH_4^+]} \qquad (2)$$

The exponential form of Eq. (2), given below, is more useful when calculating concentrations:

$$\frac{[NH_4^+]}{[NH_3]} = 10^{pKab - pH} \qquad (3)$$

The pK_{ab} determined in blood of man and dog at various ammonia levels is 9.13–9.15 (Bromberg *et al.*, 1960). This agrees with the value of 9.25 given by Jacobs (1940) in his classical formulation of diffusion of weak electrolytes.

The effects of pH in determining the relative proportions of ionized and nonionized fractions in solution are evident from Eq. (3). A change of one pH unit produces a tenfold change in the ratio of concentrations of ammonium ion and free base. Accordingly, the concentration of free base as a fraction of the ammonium ion concentration is approximately 10% at pH 8 (alkaline urine), 1% at pH 7 (blood), 0.1% at pH 6 (modestly acid urine), and 0.01% at pH 5 (very acid urine). Expressed differently, at pH 8, one of every 10 molecules is NH_3, nine are NH_4^+. In contrast, at pH 5 one of every 10,000 molecules is NH_3, the remainder are NH_4^+.

It follows from these considerations that acidification of a solution containing ammonia decreases the fraction of the readily diffusible base and increases that of the relatively impermeant ammonium ion. In contrast, alkalinization elevates the fraction present as free base and diminishes that of ammonium ion. Consequently, if a membrane permeable to the free base separates two identical solutions of ammonia, acidification of one favors accumulation of ammonia, whereas alkalinization of one favors diffusion of ammonia.

B. Factors Determining Ammonia Transfer into Urine and Renal Venous Blood

Ammonia, formed within renal tubular cells from precursor amino acids, is released into luminal fluid and peritubular blood. The factors determining rates of transfer from cells (C) into urine (U) are illustrated in Fig. 1. Similar factors applying to movements between cells and blood are not included in the diagram to avoid undue complication. Symbol sizes roughly indicate relative concentrations and partial pressures of free base (NH_3), and concentrations of ammonium ion (NH_4^+) and of hydrogen ion (H^+) within each phase and between the two phases. K, the permeability constant, includes permeability coefficients of each chemical species, thickness, and area of the membrane.

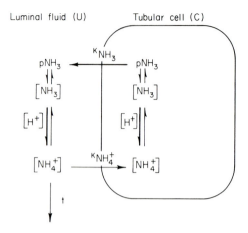

FIG. 1.   Factors determining transfer of ammonia between tubular epithelial cells (C) and urine (U). Relative concentrations ($[NH_3]$) and partial pressures (pNH_3) of free base, concentrations of ammonium ions ($[NH_4^+]$), and of hydrogen ions ($[H^+]$) within each phase and between the two phases, are indicated by different symbol sizes. Permeability coefficients, thickness, and area of the membrane are included in K. Time available for diffusion is t.

Although no membrane is completely impermeable to ammonium ion, poor permeability to this species is exaggerated in Fig. 1 to emphasize the difference in speed of transfer of the two forms of ammonia. Time available for diffusion is indicated by t. This factor depends on rates of urine flow and renal blood flow.

In the dog in chronic metabolic acidosis, steep concentration gradients of ammonia are established between urine and renal venous blood. Thus, in conditions of normal arterial blood ammonia levels of approximately 0.04-0.06 μmoles/ml, urine flow of 1-2 ml/min, and urine pH of 5.4-5.9, concentration in urine is over 30 μmoles/ml, whereas that in renal venous blood is 0.06-0.09 μmoles/ml (Stone et al., 1967). In terms of rates, however, urine excretion exceeds modestly, or may even equal, venous outflow in dog (Stone et al., 1967) and in man (Owen and Robinson, 1963). This is due to the fact that renal blood flow exceeds urine flow by several-fold. Total production is the sum of excretion and renal venous outflow rates minus arterial inflow rate of ammonia. To illustrate, in the chronically acidotic dog, commonly observed rates of ammonia production are 30-40 μmoles/minute per kidney, calculated from excretion of 25-35 μmoles/minute, venous outflow of 15-25 μmoles/minute, and arterial inflow of 10-20 μmoles/minute (Stone et al., 1967).

Although intracellular pH of renal epithelium has not been measured directly, one can safely assume it is below 7.40. Hence, most of the ammonia formed within cells is in the acid form in equilibrium with small amounts of free base. The latter diffuses passively into luminal and peritubular fluid according to the existing gradients of concentrations or partial pressures, and to the permeability constant. Accordingly, transfer rates are given by Fick's law of diffusion, using either concentrations [Eq. (4)] or partial pressures [Eq. (5)]. No energy is required for the process since ammonia moves down chemical gradients. Although these are extremely small, fast diffusion is ensured by very high permeability of tubular epithelial membranes to the free base.

$$\frac{d\mathrm{NH}_3}{dt} = K_{NH_3} \, (\, [\mathrm{NH}_3] \, _C - [\mathrm{NH}_3] \, _U) \tag{4}$$

$$\frac{d\mathrm{NH}_3}{dt} = K_{NH_3} \, (\mathrm{pNH}_{3C} - \mathrm{pNH}_{3U}) \tag{5}$$

In luminal and peritubular fluids ammonia is converted to the acid form in proportion to the hydrogen ion concentrations in each phase. This process helps maintain favorable gradients for diffusion of free base out of cells and establishes steep concentration differences of total ammonia ($\mathrm{NH}_3 + \mathrm{NH}_4^+$) between cells and acid urines, and between blood and acid urines, for the poorly permeant charged form is "trapped" in acid urine. These processes of ammonia transfer are aptly designated by the terms "nonionic diffusion," indicating movement of the un-ionized molecule, and "diffusion trapping," indicating asymmetric accumulation across cell membranes according to H^+ ion concentrations.

It follows from the above considerations that constant release of ammonia into urine and renal venous blood necessitates adequate production rates to meet the demands established by the pH values in luminal and peritubular fluids, as well as removal of the free base from the extracellular phases to maintain adequate diffusion gradients. In acid urines, the latter are ensured by conversion of free base to ammonium ions. In peritubular fluid and in alkaline urines, they are maintained by removal from the diffusion sites; thus, flow rates of alkaline urine and of renal blood are important. About 60–70% of the total ammonia produced in acidosis leaves the kidney in the urine, 30–40% in renal venous blood. In urine, ammonia is put out at high concentrations compared to levels in renal venous blood due to greater "diffusion trapping" in the relatively more acid urine.

In summary, then, the factors influencing renal release of ammonia include chemical gradients of the free base between cells and luminal fluid, and between cells and peritubular fluid, hydrogen ion concentrations in these three phases, rates of production within tubular epithelium, and rates of urine flow and renal blood flow.

C. Nonionic Diffusion

The characteristics of ammonia transfer across renal tubular epithelium conform with the general nature of the movement of weak electrolytes as formulated by Jacobs (1940). The theoretical aspects of the process have been thoroughly reviewed by Milne, Scribner, and Crawford (1958) and by Orloff and Berliner (1956). Ample experimental evidence substantiates the view that renal transfer of ammonia observes the basic tenets of nonionic diffusion of a weak base. These are (a) movement of the free base according to diffusion laws, (b) net direction of movement from the less acid to the more acid phase, and (c) accumulation across cell membranes according to the hydrogen ion concentration (Orloff and Berliner, 1956; Balagura and Pitts, 1962; Denis *et al.*, 1964; Owen and Robinson, 1965; Stone *et al.*, 1967).

Nonionic diffusion may readily be tested by studying the effects of urine pH changes on ammonia excretion. Predictably, acidification of urine by one pH unit should increase the concentration ratio of ammonium ion to free base by a factor of 10 [Eq.(3)], as the latter is converted into the acid form. Accordingly, ammonia transfer into urine should be favored in the same proportion [Eqs. (4) and (5)]. Therefore, a tenfold increase in ammonia concentration is expected as urine pH decreases by one unit provided that (1) back-diffusion of ammonium ions is nil; (2) time available for diffusion is adequate; (3) cell and urine pH are constant; (4) ammonia production rates are adequate to meet the increased demands.

Much evidence undoubtedly indicates that ammonia excretion conforms to general principles of nonionic diffusion. The effects of urine pH on excretion of ammonia and other weak bases have been thoroughly studied in the dog by Orloff and Berliner (1956). Figure 2, from their work, illustrates that, in effect, there exists an inverse correlation between urine pH and excretion rates of ammonia, Sn-8439, and quinine, in the manner expected from nonionic diffusion.

Deviations from the theoretical slope of unity are observed, for the conditions stated above hold only to a certain extent. It was already mentioned that permeability to ammonium ion is finite, albeit low. Furthermore, urine pH varies due to buffering by ammonium ions. But aside from these factors, production rate is what ultimately determines accumulation of ammonia, and thus excretion, in acid urines. Figure 3,

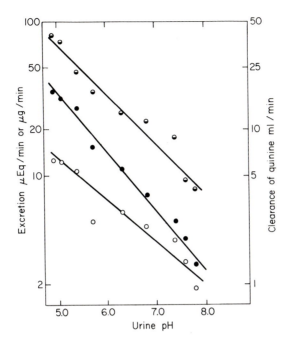

FIG. 2. The effect of the infusion of NaHCO$_3$ on urine pH and the excretion of ammonia, Sn-8439, and the clearance of quinine in dog S: ammonia excretion (μEq/min) is indicated by filled circles; Sn-8439 excretion (μg/min), by open circles; and quinine clearance, by half-filled circles. From Orloff and Berliner (1956).

from the work of Leonard and Orloff (1955) in the rat, shows that excretion rates of ammonia and atabrine, also a weak base, become lower than predicted when urine is acidified. Deviations from the theoretical straight line relation at urine pH values below 6.8 also occur in dog (Sullivan and McVaugh, 1963). Preservation of the theoretical relation when urine pH decreases by two units requires a hundredfold increase in diffusion of ammonia. Under these conditions production rates presumably become limiting in providing adequate amounts of free base to meet the extraordinary demands. Studies by Sullivan (1965) on dog in conditions of stopped flow provide support for this view. At urine pH below 6.0, infusion of glutamine, the major source of ammonia, enhances ammonia excretion. Under these conditions, the theoretical slope is approached. In general, excretion rates of weak bases into acid urines are lower than predicted. Since all weak bases except ammonia are foreign to the body, limitation in diffusion rates, not in production, account for the deviations at low urine pH, as depicted in Fig. 3 for atabrine (Orloff and Berliner, 1956).

Permeability of cell membranes to the free base is very high, of the order of at least 1×10^{-2} cm/sec in cortical segments of the nephron (Oelert *et al.*, 1968). This allows for net transfer of free base down extremely small pNH_3 gradients. When urine is acid, continued diffusion of the free base from renal cells is ensured by trapping by hydrogen ions. In contrast, when ammonia diffuses into neutral or alkaline urines, less trapping occurs. Consequently, maintenance of diffusion depends on urine flow for removal of ammonia. Increased excretion has in effect been observed in dogs during mannitol diuresis at urine pH of 6.9–7.2 (Orloff and Berliner, 1956).

Major aspects of ammonia excretion confirming nonionic diffusion are summarized in Figs. 4 and 5 from studies on the dog (Balagura and Pitts, 1962), using the Chinard (1955) method. The excretion of ammonia is compared to that of creatinine, a "glomerular substance," after a rapid injection of both compounds into one renal artery. In metabolic acidosis (Fig. 4) appearance of ammonia in urine and peak excretion precede those of creatinine (I). Accordingly, ammonia diffuses from blood into acid urine across the tubule at some point distal from the glomerulus. Ammonia in peritubular blood reaches this point faster than ammonia in the filtrate, due to differences in flow rates of luminal and peritubular fluids. Percent excretion of ammonia below that of creatinine (II) indicates movement of ammonia in the opposite

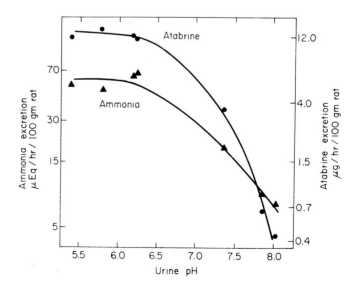

Fig. 3. Relationship between urine pH and excretion of ammonia and atabrine in rat during infusion of sodium bicarbonate. From Leonard and Orloff (1955).

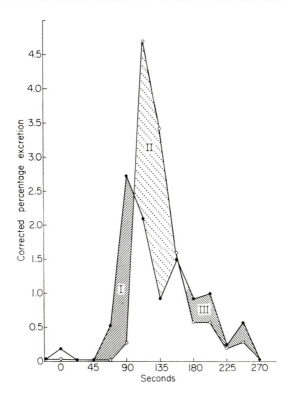

Fig. 4. Pattern of renal excretion of creatinine (open circles) and ammonia (filled circles) during acidosis. Each sample represents a collection of 22.5 seconds. From Balagura and Pitts (1962).

direction, from urine into blood or at least into tubular cells. Finally, prolonged excretion of ammonia relative to creatinine (III) indicates release from a tubular store or "sink" of ammonia accumulated from peritubular blood and tubular urine. Strikingly different results are seen in metabolic alkalosis (Fig. 5). Excretion of injected ammonia is nil; therefore, filtered ammonia must have diffused into more acid phases, namely, cells and peritubular blood. Ammonia in peritubular blood probably diffuses into the more acid cells and eventually back to blood.

Studies in the dog by Sullivan and McVaugh (1963) further support the view that net movement of ammonia across the renal tubular epithelium occurs in the direction of the more acid phases. Following injections of alkalinizing or acidifying solutions into a renal artery, changes in pH of renal venous blood precede changes in urine pH. Injection of sodium bicarbonate initially increases urine ammonia con-

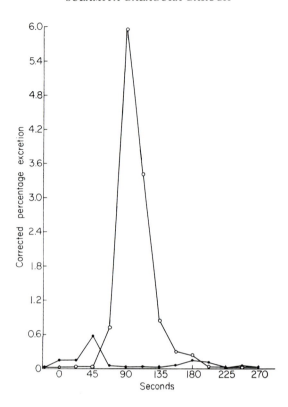

Fig. 5.   Pattern of renal excretion of creatinine (open circles) and ammonia (filled circles) during alkalosis. Each sample represents a collection of 22.5 seconds. From Balagura and Pitts (1962).

centration, as a portion previously diffusing into blood is shifted into the less alkaline urine. Thereafter, urine ammonia concentration decreases as urine is alkalinized. Similarly, when acidification of blood precedes that of urine after injection of sodium ferrocyanide, urine ammonia concentration decreases, as a portion previously diffusing into urine is shifted into the more acid blood. Thereafter, urine ammonia concentration increases as urine is acidified.

Similar results obtained in studies on man by Owen *et al.* (1960) lend support to the view that in human kidney ammonia is also transferred by nonionic diffusion. Thus, in patients with liver disease but normal renal function, these authors observed that following intravenous injection of acetazolamide there is rapid decrease of ammonia excretion, associated with alkalinization of urine, and rapid increase of arterial ammonia concentration, associated with acidification of blood. Since the excess amount of ammonia released into renal venous blood approximated the decrement of excretion, they concluded that changes of the pH gradient between urine and blood produce shifts in the partition of ammonia produced by kidney between the two fluids. Thus, the relative proportions of ammonia leaving the kidney in urine and in renal venous blood depend ultimately on the pH gradients between the two phases, provided constancy of other factors such as urine flow, renal blood flow, and cell pNH_3.

D. Diffusion Equilibrium for Ammonia

The observations described above provide conclusive evidence for nonionic diffusion of ammonia in the kidney. They show that ammonia moves from less acid to more acid phases in renal tissue (Balagura and Pitts, 1962; Sullivan and McVaugh, 1963) and that excretion proceeds in accord with laws of nonionic diffusion of weak bases (Jacobs, 1940; Orloff and Berliner, 1956). An assumption implied, although not proven in these studies, is that the free base distributes evenly throughout renal cells and fluids. Observations by Denis *et al.* (1964) in the dog suggest that indeed the free base may attain diffusion equilibrium among all cortical phases, since measured pNH_3 of renal venous blood approximates calculated pNH_3 of cortical cells.

Figure 6, from the work of these authors on dog in chronic metabolic acidosis, shows the changes in ammonia excretion and in arterial and renal venous pNH_3 when arterial ammonia concentration is raised by infusion of ammonium lactate. Under control conditions at average values of arterial ammonia of 0.041 μmole/ml blood, and of arterial pNH_3 of 22.4×10^{-6} mm Hg the renal venous pNH_3 has a mean value of 42.3×10^{-6} mm Hg. In the absence of differences of pH between arterial and renal venous blood, higher pNH_3 in the latter is due to greater ammonia concentration. Urinary ammonia excretion is high, about 31.2 μmoles/minute per kidney.

At arterial ammonia concentration twice the control level due to infusion of ammonium lactate, arterial pNH_3 increases. However, renal venous pNH_3 remains essentially at the original value. Further elevations in arterial total ammonia levels result in reversal of the initial arteriovenous pNH_3 gradient, i.e., arterial pNH_3 exceeds renal venous pNH_3. Ammonia in arterial blood diffuses into cells and then into urine. Excretion increases progressively.

At the point of intersection of the arterial and renal venous lines, there is no diffusion gradient. Ammonia formed in tubular cells is released into urine (excretion increases), not into renal venous blood.

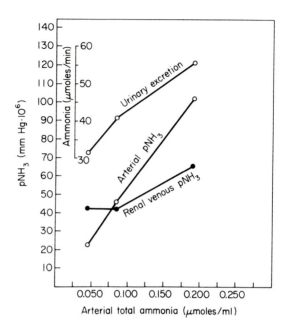

Fɪɢ. 6.   The relationships among arterial and renal venous pNH₃, ammonia excretion, and arterial ammonia concentration in dogs in chronic metabolic acidosis. Curves represent the mean of four experiments. The arterial ammonia concentration was increased by the infusion of ammonium lactate at rates of 100 and 300 μmoles/minute. From Denis *et al.* (1964).

This must mean, then, that the pNH₃ at the intersection represents the pNH₃ of tubular cells, since no net transfer occurs at this point between cells and peritubular blood, i.e., arterial and renal venous pNH₃ are equal. It is clear from the figure that the pNH₃ at this point scarcely differs from the renal venous pNH₃ in control conditions. In fact, the difference is less than 1×10^{-6} mm Hg.

Figure 7 illustrates the results obtained when similar observations are performed on dogs in chronic metabolic alkalosis. Raising blood ammonia levels by infusion of ammonium lactate produces proportional elevations in arterial and renal venous pNH₃. At all arterial concentrations, the kidney adds ammonia in net amounts to renal venous blood, as indicated by renal venous pNH₃ values always exceeding arterial levels. In these experiments in alkalosis it is not possible to establish whether diffusion equilibrium occurs, although there are no reasons to doubt its existence.

It was previously mentioned that urine flow and renal plasma flow become important determinants of renal ammonia release in conditions of alkalosis. As seen in these experiments in which urine pH and blood pH were equal, the greater flow rate of peritubular fluid than of luminal fluid probably accounts for addition of ammonia, formed in renal epithelium, to peritubular fluid, not to urine. Excretion remained negligible at all times.

In consequence, then, a main conclusion from these studies on dogs is that the pNH_3 of renal venous blood approximates that of cortical tubular cells. This is due to attainment of diffusion equilibrium for ammonia between proximal and distal tubular cells and peritubular blood. A similar situation exists in the rat kidney, as shown by Oelert *et al.* (1968) in micropuncture studies. Values of pNH_3 of renal venous blood equal those of luminal fluid from proximal tubules and from distal tubules.

Incontrovertible evidence supporting the view of diffusion equilibrium of ammonia among all cortical phases, further extending it to include all phases in the kidney along the whole length of the nephron,

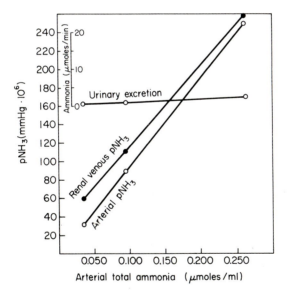

FIG. 7. The relationships among arterial and renal venous pNH_3, ammonia excretion, and arterial ammonia concentration in dogs in chronic metabolic alkalosis. Curves represent the mean of 7 experiments. The arterial ammonia concentration was increased by the infusion of ammonium lacate at rates of 100 and 300 μmoles/minute. From Denis *et al.* (1964).

has been given by Stone *et al.* (1967) in dogs in chronic metabolic acidosis. The diagram in Fig. 8 illustrates the rationale of the methods employed to assess in a more direct fashion the characteristics of ammonia transfer discussed above. Diffusion equilibrium for ammonia in the kidney necessitates rapid and even distribution of the free base throughout all phases: blood, interstitial fluid, proximal and distal tubular cells, and tubular urine along the whole length of the nephron. Accordingly, if ^{15}N-ammonia is injected into one renal artery, it should mix rapidly and evenly with unlabeled ^{14}N-ammonia synthesized within epithelial cells. If true, and provided that all ammonia in urine and renal venous blood derives from this well-mixed pool, the degree of labeling of ammonia throughout the kidney, i.e., in urine, in renal venous blood, and in the cellular "pool," should be identical.

Pool specific activity can be calculated from the ^{15}N infusion rate and the pool turnover rate (Fig. 8). The latter equals the sum of the output of ammonia determined in urine and in renal venous blood (Table I). The specific activity of ammonia ($^{15}N/^{14}N + ^{15}N$) in urine can be measured directly. The agreement found between calculated specific ac-

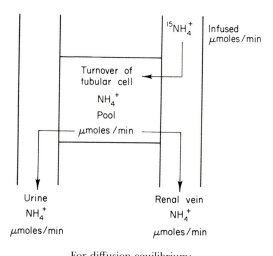

For diffusion equilibrium:

Measured	Calculated
$\dfrac{\text{Urine}}{\dfrac{^{15}N}{^{14}N + ^{15}N}}$	$= \dfrac{^{15}NH_4^+ \text{ infusion rate}}{\text{Pool turnover rate}}$

FIG. 8. Schematic representation of the renal ammonia pool and the method for assessment of diffusion equilibrium. From Stone *et al.* (1967).

TABLE I

COMPARISON BETWEEN CALCULATED AND MEASURED SPECIFIC ACTIVITIES OF AMMONIA IN THE KIDNEY OF THE ACIDOTIC DOG[a]

Ammonia			Specific activity		
Venous out	Urine out (μmoles/minute)	Pool turnover	Pool (atom % excess ^{15}N)	Urine (L-R)	Urine pool
Infuse ^{15}NH$_4$Cl -1.85 μmoles/minute					
21.2	37.6	58.8	3.16	3.30	1.04
17.4	37.7	55.1	3.36	3.35	1.00
15.1	37.2	52.3	3.45	3.44	1.00
Infuse ^{15}NH$_4$Cl -9.27 μmoles/minute					
20.4	40.0	60.4	15.35	15.39	1.00
19.1	39.0	58.1	15.95	15.85	.99
17.0	41.3	58.3	15.90	15.91	1.00

[a]Modified from Stone et al. (1967).

tivity of ammonia in the renal "pool" and measured specific activity of ammonia in urine, indicated in Table I by a quotient of unity (last column), proves diffusion equilibrium.

Accordingly, ammonia within renal epithelial cells exists in a well-mixed pool formed from preformed ammonia entering the kidney in arterial blood and that newly synthesized from precursor amino acids. This pool is small in size (Robinson and Owen, 1965) but turns over rapidly. Half-time is about 1 minute, and equilibrium is attained in less than the transit time of blood through the kidney. Ammonia diffuses from this cellular pool into urine and renal venous blood and accumulates in each phase according to the respective H$^+$ ion concentrations. In the dog kidney there are no provisions for significant utilization of ammonia by alternate routes, since ammonia fixation in synthesis of urea (Van Slyke et al., 1943), of glutamate (Stone and Pitts, 1967), or of glutamine (Lyon and Pitts, 1967) does not occur in the dog kidney. In the rat kidney, in contrast, ammonia is utilized for synthesis of glutamate and glutamine (Pitts, 1968b). No information is available on human kidneys in this respect.

The experimental evidence demonstrating diffusion equilibrium of free base in the dog kidney precludes a major contribution of active transport to ammonia secretion. If it does indeed occur, its role must certainly be minor because an active transport system could hardly account for equilibrium of the free base along the whole length of the nephron, among heterogeneous phases of unequal hydrogen ion concentrations.

E. Sites of Production and Secretion of Ammonia

Assessment of the sites of production and secretion of ammonia in the kidney requires information derived from diverse experimental approaches, such as stop-flow studies, micropuncture procedures, and biochemical techniques for identification of enzymes involved in ammonia formation in sections of renal cortex and medulla. High ammonia concentration in a sample obtained from a given tubular segment indicates diffusion trapping in a region of high acidity rather than production in that particular site of the nephron. This follows from the fact that ammonia distributes in all phases of the kidney following principles of nonionic diffusion of weak bases, as discussed in the previous section.

Accordingly, the degree to which ammonia accumulates in luminal fluid in each portion of the nephron is expected to parallel the degree to which hydrogen ions are secreted in each segment. In effect, micropuncture studies on amphibia have established that neither significant acidification (Montgomery and Pierce, 1937) nor ammonia secretion (Walker, 1940) occur in proximal tubules. In the frog, urine ammonia derives from that secreted in the last two-thirds of the distal tubules and the early part of collecting ducts (Walker, 1940). Similarly, the collecting ducts are major sites of acidification (Ullrich and Eigler, 1958) and ammonia secretion (Ullrich *et al.*, 1958) in the golden hamster.

The contribution of proximal tubules to urine ammonia in mammalian kidneys was first demonstrated on the rat by Glabman, Klose, and Giebisch (1963). The findings have been confirmed by Hayes *et al.* (1964). In micropuncture studies on normal, alkalotic, and acidotic rats, these authors found that net ammonia secretion occurs in the proximal tubule, that all parts of the nephron add ammonia to luminal fluid, and that in acidosis, the proximal tubule may contribute as much as 50 to 70% of total urine ammonia. Similar characteristics of hydrogen ion secretion have been found as follows. In rat kidney, progressive acidification occurs in the proximal tubule (Litchfield and Bott, 1962; Bank and Aynedjian, 1963), distal tubule, and collecting ducts (Gottschalk *et al.*, 1960). Furthermore, it has been estimated that about 52% of the titratable acidity in urine generates in proximal tubules (Bloomer *et al.*, 1963), a value in agreement with the calculated contribution of this segment to urine ammonia.

In the dog, results from stop-flow studies indicate that the sites of ammonia secretion and urine acidification are coextensive in the distal portion of the nephron (Pitts *et al.*, 1958; Sullivan *et al.*, 1960). In micropuncture studies on normal dogs, neither ammonia secretion (Clapp *et al.*, 1965) nor acidification (Bernstein and Clapp, 1968) are apparent in proximal tubule, in contrast with findings on normal rats. However, both become evident in chronic metabolic acidosis. The possibility of proximal contribution to urine ammonia in the normal state cannot be discarded, for even if substantial, it could still be below 0.3 mM, the limit of sensitivity for analytical detection. Late proximal acidification has also been found in the *Rhesus* monkey (Bennett *et al.*, 1968), but there is no information on ammonia secretion in this form.

Since in the dog, reabsorption of precursor amino acids takes place in the proximal tubule (Ruszkowski *et al.*, 1962), it is reasonable to assume that ammonia is produced in proximal epithelial cells. Renal uptake of glutamine, the major ammonia precursor, exceeds reabsorption. Thus, glutamine enters renal cells from peritubular blood as well as from luminal fluid (Shalhoub *et al.*, 1963). It is not known in what parts of the nephron this peritubular transfer occurs.

Glutaminase I, the enzyme system which accounts for most of the ammonia produced in the kidney, is distributed throughout the cortex and medulla in man (Holmgård, 1962), dogs, rats, guinea pigs (Richterich and Goldstein, 1958), and golden hamsters (Karnovsky and Himmelhoch, 1961). Activity in collecting ducts is high enough to account for maximal ammonia secreted by most species (Richterich and Goldstein, 1958). However, some attribute this function exclusively to proximal convoluted tubules because, in the rat, enhanced ammonia production in chronic metabolic acidosis is associated with increments of glutaminase activity only in proximal tubules, not in any other renal segments (Weiss and Longley, 1960; Karnovsky and Himmelhoch, 1961).

Studies by Robinson and Owen (1965) on the distributional pattern of concentration of ammonia in renal tissue suggest a medullary countercurrent exchange system in the distribution of ammonia. This concept derives from the following findings on dog: In conditions of mannitol diuresis, renal ammonia concentration is equal in cortical and medullary tissue (0.7–2.7 mM). In conditions of antidiuresis, in contrast, it increases progressively towards the medulla, reaching values of about 12 mM in the papilla. This corticomedullary gradient in antidiuresis is independent of urine pH, for it is only slightly less pronounced in alkaline urines than in neutral or acid urines.

The total ammonia ($NH_3 + NH_4^+$) entering Henle's loop, a mixture of ammonia filtered and secreted along the proximal tubule, is progressively concentrated as fluid moves down the descending limb, an effect of water reabsorption. In addition, as the fluid becomes alkaline in this region (Gottschalk *et al.*, 1960), the proportion of diffusible free base

(NH_3) rises. Consequently, ammonia diffuses out from descending to ascending limbs, and back into descending limbs due to its high permeability. Furthermore, diffusion includes transfer to all medullary structures, namely, interstitial fluid, vasa recta blood, and collecting duct fluid. Diffusion equilibrium occurs; accumulation of ammonia as the ion (NH_4^+) depends on the pH existing in each phase. In acidosis, great accumulation occurs in collecting ducts since the free base is trapped as the ionized form. During diuresis, the corticomedullary gradient is not established because less subtraction of water and less alkalinization along the descending limb minimize the increased concentration in total ammonia as well as the increased concentration of diffusible nonionized ammonia in this segment. Such a scheme of countercurrent distribution of ammonia may explain why the concentration ratio of urine ammonia to blood ammonia exceeds the corresponding concentration ratio of hydrogen ions when urine pH is above 6.0. This would be explained by the existence of diffusion equilibrium of ammonia in all regions of medullary tissue. In consequence, ammonia in collecting duct fluid equilibrates with that in loop fluid, which is concentrated above that in cortical fluids due to countercurrent exchange diffusion (Sullivan, 1965).

To summarize, all parts of the nephron contain glutaminase I, and may thus produce ammonia. Secretion, however, only occurs in those segments where acidification takes place. This is a consequence of diffusion equilibrium of the free base and of net transfer from the less acid to the more acid sites. Thus, in amphibia, urine ammonia derives from that secreted in late distal tubules and early collecting ducts. In mammals, all parts of the nephron possibly contribute to urine ammonia, in the same degree that they contribute to urine acidification.

F. Summary

Ammonia is a weak electrolyte which dissociates, according to the H^+ ion concentration of the solution, into a nonionized form, the free base (NH_3), and an ionized form, ammonium ion (NH_4^+). Dissolved free base is in equilibrium with gaseous ammonia. Thus, the chemical nature of the ammonia system ensures rapid movement in all directions across tubular cells, as well as development of steep concentration gradients of total ammonia between blood and acid urine. The free base (NH_3) has high lipid solubility, is freely permeant, and distributes rapidly and evenly according to diffusion laws throughout all phases of the kidney, namely, epithelial cells, interstitial fluid, luminal fluid, and peritubular blood. Ammonium ion (NH_4^+) is water-soluble, poorly permeant, and accumulates in each phase according to the respective H^+ ion concentrations. The metabolic cost of renal ammonia transfer itself is nil, i.e., no extra energy is required besides that needed for secretion of hydrogen ions that leads to accumulation of ammonia. The terms commonly used in referring to ammonia transfer best describe its characteristics: "nonionic diffusion" stresses movement of the un-ionized free base; "diffusion trapping" designates accumulation as ammonium ion, the impermeant form trapped by hydrogen ions.

Preformed ammonia in arterial blood and that synthesized within renal epithelial cells from precursor amino acids form a homogeneous cellular pool. The free base distributes rapidly and evenly among cells, luminal fluid, interstitial fluid, and peritubular blood. Transfer into urine and renal venous blood occurs according to diffusion laws, down extremely small concentration gradients of free base. Net direction of movement is from the less acid to the more acid phases, and accumulation in each phase is determined by the respective H^+ ion concentration.

III. Origin of Urinary and Renal Venous Ammonia

A. Experimental Approach

Various experimental approaches have been used for elucidating the pathways operating in ammonia production by the kidney. In studies *in vitro*, metabolic reactions in renal tissue are identified by measurements of ammonia production by renal slices or homogenates incubated with a particular substrate. Enzyme activity is expressed in terms of ammonia produced per unit time, per unit tissue weight, or per unit tissue protein.

The values obtained depend to a great extent on the composition of the incubating media. Thus renal tissue forms little ammonia from glutamine in the absence of phosphate. Upon addition of this ion, ammonia production increases severalfold (Errera and Greenstein, 1949; Sayre and Roberts, 1958), a fact that has led to characterization of phosphate-dependent and phosphate-independent glutaminase I enzyme systems. However, the activation effect is not solely induced by phosphate. Other ions, such as sulfate, arsenate, pyrophosphate (Klingman and Handler, 1958), acetate, and Krebs cycle intermediates (O'Donovan and Lotspeich, 1966), enhance ammonia production from glutamine by kidney homogenates. Clearly, then, identification of a reaction in studies *in vitro* only suggests its potential existence in the intact functioning kidney, but does not prove its operation under the conditions prevailing in the intracellular milieu.

In studies *in vivo*, ammonia precursors are generally identified by observing the effects of oral or intravenous administration of single amino acids on urine ammonia output. Under these conditions, increased excretion suggests, but does not prove, derivation of ammonia from the presumed precursor in the kidney. The effect could be mediated by increased blood ammonia levels produced by amino acid loading (Du Ruisseau *et al.*, 1956; Wergedal and Harper, 1964) and/or by conversion into a different amino acid at extrarenal sites (Duda and Handler, 1958). A more refined approach is used in balance studies in which arteriorenal venous concentration differences are measured to correlate renal extraction of individual amino acids and/or α-amino and amide nitrogen with renal production of ammonia nitrogen.

Evidently, neither approach mentioned provides means for assessment of the relative contributions of ammonia precursors to urine ammonia, or of the metabolic pathways actually operating in the intact kidney and leading to synthesis of ammonia. All information on these processes available at present derives from a series of studies by Pitts and co-workers. The approach used entails administration of ^{15}N-labeled precursors and measurements of specific activities of nitrogen in urine ammonia and in the precursor in arterial plasma. The ratio between the two values represents the exact proportion of ammonia derived from the labeled compound. This approach has represented a major contribution to the field. Without it little would be known on renal ammonia metabolism in the intact functioning kidney.

The rationale of the procedure (Pitts, 1966), illustrated in Fig. 9, is as follows: A ^{15}N-labeled amino acid is injected at constant, known, and low rates into a renal artery. For example, in Fig. 9, intraarterial infusion of glutamine, with 95% of its amide nitrogens of the ^{15}N variety, is shown. Amide ^{15}N-glutamine is represented by capital G, and ^{14}N-glutamine, the normally present variety, by small g. The ureters are individually catheterized for collection of urine separately from each kidney. If ammonia in urine from the infused kidney derives from the amide nitrogen of glutamine, it should be labeled. The degree of labeling depends on the proportion of urine ammonia drawn from amide glutamine.

Urine ^{15}N-ammonia is represented by capital A, and ^{14}N-ammonia, the normally occurring variety, by small a. Part of the injected labeled glutamine recirculates and is extracted by both kidneys. Thus the urine from the noninfused kidney also contains some ^{15}N-ammonia. Subtraction of the atoms percent excess of ^{15}N(specific activity) in ammonia

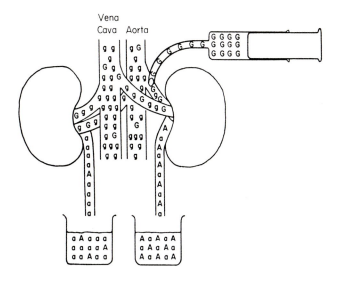

FIG. 9. Diagram illustrating the use of ^{15}N-labeled amino acids in studies on the origin of urinary ammonia. From Pitts (1966). (G), ^{15}N amide glutamine; (g), ^{14}N glutamine; (A), ^{15}N ammonia; and (a), ^{14}N ammonia.

excreted by this kidney from that excreted by the infused kidney is the specific activity of the ammonia derived exclusively from the ^{15}N-amide glutamine given into the renal artery.

The total glutamine load to the kidney is the sum of the load infused and that normally present. The latter is the product of renal plasma flow and arterial glutamine concentration. The specific activity of arterial glutamine is, thus, the ratio between the rate of infusion of ^{15}N and the total glutamine load. Subtraction of the corresponding value for the noninfused kidney from the value for the infused kidney corrects for recirculation of ^{15}N in any form. The ratio between the corrected specific activity of urine ammonia and that of arterial plasma glutamine represents the fraction of urine ammonia derived from the amide nitrogen of glutamine. In the more general case,

$$\frac{\text{Corrected specific activity of urine ammonia}}{\text{Corrected specific activity of arterial plasma precursor}} \times 100$$

= Percent of urinary ammonia derived from precursor in arterial plasma

The feasibility of applying all methods described in any one species and in each state of acid–base balance is limited. Hence, general conclusions on ammonia metabolism are drawn from data collected in independent studies on different animal forms. From the information accumulated at present, it is becoming evident that there are quantitative differences among species relating to determinant factors in ammonia metabolism, such as precursor supply, tubular permeability to amino acids, and metabolic pathways selected in normal and altered acid–base balance.

The source of ammonia in urine and renal venous blood is a single homogeneous ammonia pool within the renal tubular epithelium. This pool is formed by the nitrogen groups of glutamine and other amino acids, and by preformed blood ammonia. Since arterial ammonia mixes thoroughly and evenly with that newly synthesized in renal cells, i.e., diffusion equilibrium exists, precursors contribute in identical proportions to ammonia released into urine and into renal venous blood.

These proportions, as illustrated in Fig. 10, apply to dogs in chronic metabolic acidosis. Data are taken from studies by Pitts and co-workers (Pitts *et al.*, 1965; Pitts and Pilkington, 1966; Pitts and Stone, 1967a,b; Stone and Pitts, 1967; Stone *et al.*, 1967). About 33–50% of urinary ammonia derives from the amide nitrogen of glutamine. The remainder is drawn in approximately equal proportions from the amino nitrogen of glutamine and from preformed blood ammonia. A small fraction, 2 to 8%, originates from the amino nitrogen of alanine. Accordingly, over 90% of the ammonia synthesized in the renal epithelium derives from a single amino acid, glutamine.

The extent to which these values can be applied to man and other animal species in diverse states of acid–base balance remains to be ascertained. However, it is generally conceded that mammalian kidney derives the vast majority of ammonia from glutamine, and that it contains adequate metabolic reactions to use additional amino acids for

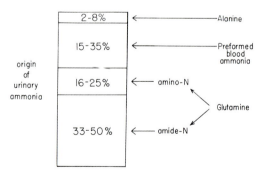

FIG. 10. Sources of ammonia released by the kidney into urine and renal venous blood. The proportions derived from each precursor apply to the dog in chronic metabolic acidosis.

ammonia production. The relative contribution of a potential precursor to urine ammonia depends on factors such as availability in plasma, permeability of renal tubular epithelium and mitochondria, and occurrence of adequate metabolic reactions in the kidney. These factors determine species differences with respect to predominant sources of ammonia, as well as relative efficacy of amino acids as ammonia formers in a single species.

B. Glutamine as Ammonia Precursor

In 1943 Van Slyke and co-workers established in the dog that glutamine is the major precursor of ammonia in urine and in renal venous blood. Their discovery ended a long-standing dispute concerning the role of urea in renal production of ammonia (Barnett and Addis, 1917). Van Slyke and associates did balance studies correlating net renal extraction of amide and amino nitrogens with net renal production of ammonia nitrogen. Their conclusions as originally stated, that renal extraction of the amide nitrogen of glutamine can account for all ammonia released into renal venous blood and for 60% or more of that released into urine, deserve a word of caution. They should be interpreted in terms of net rates in balance studies, not in terms of relative contribution of precursors to urinary and renal venous ammonia.

Compared to liver and other tissues, the kidney ranks high in its ability for accumulating a variety of infused amino acids (Friedberg and Greenberg, 1947a,b; Kamin and Handler, 1951a). However, at normal endogenous plasma levels, net renal extraction of glutamine exceeds by far that of any other amino acid. The difference in glutamine concentration between arterial and renal venous plasma is 6 times greater than that of glycine, the only other amino acid extracted in quantitatively significant amounts in the acidotic dog (Shalhoub et al., 1963).

Glutamine enters renal tubular cells from peritubular blood across antiluminal membranes and from filtered fluid across luminal membranes (Shalhoub et al., 1963). Since urinary excretion in man (Meister, 1956) and dog (Shalhoub et al., 1963) is vanishingly low, reabsorption must be active. In all probability, peritubular movement is also by active transport. In addition to high extraction rates, plentiful supply of glutamine for renal ammonia production is ensured by its high arterial concentration which constitutes 18 to 25% of total concentration of free α-amino acids in human and dog plasma (Hamilton, 1945; Meister, 1956).

Notwithstanding availability and renal epithelial permeability to amino acids, what ultimately determines the predominant sources of ammonia is the occurrence of adequate metabolic reactions within the kidney. In this respect also, abundant and ubiquitous distribution of renal glutaminases ensures preferential derivation of ammonia from glutamine throughout the animal kingdom.

C. Other Precursor Amino Acids

Although the bulk of ammonia formed in the kidney derives from glutamine, other amino acids as well are potential precursors. This effect becomes discernible as ammonia output increases in man (Madison and Seldin, 1958) and dog (Bliss, 1941; Lotspeich and Pitts, 1947) during administration of various individual amino acids. In fact, in the normal dog asparagine, alanine, and histidine are as effective as glutamine in augmenting ammonia excretion when comparable doses are given intravenously (Kamin and Handler, 1951b).

Amino acids are usually grouped according to potency for increasing urine ammonia as shown in Table II. The classification is taken from studies in the dog in normal acid–base balance (Kamin and Handler, 1951b) and in chronic metabolic acidosis (Lotspeich and Pitts, 1947) during intravenous infusion of amino acids. It is useful insofar as it points out possible ammonia precursors and indicates which amino acids should be included when increased ammonia excretion is desired by exogenous administration of precursors.

At endogenous plasma levels reabsorption of filtered amino acids is essentially complete, suggesting active transport. Saturation (Tm) occurs at a different plasma concentration for each amino acid, a factor which may be influential in determining the efficacy for ammonia formation (Lotspeich and Pitts, 1947). An additional and not less significant factor in this connection is the permeability of mitochondrial membranes to the individual amino acids, since deamidation (Goldstein and Schooler, 1966; Katunuma et al., 1966), deamination (Bendall and

TABLE II

CLASSIFICATION OF AMINO ACIDS ACCORDING TO POTENCY FOR ENHANCING URINARY EXCRETION OF AMMONIA[a,b]

High	Moderate	Low or none
Glutamine (N)	Methionine (N)	Glutamate (N,A)
Asparagine (N)	Cysteine (N)	Lysine (N)
Histidine (N)	Aspartate (N,A)	Arginine (N)
Alanine (N,A)	Leucine (N,A)	
Glycine (A)	Glycine (N)	

[a]N = dogs in normal acid–base balance (Kamin and Handler, 1951b).
[b]A = dogs in chronic metabolic acidosis (Lotspeich and Pitts, 1947).

De Duve, 1960), and transamination by the GOT reaction (Eichel and Bukovsky, 1961) are intramitochondrial reactions.

These considerations are exemplified by the insignificant effects of administered glutamate on ammonia excretion. The kidney can certainly deaminate glutamate present in renal tissue (Stone and Pitts, 1967). However, a meager fraction of 1–2% of urine ammonia derives from exogenous glutamate during exaggerated conditions of arterial loads 300% above endogenous levels. Since only a fraction of the glutamate reabsorbed is actually deaminated, it follows that low mitochondrial permeability possibly accounts for the weak efficacy of this amino acid in enhancing urinary output of ammonia (Pitts *et al.*, 1965). Studies *in vitro* support this reasoning, for the activation of glutamate dehydrogenase, which is a latent mitochondrial enzyme, by such procedures as freezing and thawing of mitochondria has been interpreted as resulting from increased permeability of the mitochondrial membranes to glutamate (Bendall and De Duve, 1960).

The contribution of a precursor to urine ammonia under normal conditions seems to be determined by the arterial load to the kidney rather than by the levels in renal tissue itself. This view is illustrated by consideration of the corresponding values for glutamine and glutamate. In the dog, concentration of glutamine in the kidney, although 3 to 4 times greater than in the plasma, represents only 4 to 7% of the total free α-amino acid concentration (Hamilton, 1945; Shalhoub *et al.*, 1963). Plasma glutamine levels, in contrast, constitute the largest fraction of free plasma nitrogen from a single source. Similarly, glutamine is the largest nitrogen donor to urine ammonia.

The extremely low contribution of glutamate to urine ammonia (Pitts *et al.*, 1965) correlates with very low plasma levels rather than with a kidney concentration that surpasses that of any other amino acid. In fact, it is 4 to 7 times greater than that of glutamine in the dog (Shalhoub *et al.*, 1963) and rat (Meister, 1956). Good correlation between the relative proportions of amino acids in plasma and their renal utilization for ammonia production is also suggested by studies in amphibia (Balinsky and Baldwin, 1962) and reptiles (Coulson and Hernandez, 1959). In these species, plasma concentrations of alanine and glycine exceed those of other amino acids, and they seem to be predominant sources of urine ammonia.

D. Metabolic Pathways in Ammonia Production

Aside from the general aspects of availability and permeability discussed above, what ultimately determines whether ammonia is formed in the kidney from a given amino acid is the adequacy of metabolic reactions. Most significant among these are (1) deamidation of glutamine, (2) oxidative deamination of glutamate and other amino acids, and (3) transamination reactions (Meister, 1965).

1. DEAMIDATION OF GLUTAMINE

The amide group of glutamine, indicated by N· in the reactions below, is liberated by the independent action of two enzyme systems: glutaminase I and glutaminase II. The latter is alternately known as glutamine-keto-acid transaminase ω-amidase, and abbreviated as GKA.

Glutaminase I

$$H_2N\cdot—C—CH_2—CH_2—CH—COOH \xrightarrow[H_2O]{\text{Glutaminase I}}$$
$$\quad\quad\quad \|\quad\quad\quad\quad\quad\quad\quad |$$
$$\quad\quad\quad O\quad\quad\quad\quad\quad\quad\quad NH_2$$

Glutamine

$$HOOC—CH_2—CH_2—CH—COOH + N\cdot H_3$$
$$\quad\quad\quad\quad\quad\quad\quad\quad |$$
$$\quad\quad\quad\quad\quad\quad\quad\quad NH_2$$

Glutamic acid   Ammonia

Glutaminase II (GKA)

$$H_2N\cdot—C—CH_2—CH_2—CH—COOH + R—C—COOH$$
$$\quad\quad\quad \|\quad\quad\quad\quad\quad\quad |\quad\quad\quad\quad\quad \|$$
$$\quad\quad\quad O\quad\quad\quad\quad\quad\quad NH_2\quad\quad\quad\quad O$$

Glutamine   α-Keto acid (α-ketoglutarate,
                                         pyruvate or oxaloacetate)

$$\xrightarrow{\text{α-Keto-acid transaminase}} H_2N\cdot—C—CH_2—CH_2—C—COOH +$$
$$\quad\quad\quad\quad\quad\quad\quad\quad\quad\quad\quad \|\quad\quad\quad\quad\quad\quad \|$$
$$\quad\quad\quad\quad\quad\quad\quad\quad\quad\quad\quad O\quad\quad\quad\quad\quad\quad O$$

α-Ketoglutaramic acid
$$R—CH—COOH$$
$$\quad\quad |$$
$$\quad\quad NH_2$$
α-Amino acid (glutamate,
alanine, or aspartate)

α-Ketoglutaramic acid $\xrightarrow{\text{ω-Amidase}}$
$$HOOC—CH_2—CH_2—C—COOH + N\cdot H_3$$
$$\quad\quad\quad\quad\quad\quad\quad\quad \|$$
$$\quad\quad\quad\quad\quad\quad\quad\quad O$$

α-Ketoglutaric acid   Ammonia

Although both systems are glutaminases, i.e., they catalyze deamidation, when not specified, the term "glutaminase" is generally used in reference to glutaminase I for two reasons: its recognition (Krebs, 1935) well anteceded that of glutaminase II in the kidney

(Goldstein *et al.*, 1957a), and it is quantitatively the most important enzyme system for ammonia production (Goldstein, 1967). The distribution of glutaminases in renal tissue is ubiquitous in the animal kingdom. Both systems are found in kidney cortex; in addition, glutaminase I is present in inner medulla, and glutaminase II in outer medulla (Richterich and Goldstein, 1958). Of lesser importance but also present in renal tissue is asparaginase, which acts on asparagine in a manner similar to the action of glutaminase I on glutamine (Meister, 1965).

Activity of renal glutaminase I is highest in dog, rat, mouse, and pig; intermediate in man; moderate in guinea pig; and extremely low in rabbit (Errera and Greenstein, 1949; White and Rolf, 1952; Klingman and Handler, 1958; Richterich and Goldstein, 1958; Holmgård, 1962). Interestingly enough, the distribution of glutaminase I is not restricted to tissues that produce glutamine. Thus, it is also found in kidneys of dogs, cats, and pigs, which do not contain glutamine synthetase (Krebs, 1935; Rector and Orloff, 1959; Lyon and Pitts, 1969). This enzyme catalyzes formation of glutamine from glutamate, ammonia, and ATP.

Kidney slices or homogenates incubated with L-glutamine produce more ammonia when phosphate is added. This has led to the characterization of glutaminase I as phosphate-dependent (PDG) and phosphate-independent (PIG) glutaminase. PDG has a pH optimum of 7.9–8.1, is inhibited by the end products of the reaction, namely, ammonia and glutamate, is not resistant to acid, heat, and cold, and is distributed in cortex and inner medulla. In contrast, PIG has a pH optimum of 7.4–7.6, is not inhibited by the end products, is resistant to physical agents, and is found only in cortex. In general, PDG is considered more important than PIG in renal ammonia production, although there are marked species differences in the relative activities in kidney (Krebs, 1935; Errera and Greenstein, 1949; Goldstein *et al.*, 1957a,b).

The activity of glutaminase II (GKA), compared to that of glutaminase I, is a small fraction in rat kidney (Goldstein, 1967) and a minimal fraction in dog kidney (Richterich and Goldstein, 1958). As glutaminase I, the enzyme is widely distributed in the animal kingdom. Optimal pH of 8.6–8.8, absence of end-product inhibition, and activation by keto acids, differentiate glutaminase II from phosphate-dependent glutaminase I (Goldstein *et al.*, 1957a,b). *In vitro*, several keto acids are active in the transamination step, especially α-ketoglutarate and pyruvate, but not oxaloacetate (Meister, 1954). However, from results of studies *in vivo*, described in pages 288–89, it appears that oxaloacetate may also participate in the reaction (Stone and Pitts, 1967).

2. Oxidative Deamination of Glutamate and Other Amino Acids

Glutamic acid is the end product in the glutaminase I reaction; it is also an end product in the glutaminase II reaction when α-ketoglutarate is the keto acid transaminated. Alternately, this may be pyruvate or oxaloacetate which convert into alanine or aspartate, respectively. Thereafter, each transaminates with α-ketoglutarate to yield glutamate. Consequently, in all cases the amino group of glutamine appears in glutamate. The glutamate dehydrogenase enzyme system (GDH) catalyzes oxidative deamination of glutamate to α-ketoglutarate. In this reaction ammonia is liberated and NAD$^+$ or NADP is reduced to NADH or NADP·H (Krebs *et al.*, 1948; Olson and Anfinsen, 1953; Papa *et al.*, 1967), as follows:

$$\text{HOOC—CH}_2\text{—CH}_2\text{—CH—COOH} \xrightarrow[\text{NADH}]{\text{NAD}^+}$$
$$\underset{\text{NH}_2}{|}$$

Glutamic acid

$$\text{HOOC—CH}_2\text{—CH}_2\text{—C—COOH} + \text{NH}_3$$
$$\underset{\text{O}}{\|}$$

α-Ketoglutaric acid   Ammonia

Glutamate dehydrogenase has been identified in enzyme assays in dog and rat kidney (Rector and Orloff, 1959; Rogulski *et al.*, 1962; Pollak *et al.*, 1965). *In vivo* studies indicate that in dog kidney the reaction occurs to a significant degree only in the direction of deamination, not of reductive amination of α-ketoglutarate (Stone and Pitts, 1967).

Natural or L-amino acids and unnatural or D-amino acids are oxidatively deaminated to the corresponding keto acids and ammonia by L- and D-amino-acid oxidases.

$$\text{R—CH}_2\text{—COOH} \xrightarrow{\text{L- or D-Amino-acid oxidase}} \text{R—C—COOH} + \text{NH}_3$$
$$\underset{\text{NH}_2}{|} \qquad\qquad\qquad \underset{\text{O}}{\|}$$

α-Amino acid α-Keto acid   Ammonia

A seemingly contradictory situation exists in relation to D- and L-amino-acid oxidases: D-amino acid oxidase in the kidney is ubiquitous in the animal kingdom (Meister, 1965). In contrast, L-amino-acid oxidase, with highest specificity for the naturally occurring amino acids, is found solely in the rat kidney (Blanchard *et al.*, 1944).

Oxidation of glycine is catalyzed by glycine oxidase, which in contrast with L-amino-acid oxidase, is absent from rat kidneys and present in most species studied (Ratner *et al.*, 1944).

$$CH_2—COOH \xrightarrow{\text{Glycine oxidase}} CH—COOH + NH_3$$
$$| \qquad\qquad\qquad\qquad ||$$
$$NH_2 \qquad\qquad\qquad\qquad O$$

Glycine   Glyoxylic acid   Ammonia

3. TRANSAMINATION REACTIONS

Transamination of glutamine with keto acids in the initial step of the glutaminase II (GKA) reaction has already been described (pages 282–83). In addition, other transamination reactions are important in ammonia production. In some instances they represent the only means by which the amino group of an amino acid may become a source of ammonia by transamination to glutamate, followed by oxidative deamination in the glutamate dehydrogenase reaction. Of particular interest in renal ammonia metabolism are the reactions listed below:

Alanine amino transferase or glutamic-pyruvic transaminase (GPT)
Alanine + α-Ketoglutarate $\rightleftharpoons$ Pyruvate + Glutamate
Aspartate amino transferase or glutamic-oxaloacetic transaminase (GOT)
Aspartate + α-Ketoglutarate $\rightleftharpoons$ Oxaloacetate + Glutamate

Table III contains the distribution of enzyme systems concerned with ammonia production in kidneys of several animal forms. The actual functioning of many of the enzyme systems described has been verified in the intact dog kidney (Section III, E) and may be inferred to occur in the human kidney from studies of ammonia excretion in man during administration of a variety of amino acids (Madison and Seldin, 1958). The occurrence of glutaminase I, glutamate dehydrogenase, GOT, and GPT has been corroborated in assays in biopsies from human kidney (Holmgård, 1962).

E. General Characteristics Observed *in Vivo* of Reactions Involved in Ammonia Production

When ^{15}N-ammonium chloride or ^{15}N-amide glutamine is injected into a renal artery in dog, the ^{15}N label appears in urine ammonia equally fast, the periods from injection to peak excretion are identical, and the mean transit times are the same. When ^{15}N-amino glutamine is injected the corresponding times are slightly longer (Fulgraff and Pitts, 1965). In conditions of sustained infusion into one renal artery of either ^{15}N-ammonium chloride (Stone *et al.*, 1967) or ^{15}N-amide glu-

TABLE III

Distribution of Enzyme Systems Important in Ammonia Metabolism in the Mammalian Kidney[a]

Species	Glutaminase I (L-Glutamine)	Glutaminase II (L-Glutamine)	Glutamate dehydrogenase (Glutamate)	Glycine oxidase (Glycine)	Amino acid oxidases (L-Amino acids)	(D-Amino acids)	Not specified	Transaminases	Glutamine synthetase (Glutamate + ammonia)
Man									
vv	Present[b]	—	Small[b]	Present[b,d]	Present[b,d]	Present[b]	—	Present[b,d]	—
vt	Present[c]	—	—	Present[e]	—	—	—	—	—
Dog									
vv	Present[f]	Present[k,j]	Present[l,m]	Present[f,n,o]	—	Present[q]	Present[m,q]	Present[f,k,l,q]	Absent[r]
vt	Present[g,j,h,i]	Present[g,i,h]	Present[o,h]	Present[e]	Little[p]	Present[g]	—	Present[g,h]	Absent[h]
Rat									
vv	Present[g]	—	—	Absent[e]	Present[p,t]	—	—	Unimportant[bb]	Present[h,i]
vt	Present[h,i,l,r,u,r,w]	Present[h,i,u,w]	Present[h,z]	Present[t]	Present[p,t]	Present[aa,v]	—	Present[h,t]	Present[h,i]
Guinea pig									
vv	—	—	—	—	—	—	—	—	Present[r]
vt	Present[cc,dd,ee,i]	Present[i,cc,ff]	—	—	—	—	—	—	Present[i,cc]
Rabbit									
vt	Little[c,gg,hh]	Little[i]	Present[c]	—	Little[p]	—	—	Present[c]	Present[i]
Pig									
vt	Present[ii]	—	—	Present[e]	Little[p]	—	—	—	—
Cat									
vv	—	—	—	—	Little[p]	—	—	—	—
vt	—	—	—	Present[e]	Little[p]	—	—	—	Absent[r]
Golden hamster									
vt	Present[jj]	—	—	—	—	—	—	—	—
Lamb, ox									
vt	—	—	—	Present[e]	Little[p]	—	—	—	—

[a] vv = Information from studies *in vivo*, vt = information from studies *in vitro*. Substrates of the reactions are given in parentheses in the column heads.
[b] Madison and Seldin (1958).
[c] Holmgård (1962).
[d] Wu and Sendroy (1959).
[e] Ratner et al. (1944).
[f] Kamin and Handler (1951b).
[g] Pollak et al. (1965).
[h] Rector and Orloff (1959).
[i] Richterich and Goldstein (1958).
[j] Sayre and Roberts (1958).
[k] Pitts and Stone (1967a).
[l] Stone and Pitts (1967).
[m] Pitts and Stone (1967b).
[n] Lotspeich and Pitts (1947).
[o] Pitts and Pilkington (1966).
[p] Blanchard et al. (1944).

[q] Bliss (1941).
[r] Lyon and Pitts (1969).
[s] Portwood and Madison (1956).
[t] Davies and Yudkin (1952).
[u] Goldstein (1967).
[v] Iacobellis et al. (1954).
[w] Rector et al. (1955).
[x] Weiss and Longley (1960).
[y] Goldstein (1964).
[z] Rogulski et al. (1962).
[aa] Handler et al. (1949).
[bb] Portwood and Madison (1958).
[cc] Goldstein et al. (1956).
[dd] Goldstein (1958).
[ee] Goldstein and Kensler (1960).
[ff] Goldstein et al. (1957a).
[gg] Errera and Greenstein (1949).
[hh] White and Rolf (1952).
[ii] Klingman and Handler (1958).
[jj] Karnovski and Himmelhoch (1961).

tamine (Pitts *et al.*, 1965) a plateau in specific activity of urine ammonia is attained at equal times. These observations, and an estimated half-time of less than 2.5 minutes for constancy of labeling of the intrarenal glutamine pool (Pitts *et al.*, 1965), indicate that the turnover rate of the amide nitrogen of glutamine in the kidney must certainly be very fast, and that ammonia formation from this amino acid occurs at extremely high rates in the chronically acidotic dog.

There is consensus that the system chiefly responsible for deamidation of glutamine is phosphate-dependent glutaminase I. The activity of this enzyme surpasses that of glutaminase II in dog kidney by a factor of 20 (Richterich and Goldstein, 1958). From these observations *in vitro*, little importance had been ascribed to glutaminase II until Stone and Pitts (1967) suggested that in dogs in chronic metabolic acidosis, it may account for a significant fraction of urine ammonia. Participation of glutaminase II in ammonia metabolism is clearly indicated in Fig. 11A, which illustrates that during infusion of ^{15}N-amino glutamine into one renal artery, labeling in kidney aspartate exceeds that in kidney glutamate and alanine. This finding suggests that aspartate derives its label from the highly labeled glutamine rather than from glutamate. Transamination of glutamine with oxaloacetate in the initial step of the reaction may account for transference of the labeled amino group from glutamine to aspartate. Had glutamine transaminated only

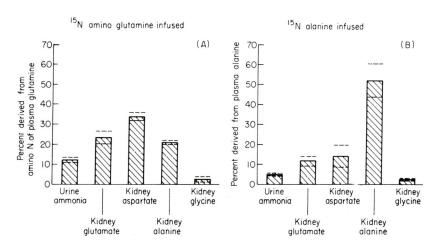

FIG. 11.   Percentages of urinary ammonia and of free alanine, aspartate, glutamate, and glycine in kidney tissue derived from circulating plasma precursors. (A) Percentages derived from amino nitrogen of glutamine. (B) Percentages derived from amino nitrogen of alanine. From Stone and Pitts (1967).

with α-ketoglutarate, labeling in kidney aspartate should be equal to or lower than that in glutamate, certainly not higher. Alternately, aspartate might have derived its label from glutamate by transamination of oxaloacetate, catalyzed by the GOT reaction within mitochondria. The glutamate used would be more highly labeled than the total kidney glutamate shown in Fig. 11A. This explanation is based on the existence of separate cellular pools of glutamate. Although compartmented cellular pools of glutamate have been suggested for cerebral cortex (Berl et al., 1962a), their existence in renal cells remains to be ascertained.

When the infused ^{15}N-label is contained in alanine (Fig. 11B) kidney glutamate and aspartate become labeled to the same extent. Glutamate probably derives from alanine by transamination with α-ketoglutarate (GPT reaction), and aspartate from glutamate transaminating with oxaloacetate (GOT reaction). As seen in Fig. 11B, 52% of total kidney alanine has its source in plasma alanine. The remaining 48% is synthesized in renal cells. The nitrogen derives mainly from the amino group of glutamine appearing in glutamate and transferred to pyruvate in the GPT reaction.

The label in urine ammonia when either ^{15}N-amino glutamine or alanine-^{15}N is infused is accounted for by oxidative deamination of glutamate catalyzed by glutamate dehydrogenase. It is interesting that even if the equilibrium of the latter reaction favors reductive amination of α-ketoglutarate (Olson and Anfinsen, 1953), this step is of minor importance in the intact functioning kidney of the acidotic dog, since kidney amino acids do not acquire a label during infusion of ^{15}N-ammonium chloride into one renal artery (Stone and Pitts, 1967). Whether fixation of ammonia by the GDH reaction occurs in the intact kidney of other animal species remains to be determined. The reaction is present in renal preparations from sheep (Krebs et al., 1948), pig (Dewan, 1938), and rat (Krebs et al., 1948; Rogulski et al., 1962), and in the perfused rat kidney (Pitts and Krebs, 1968, personal communication).

It was previously mentioned that increasing the arterial supply of any precursor amino acid results in enhanced ammonia excretion. This suggests that enzyme systems are present in excess amounts and that ammonia production is limited by precursor supply and membrane permeability to amino acids rather than by renal enzyme content. The following examples illustrate this view: When glutamine concentration in arterial plasma is increased to levels approximately 4 times above normal, ammonia excretion rises by about 70% in the chronically acidotic dog. Even during these exaggerated conditions of elevated precursor supply, the relative proportions of urine ammonia derived from each nitrogen of glutamine are identical to those at normal plasma levels (Pitts and Pilkington, 1966).

When alanine concentration in arterial plasma is progressively increased in the chronically acidotic dog, ammonia excretion rises. As shown in Fig. 12 (left panel) from the work of Pitts and Stone (1967b), the percent of urinary ammonia derived from alanine progressively increases from 2 to 8% in control conditions, to as high as 20% at plasma levels 5 times greater than normal. Evidently (right panel), infusion of alanine enhances the quantity of urinary ammonia derived from plasma alanine.

F. Summary

Preformed ammonia entering the kidney in arterial blood mixes rapidly and evenly with ammonia newly synthesized within tubular epithelium. The pool thus constituted is homogeneous, small, and turns over rapidly. It is the source of all ammonia released into urine and renal venous blood.

Since renal epithelium is richly supplied with enzymes involved in deamidation, deamination, and transamination reactions, several amino

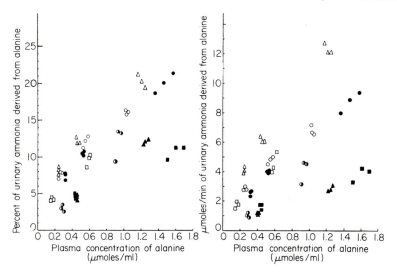

Fig. 12. *Left*: Relationship between arterial plasma concentration of alanine and the percent of the urinary ammonia derived from plasma alanine. *Right*: Relationship between arterial plasma concentration of alanine and the quantity of urinary ammonia derived from plasma alanine. Each of seven experiments is represented by a different symbol. Arterial plasma alanine was increased above control value of 0.2 to 0.4 μmoles/ml by the intravenous infusion of unlabeled alanine. From Pitts and Stone (1967).

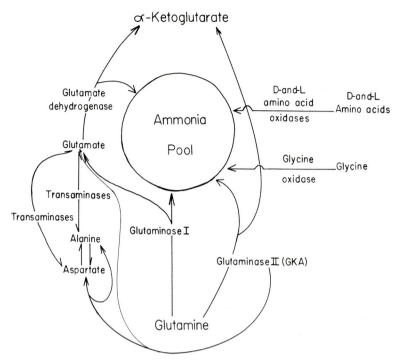

FIG. 13.   Diagram illustrating the metabolic pathways in synthesis of ammonia from precursor amino acids in the kidney. Preformed arterial ammonia mixes readily and evenly with that newly formed, constituting a homogeneous pool within the renal tubular epithelium.

acids are potential ammonia precursors (Fig. 13). However, the predominant source of ammonia nitrogen is glutamine, due to the combination of ample arterial supply to the kidney, high permeability of tubular epithelium and mitochondria, abundant renal content of adequate enzyme systems, and fast intrarenal turnover rates. These factors determine the sources of ammonia produced in the kidney in the various animal species and in a given species under different conditions.

Direct deamidation of glutamine, catalyzed by glutaminase I, and transamination coupled with deamidation, catalyzed by glutaminase II, provide the amide group of glutamine for the ammonia pool (Fig. 13). The amino group appearing in glutamate becomes available via oxidative deamination catalyzed by glutamate dehydrogenase. The carbon skeleton of glutamine thus enters the Krebs cycle as α-ketoglutarate. The amino nitrogens of alanine and aspartate may contribute to the ammonia pool by transamination to glutamate, and those in other amino acids via oxidative deamination catalyzed by D- and L-amino-acid oxidases.

In dog in chronic metabolic acidosis, about 50% of ammonia released by the kidney derives from the amide nitrogen of glutamine, 16–25% from its amino group, 16–25% from preformed arterial ammonia, and 2–8% from the amino nitrogen of alanine. Although similar sources are presumed to contribute to urine ammonia in man and other species, a definite assertion awaits further investigation.

IV. Effects of Acid–Base Balance of the Body on Renal Ammonia Production

A. Role of Ammonia in Nitrogen Metabolism and in Acid–Base Equilibrium

In man, 60% of the total nitrogen derived from protein metabolism is excreted as urea, 20% as ammonia, and the remainder mainly as creatinine. Urea and ammonia are formed from precursor amino acids, the former in liver, the latter in kidney. Synthesis of ammonia is metabolically inexpensive, for deamidation and deamination are not energy-requiring reactions. Consequently, when external conditions ensure adequate removal of ammonia, which is highly toxic to the body, animal species channel the nitrogen wastes into ammonia rather than into urea. This is found in completely aquatic forms, including fish, some amphibia, and reptiles. Removal of ammonia is ensured by means of urinary excretion and/or diffusion through gills or skin into the ample water surroundings (Coulson *et al.*, 1950; Cragg *et al.*, 1961; Balinsky *et al.*, 1961; Fromm, 1963; Fanelli and Goldstein, 1964).

In contrast, urea is the main nitrogen waste product normally occurring in all terrestrial forms and in aquatic forms during water shortage. Adaptation of partly terrestrial amphibia that normally excrete urea to aquatic media, involves decreased excretion of urea and increased excretion of ammonia, the least costly product (Balinsky *et al.*, 1961).

In man on a normal mixed diet, some 40–80 mEq of acid, formed from metabolism of foodstuffs, are excreted daily in two forms: combined with ammonia, 30–50 mEq, and as titratable acid, 10–30 mEq. When acid production in the body increases, acid excretion rises. If the increments are equal, acid–base balance is preserved. When compensation is inadequate, acidosis supervenes. To remove excess acid, titratable acidity and ammonia output increase to levels even 5 to 10 times greater than normal. This situation is not uncommon in diabetes, when excessive amounts of phosphoric and sulfuric acids, and in addition, β-

hydroxybutyric and acetoacetic acids are formed. Under these conditions, some 300–500 mEq of acid are excreted each day combined with ammonia, 75–250 mEq as titratable acid. The sum of the two rates represents replenishment of buffer reserves to the body by the kidney (Pitts, 1968a).

B. Adaptation of Ammonia Production in Chronic Metabolic Acidosis

It is not surprising that changes of the acid–base balance of the body, hence of urine pH, affect ammonia excretion. According to the principles of nonionic diffusion of weak bases (page 262), increased output in acidosis and decreased output in alkalosis are expected. What is surprising though is that, at comparable values of urine pH, rates in chronic acidosis exceed the rates in normal acid–base balance, and even those in acute acidosis. Ever since Pitts (1948) first demonstrated this effect, the subject has proved enticing and rewarding for research. The intense investigative efforts directed at finding the causes of adaptive increase in ammonia excretion have not succeeded in the original aim. However, they have disclosed intriguing aspects of regulation in biological systems.

The experiment by Pitts (1948) on dogs in normal acid–base balance, given in Fig. 14, shows that ammonia excretion decreases linearly as urine pH is alkalinized by intravenous infusion of sodium bicarbonate. An identical reciprocal linear relation is observed when the same procedure is repeated in the same animal in chronic metabolic acidosis, induced by daily oral administration of ammonium chloride. However, the absolute rates of ammonia excretion, at any given value of urine pH, are strikingly higher in the chronically acidotic dog than in the normal dog. These observations are the basis for the view of "adaptation" of ammonia excretion in chronic metabolic acidosis.

The role of the adaptive increase of ammonia excretion in the preservation of acid–base balance of the body is best illustrated in Fig. 15, from observations on man by Sartorius, Roemmelt, and Pitts (1949). Urinary excretion of various ions was studied daily under control conditions of constant salt and caloric intake (left panel), during daily intake of ammonium chloride (center panel), and in the period of recovery from ingestion of the ammonium salt (right panel).

The differences in urinary excretion of ions, mainly sodium, between the 1st and 5th days of acidosis indicate the role of the adaptive increase of ammonia excretion in preservation of homeostasis. Thus, whereas initially sodium loss is notable as it is excreted with excess chloride, in the 5th day of acidosis sodium balance has become positive and stays

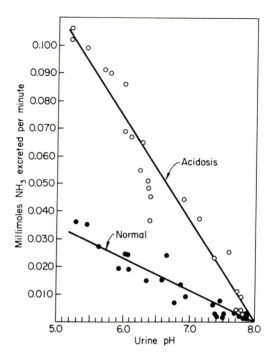

Fig. 14.   Relationship between the rate of excretion of ammonia and urine reaction in a normal dog and in a dog rendered acidotic for 48 hours. From Pitts (1948).

so for 4 days in the recovery period. Consequently, even overcompensation in plasma pH and in sodium and bicarbonate concentrations occurs.

The defense mechanisms against acidosis involve increase of urine titratable acidity, and, most important, progressive elevation of ammonia excretion. In the 5th day, the rates exceed those in the 1st day by a factor of 5. Instead of sodium chloride, ammonium chloride is excreted. Furthermore, during recovery, ammonia excretion declines progressively, not sharply, to attain control levels only around the 5th day. Thus elevation of ammonia output in acidosis serves to eliminate excess acid as ammonium ion, to prevent sodium loss, and to restore blood levels of sodium, bicarbonate, and pH to normal.

The acid-induced rise of ammonia excretion is universal in the animal kingdom. It occurs in most species, including birds (Milroy, 1904; Wolbach, 1955), amphibia (Yoshimura et al., 1961a), guinea pigs (Goldstein and Kensler, 1960), rats (Rector et al., 1954a, 1955; Lotspeich, 1965), dogs (Pitts, 1948), and man (Ryber, 1948; Pitts, 1948;

Madison and Seldin, 1958). In most, the time course is similar: as acidosis develops during daily administration of ammonium chloride, ammonia excretion rises steeply in the first day or two, slowly tapers off, and finally reaches maximal values between the 4th and 6th days. During recovery in man and dog, high urine ammonia persists for several days (Pitts, 1948; Sartorius et al., 1949). In contrast it drops sharply in rat (Dies and Lotspeich, 1967).

The causes for the three phases in this response, namely, the delay in attaining plateau levels, the attainment of these, greatly exceeding those in acute acidosis, and the persistence of elevated excretion during recovery in some species, are not clear at present.

Although the magnitude of the maximal rates is proportional to the degree of acidosis developed, once attained, they do not increase despite continued acidosis. However, further substantial elevations in the plateau levels may be induced by acute administration of amino acids in

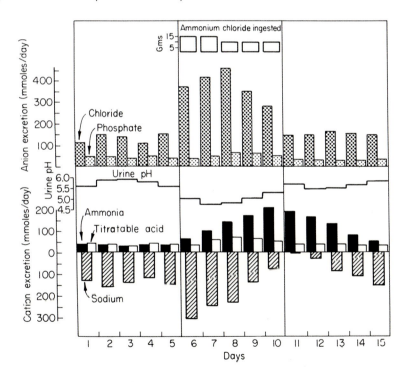

FIG. 15. Rates of excretion of ions prior to, during, and after a period of acidosis induced by the ingestion of ammonium chloride. Subject, a normal young adult. From Pitts (1948).

man (Madison and Seldin, 1958) and dog (Lotspeich and Pitts, 1947). These observations are consonant with the view that neither the renal concentrations of deamidating and deaminating enzymes nor the tubular transport of precursor amino acids seem to be rate-limiting processes in ammonia production.

A great deal of research has been devoted to discerning the causes of adaptation in acidosis. In theory, logical causative factors include acid-induced elevations in enzyme activity, particularly of glutaminase. Thus, the findings of Davies and Yudkin in 1952 of increased activity of renal glutaminase, glycine oxidase, and L-amino acid oxidase in rats fed ammonium chloride for 3 months were almost expected. The association of enhancement of ammonia excretion and of renal glutaminase activity in chronic metabolic acidosis in the rat (Leonard and Orloff, 1955; Muntwyler et al., 1956) and the guinea pig (Richterich and Goldstein, 1957), as well as depression in both enzyme activity and ammonia excretion in chronic metabolic alkalosis in the rat (Davies and Yudkin, 1952; Muntwyler et al., 1956), have been extensively documented. However, the relation between changes in glutaminase activity and urine ammonia is deceptive, as will be discussed in Section V, B, 1. Suffice it to say that adaptation of ammonia excretion occurs in the acidotic dog without increase in glutaminase activity (Pollak et al., 1965). Furthermore it is present in the acidotic rat even when glutaminase adaptation is suppressed by inhibitors of protein synthesis (Goldstein, 1965).

C. Factors Influencing Adaptation

1. EXTRACELLULAR FACTORS: pH, BICARBONATE

Much research has focused on exploring which factors in extracellular and intracellular fluids are responsible for changes in renal ammonia production during alterations of acid–base balance of the body. Most observations suggest lack of correlation between adaptation of ammonia production and extracellular fluid factors, such as blood pH and plasma bicarbonate. Thus, in the rat, adaptive increases in ammonia excretion and glutaminase activity are seen at low plasma bicarbonate levels in chronic metabolic acidosis (Rector et al., 1954a), as well as at high plasma bicarbonate in hypokalemic alkalosis (Iacobellis et al., 1954; Seldin et al., 1954), and at normal plasma bicarbonate concentrations during administration of small acid loads (Rector et al., 1955). Furthermore, adaptation occurs in response to ammonium chloride, not to acid phosphate, despite equal degrees of extracellular acidosis developed (Seldin *et al.*, 1957). Similarly in man, substantial increases of ammonia output have been observed without changes in serum electrolytes and pH upon infusion of sodium sulfate to individuals given a low sodium diet and compound F acetate (Schwartz *et al.*, 1955). It follows from these observations that rates of ammonia excretion cannot be predicted solely on the basis of values of pH and bicarbonate concentration in extracellular fluid.

2. RENAL INTRACELLULAR FACTORS: pH, POTASSIUM

Much better correlation exists between adaptive increase of ammonia excretion and renal intracellular factors, such as concentrations of potassium and hydrogen ions. Although neither has been determined in the kidney, the view is inferential from observations of changes observed in plasma electrolytes during chronic metabolic acidosis (Yoshimura *et al.*, 1961b) and of pH of muscle cells calculated from DMO distribution during potassium deficiency (Sanslone and Muntwyler, 1966). These two conditions lead to adaptation not correlated with blood pH, which is low in the first, high in the second. In both states, however, the intracellular milieu is acid and low in potassium. In both, adaptive increases of ammonia production and of renal glutaminase activity in rat are well known effects (Iacobellis *et al.*, 1954; Rector *et al.*, 1954b; Seldin *et al.*, 1954; Muntwyler *et al.*, 1956; Iacobellis *et al.*, 1957). The view that renal intracellular potassium levels exert regulating effects on ammonia production is strengthened by studies on dogs. Combinations of low-potassium diets and administration of DOCA, besides stimulating ammonia excretion, cause glutaminase induction (Iacobellis *et al.*, 1955), an effect which even chronic acidosis fails to produce in dog kidneys (Rector and Orloff, 1959; Pollak *et al.*, 1965).

D. Effects of Respiratory Disturbances of Acid–Base Balance

From the above considerations it follows that there is consensus favoring intracellular acid–base alterations as factors intimately related with adaptation in renal ammonia production. Since CO_2 crosses cell membranes more readily than bicarbonate ion, variations in extracellular pCO_2 levels in all likelihood affect intracellular pH more intensely than changes in extracellular bicarbonate concentrations (Wallace and Hastings, 1942; Wallace and Lowry, 1942). Hence, it is seemingly confusing that respiratory acidosis and alkalosis exert lesser influences on ammonia excretion than their metabolic counterparts, a fact illustrated by the examples that follow.

In rats breathing 10–15% CO_2 for over a week, titratable acidity and urine ammonia rise during the first 2 days and then fall to levels slightly above control. Renal glutaminase activity remains unchanged (Carter *et al.*, 1959). Similarly, in dogs (Fuller and MacLeod, 1956; Cade *et al.*, 1961) and man (Stanbury and Thomson, 1952; Longson and Mills, 1953; Barker *et al.*, 1957) acute respiratory acidosis and alkalosis fail to induce substantial variations in ammonia excretion as those seen during metabolic acid–base alterations. Although in patients with chronic respiratory failure and CO_2 retention there seems to be a direct correlation between arterial pCO_2 and renal ammonia production, superimposed acute hypercapnia does not affect ammonia output (Aber *et al.*, 1965).

The following reason has been advanced to explain weaker and less predictable responses of ammonia production to respiratory than to metabolic acid–base changes: Plasma bicarbonate and urine pH are higher in chronic respiratory acidosis than in chronic metabolic acidosis. Accordingly, less diffusion trapping of ammonia occurs in the former state (Carter *et al.*, 1959; Schwartz *et al.*, 1965).

Stronger effects of metabolic acidosis than of respiratory acidosis extend to other aspects of renal metabolism besides ammonia production. Thus, renal hypertrophy is very pronounced in rats made acidotic with ammonium chloride, whereas it does not occur in animals breathing 8–10% CO_2 for a week (Lotspeich, 1965). Similarly, the activity of the hexose monophosphate shunt in rat kidney is greatly stimulated by metabolic acidosis, whereas it scarcely varies in respiratory acidosis (Dies and Lotspeich, 1967).

The intracellular concentration of potassium seems to influence the intensity of changes of ammonia excretion during respiratory acid–base alterations. Thus, breathing 8% CO_2 for a day raises substantially the ammonia output in potassium-deficient rats (Levitin and Epstein, 1961), contrasting with the slight changes seen in normal rats (Carter *et al.*, 1959). The differences might be due to greater cellular acidification during hypercapnia in potassium-depleted rats than in normal rats. Thus, using DMO distribution to measure muscle cell pH, Sanslone and Muntwyler (1967) found that similar increases of plasma pCO_2 produce greater cell acidification in low-potassium animals than in normal rats.

E. Summary

Prolonged acid stresses induce adaptation of ammonia excretion throughout the animal kingdom. This response occurs when acid loads are given, as well as during acidosis in such conditions as diabetes, starvation, and gastrointestinal malfunctions leading to base loss. The degree of adaptation, i.e., the magnitude of ammonia excretion, correlates with the intensity of the acid stresses.

Excretion of excess acid as ammonium salt represents a means of salvaging sodium bicarbonate to replenish body buffer reserves. Were it not for adaptation of ammonia output in acidosis, uncontrolled sodium bicarbonate loss would supervene. Even mild acid stresses would soon become fatal.

No single factor in extracellular fluid, namely, electrolyte and bicarbonate levels, or even pH, independently determines adaptation of renal ammonia production. Most likely this depends on a combination of intracellular factors in kidney, such as decreased pH and potassium concentration, a view reached by exclusion of extracellular factors rather than by direct proof of intracellular changes. The studies on ammonia production in respiratory and metabolic acidosis and alkalosis point out the complexity of the system and the need for expanded research in this area.

V. Control of Renal Ammonia Production

The concentration of ammonia in renal cells, hence the cell pNH_3, represents a balance between production rates and diffusion rates of ammonia, as illustrated in the diagram in Fig. 16. The factors determining diffusion have been discussed in Section II. Briefly, they in-

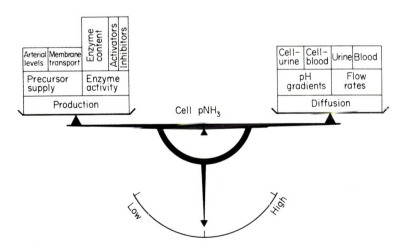

FIG. 16. Diagram illustrating factors that determine renal cellular pNH_3. Cell pNH_3 represents the balance between rates of ammonia production in renal tubular epithelium and rates of diffusion from cells into urine and renal venous blood.

clude the pH gradients between cells and luminal fluid and between cells and peritubular fluid, and the flow rates of urine and renal blood.

Production of ammonia is determined by two main factors: (a) Supply of precursors, chiefly glutamine, for ammonia synthesis in mitochondria. Consequently, supply depends on arterial levels as well as on transport of glutamine and other amino acids across epithelial and mitochondrial membranes. (b) Renal activity of enzymes involved in ammonia production, determined by the renal tissue concentration of enzymes as well as by the levels of activators and inhibitors of the reactions.

A. Supply of Precursors

1. ARTERIAL SUPPLY

Although renal tissue concentrations of amino acids are high, actually exceeding blood levels, the kidneys depend to a great extent on arterial supply of glutamine and other amino acids for ammonia synthesis. This situation is particularly apparent in the dog kidney. The excess amount of ammonia released in acidosis, compared to the control state or to alkalosis, is formed mainly at the expense of extrarenal glutamine. In dogs, chronic metabolic acidosis greatly enhances the renal extraction rates of glutamine over those in alkalosis and in normal acid-base balance (Shalhoub et al., 1963; Pilkington et al., 1970). In man, even mild chronic metabolic acidosis is sufficient to double renal glutamine uptake compared to values in the normal state (Owen and Robinson, 1963).

Alterations of the acid–base balance in dogs affect in substantial proportions solely the renal extraction of glutamine, not that of any other amino acid (Shalhoub et al., 1963). In man, in addition, acidosis changes renal release of glutamate, seen in the normal state, to extraction (Owen and Robinson, 1963). The latter observations suggest that glutamate may be a better ammonia source in human than in dog kidneys.

From the previous considerations it might be anticipated that the increased renal utilization of glutamine in acidosis would lower its concentration in arterial blood. Since in the dog plasma levels do not change or even increase (Shalhoub et al., 1963; Addae and Lotspeich, 1968a), supply of glutamine at faster rates by extrarenal sites must be postulated.

This view has been tested by Addae and Lotspeich (1968a) in dogs and rats. The results of their studies indicate that acidosis enhances hepatic production of glutamine in both species. In the dog, the increased supply of this amino acid by the liver to the kidney is sufficient to cope with the high demands for ammonia production in acidosis. Hence, a steady state exists, as indicated by extraction rates of amino and amide nitrogens matching production rates of ammonia nitrogen (Pitts *et al.*, 1963).

Most certainly, acidosis exerts independent effects on glutamine metabolism in the kidney and liver, as suggested by the following findings. In dogs, lowering of blood glutamine levels by hemodialysis results in increased hepatic production of this amino acid. However, the correlation between hepatic glutamine release and its removal by kidneys and dialysis is only half the value found during superimposed acidosis. In other words, acidosis is a more potent stimulus for hepatic glutamine production than is decreased blood glutamine concentration (Addae and Lotspeich, 1968b).

2. Membrane Transport

Glutamine enters renal epithelial cells across luminal and antiluminal membranes, probably by active transport (Shalhoub *et al.*, 1963; Pilkington *et al.*, 1970). Once inside cells, it must traverse mitochondrial membranes to become available for ammonia synthesis. A matter not established yet is whether acidosis stimulates membrane transport systems of glutamine directly, or indirectly through enhancement of its utilization.

B. Renal Activities of Enzymes Involved in Ammonia Production

Much attention has been devoted to studying changes of enzyme activity in the kidney that participate in the control of ammonia production. A brief discussion of the terms used in this connection is pertinent because the usage does not strictly conform to biochemical definitions. Thus, in enzyme kinetics, the term "adaptation" implies stimulation of enzyme synthesis. When this is caused by increased amounts of substrates, it is called "induction." When it is caused by decreased amounts of end products, it is called "derepression" (Moyed and Umbarger, 1962). In contrast, in discussions of renal ammonia metabolism, "adaptation" is used to denote greater ammonia excretion in chronic metabolic acidosis than predicted from urine pH values, not necessarily linked with elevated enzyme content. In some species the acid-induced rise of ammonia output is associated with increased renal glutaminase activity. In these cases, the term "induction" has been used. However, it should not be construed to mean that greater supply of substrate is the causative factor, as the biochemical usage would imply.

In fact, an ample supply of glutamine does not seem to be responsible for renal glutaminase induction in the chronically acidotic rat. This view is borne out by observations of renal glutaminase activity during prolonged administration of glutamine to rats: no changes are seen in the normal acid–base balance. Furthermore, although induction is found in chronic metabolic acidosis, it is less pronounced than in acidosis without administration of glutamine (Portwood and Madison, 1956). Consequently, increased supply of glutamine does not seem to be the cause of enhanced glutaminase activity in acidosis.

Besides changes in the amount of enzyme present, two additional factors may alter the activity of a reaction, namely, the levels of activators and inhibitors. Increases in the former and/or decreases in the latter will elevate enzyme activity. In all likelihood, acid–base equilibrium affects the concentrations of such factors in the intracellular milieu. If true, enzyme activity would thus be easily regulated, even on a moment-to-moment basis, by changes in supply and removal of activators and/or inhibitors. It is conceivable that these effects may not be apparent in enzyme assays in kidney slices or homogenates. However, the failure to detect changes of renal glutaminase activity in enzyme assays, exemplified by the situation in the dog, does not negate the variation of activity *in vivo* during alterations of acid–base equilibrium.

1. RENAL ENZYME CONTENT

Attempts to correlate adaptation of ammonia excretion in chronic metabolic acidosis with increased glutaminase I activity have only been successful in two species: rat (Rector *et al.*, 1955) and guinea pig (Goldstein and Kensler, 1960). However, even in these forms it seems doubtful that stimulation of enzyme synthesis is a main determinant of adaptation, as will be discussed later.

In the rat (Fig. 17), as acidosis develops during daily administration of ammonium chloride, ammonia excretion starts rising progressively from the 1st day. Plateau levels are attained around the 6th day. Similarly, renal glutaminase activity increases progressively to attain plateau levels around the 6th day. Thus, with the exception of the 1st day when glutaminase activity remains unchanged, the increases in enzyme activity and ammonia excretion follow parallel time courses (Rector *et al.*, 1955).

The effects of chronic metabolic acidosis are not restricted to renal glutaminase I activity. Table IV summarizes the changes observed in renal activities of other enzymes involved in ammonia production in dog, rat, and guinea pig. It is immediately apparent that species differ

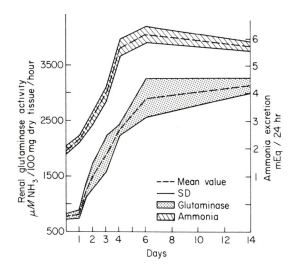

FIG. 17.   The rate of renal glutaminase adaptation and its relation to ammonia excretion in rats given 5 mEq of NH₄Cl daily. From Rector *et al.* (1955).

notably with respect to acid-induced variations in renal enzyme activity. The following aspects are noteworthy:

(a) In rat kidney the changes favor formation of ammonia, as well as decreased utilization of ammonia in glutamine synthesis. Activities of glutaminases I, II, and of glutamate dehydrogenase, are increased, whereas that of glutamine synthetase is decreased.

The activity of renal glutamine synthetase has been studied *in vivo*, for the first time, by Damian and Pitts (Pitts, 1968b) in the rat. Their approach consisted of pulse-labeling of glutamate by a single injection of α-ketoglutarate-^{14}C into a renal artery, removal and freezing of the kidneys in liquid nitrogen at 10, 15, 30, or 45 seconds after injection, and measurement of specific activities of renal glutamate and glutamine. Under these conditions the specific activity of glutamate remains constant for 30 to 45 seconds. Figure 18 illustrates the results obtained in chronic metabolic acidosis and alkalosis. The slopes of the lines are the rates of synthesis of glutamine from glutamate. The values in metabolic alkalosis (24.5 μmoles/gm wet weight per hour) are seven-fold greater than in acidosis (3.3 μmoles/gm wet weight per hour) (Damian and Pitts, 1970).

From the above considerations it is safe to conclude that a dual system of control of ammonia release exists in rat kidney. Both hydrol-

TABLE IV

EFFECTS OF CHRONIC METABOLIC ACIDOSIS ON ENZYME ACTIVITIES IN THE KIDNEY OF DOGS, RATS, AND GUINEA PIGS[a]

Enzyme	Dog	Rat	Guinea Pig
Glutaminase I	$\rightleftharpoons$[b] $\downarrow$[c]	$\uparrow$[c-f]	$\uparrow$[g,h]
Glutaminase II	$\rightleftharpoons$[b,c]	$\downarrow$[i] $\uparrow$[c,e]	$\rightleftharpoons$[g]
Glutamate dehydrogenase	$\rightleftharpoons$[b,c]	$\uparrow$[c]	—
Transaminases			
GPT	$\rightleftharpoons$[b]	—	—
GOT	$\uparrow$[b] $\rightleftharpoons$[c]	$\rightleftharpoons$[c]	—
Amino acid oxidases	$\rightleftharpoons$[b]	$\rightleftharpoons$[j]	—
Glutamine synthetase	Absent[c,k*]	$\downarrow$[c,l*]	$\rightleftharpoons$[g]

[a] Increases ($\uparrow$), decreases ($\downarrow$), and no change ($\rightleftharpoons$), refer to comparisons between observations in acidosis with those in normal or alkalotic states. Asterisks indicate observations *in vivo*.
[b] Pollak *et al.* (1965).
[c] Rector and Orloff (1959).
[d] Davies and Yudkin (1952).
[e] Goldstein (1965).
[f] Rector *et al.* (1955).
[g] Goldstein *et al.* (1956).
[h] Goldstein and Kensler (1960).
[i] Goldstein (1967).
[j] Handler *et al.* (1949).
[k] Lyon and Pitts (1969).
[l] Pitts (1968b).

ysis and synthesis of glutamine are influenced by acid–base balance. Acidosis, by promoting deamidation and retarding synthesis, favors ammonia release. Alkalosis, by exerting opposing actions, favors ammonia fixation.

(b) Dog kidney, in sharp contrast with rat kidney, does not contain glutamine synthetase, and thus lacks the possibility of regulation by means of ammonia fixation in glutamine (Krebs, 1935; Rector and Orloff, 1959; Lyon and Pitts, 1969). It is not known whether human kidney resembles dog or rat kidney with respect to the glutamine synthetase reaction. Marked species differences exist: The activity of this reaction in the kidney exceeds that of deamidation in rabbits and guinea pigs, is lower in rats and sheep, and absent in dogs, pigs, cats, and pidgeons (Krebs, 1935). Since in normal man the kidney adds glutamate to renal venous blood (Owen and Robinson, 1963), fixation of ammonia, at least in glutamate, can be conceived as an additional means of control.

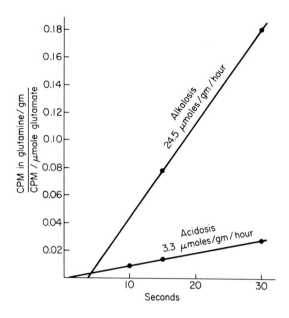

FIG. 18. Effects of chronic metabolic alkalosis and acidosis on glutamine synthetase activity in the intact rat kidney. Renal glutamate was pulse-labeled by a single injection of α-ketoglutarate-^{14}C into one renal artery. Formation of glutamine from glutamate was determined from specific activities of these substrates found in kidneys removed at 10, 15, or 30 seconds following injection. Each point is the mean value obtained in three to five rats. The slopes of the lines represent rates of synthesis of glutamine. From Pitts (1968b).

(c) In the dog kidney, glutaminase activity is not stimulated by acidosis. The only change observed in this state is increased activity of aspartate amino transferase (Pollak *et al.*, 1965). Evidently, extrapolation of this information to man and other species would not be judicious. Studies by Madison and Seldin (1958), illustrated in Fig. 19, provide suggestive evidence for adaptation of various enzymes in human kidney during chronic metabolic acidosis. These authors determined ammonia excretion after a single oral dose of various individual amino acids had been given to humans receiving daily doses of 5, 10, or 15 gm of ammonium chloride (Fig. 19). Ingestion of glycine, asparagine, glutamine, D- and L-alanine, L-leucine, and other amino acids, except L-lysine, increased urine ammonia over the already high levels in chronic acidosis. In all cases, the excess ammonia excretion produced by ingestion of amino acids progressively increased as intake of NH$_4$Cl rose from 5 to 15 gm. Hence, adaptation in renal activities of glycine oxidase, asparaginase, glutaminase, and L- and D-amino acid oxidases

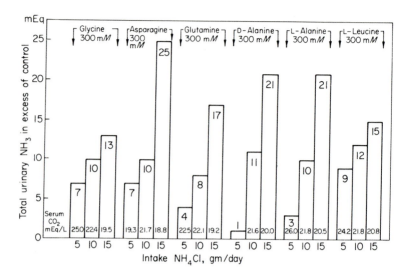

Fig. 19. Effect of different amino acids and amino acid amides on net urinary ammonia excretion following stepwise increase in the magnitude of the chronic ammonium chloride load. The numbers in the columns refer to the net increase in urinary ammonia after the substrate load. From Madison and Seldin (1958).

might be postulated by inference. However, and in agreement with the authors' comments, it is questionable whether adaptation in this study can strictly be attributed to renal enzymes. Equal effects could result from changes in permeability of tubular epithelium to amino acids, leading to increased renal uptake in proportion to the degree of acidosis developed.

Two pieces of evidence indicate that the relation between glutaminase induction in rat kidney and ammonia output is delusory. First, administration of inhibitors of protein synthesis prevents enzyme induction without altering adaptation of ammonia excretion in acidotic rats (Goldstein, 1965) and guinea pigs (Goldstein and Kensler, 1960). Second, adaptive increase of ammonia production in the dog occurs without glutaminase induction (Rector and Orloff, 1959; Pollack et al., 1965). The argument that in dogs there is no need for enzyme induction because the basal levels are very high may also be applied to rats and guinea pigs. True, renal glutaminase activity in these species is lower than in dogs. However, the basal levels are more than adequate to account for the maximal ammonia output in acidosis (Richterich and Goldstein, 1958). A completely opposite situation is found in rabbits. In this species very low basal levels of renal glutaminase activity (White and Rolf, 1952) correlate well with a vanishingly low ammonia excretion and, probably, with the inability to survive acidosis (Walter, 1877; White and Rolf, 1952).

The fact that administration of amino acids increases ammonia output even when this is at maximal rates in chronic metabolic acidosis, is consonant with the view that renal enzyme content is not rate-limiting in ammonia formation. This may even be extended to include rat kidney, as the following studies suggest. When glutamine is fed to rats receiving ammonium chloride, rates of ammonia excretion equal those in rats receiving ammonium chloride alone. In both groups, glutaminase induction occurs. However, it is less pronounced in the group given glutamine together with the ammonium salt. Thus, prolonged exposure to glutamine enhances the "efficiency" of glutaminase, i.e., more ammonia is produced per unit enzyme (Portwood and Madison, 1956). An additional point of interest brought out by this experiment is that chronic ingestion of glutamine fails to increase ammonia output in chronically acidotic rats. In contrast, elevations are observed in normal rats (Portwood and Madison, 1956) receiving glutamine for several days, as well as in chronically acidotic man (Madison and Seldin, 1958) and dog (Pitts and Pilkington, 1966) during acute administration of glutamine.

Increased "efficiency" of ammonia production has also been observed in rat kidney during administration of 5% and 50% casein diets for a week. Activity of phosphate-dependent glutaminase increases in both cases. With 50% casein, glutaminase levels are 4 times and ammonia production 7 times greater than with 5% casein (Katunuma et al., 1966). Therefore, more ammonia is produced per unit enzyme during the former diet. These studies indicate that, in addition to renal enzyme content itself, other factors determine the amount of ammonia formed at given substrate and enzyme concentrations.

Additional studies with chronic exposure to amino acids may help elucidate factors regulating ammonia production. It is possible that "latent" reactions become manifest by changes of enzyme activity and membrane permeability during continued supply of substrate. For instance, ammonia excretion, which scarcely varies in man following single oral doses of glutamate, proline, or aspartate (Madison and Seldin, 1958), greatly increases during prolonged feeding of each amino acid. Surprisingly, glutamic acid becomes as effective as glutamine in enhancing ammonia excretion in these conditions (Watts et al., 1965).

2. LEVELS OF INHIBITORS AND ACTIVATORS

One of the most common mechanisms of control in biosynthetic reactions, that of inhibition by end products, may be important in the regulation of ammonia production. Thus, the activity of phosphate-dependent glutaminase is inhibited by the two end products of the reaction: ammonia and glutamate. Ammonia interacts with glutamine in a competitive manner, glutamate in a noncompetitive manner. In addition, glutamate acts as a competitive inhibitor of phosphate (Krebs, 1935; Sayre and Roberts, 1958).

a. Glutamate. The concentration of glutamate in normal rat kidney, 7.3 μmoles/gm wet weight, is high enough to produce 55% inhibition of glutaminase activity *in vitro.* Chronic metabolic acidosis results in lowering of glutamate concentration to 5.2 μmoles/gm wet weight (Goldstein, 1966). This decrement may account adequately for a 20% increase of glutaminase activity. The enhancement of ammonia production expected by this mechanism is still below that actually seen in chronic acidosis. Thus, if the changes *in vivo* are of the same order of magnitude as those *in vitro* and affect equally enzyme activity, other factors must account for adaptive increase of ammonia excretion in acidosis.

The cause of the lowering of renal glutamate concentration, at least in rat kidney, seems to relate to faster removal of α-ketoglutarate in acidosis. Consequently, by mass action effects, oxidative deamination of glutamate in the glutamate dehydrogenase reaction is favored. Subsequent decreases of renal glutamate levels thus activate deamidation of glutamine by release of inhibition of the glutaminase I reaction. Therefore, regulation of ammonia production may reside, at least partly, in reactions in which α-ketoglutarate is consumed (Goodman *et al.*, 1966; Goorno *et al.*, 1967; Alleyne, 1968). Recent studies suggest that chronic metabolic acidosis produces similar effects in dog kidney as those described above for rat kidney. Thus, renal glutamate concentration in acidosis is 4.12 μmoles/gm wet weight, a value 60% of the normal of 6.80 μmoles/gm wet weight (Balagura-Baruch *et al.*, 1970).

b. α-Ketoglutarate. The following pieces of evidence are consonant with the view that renal levels of α-ketoglutarate may represent one of several possible control systems of ammonia production.

(1) In the experiments illustrated in Fig. 20, from studies on chronically acidotic rats by Pitts (1970), the isolated kidney was perfused with one of the following amino acids: aspartate, alanine, glycine, and leucine, in concentrations of 5 m*M.* Rates of addition of ammonia, glutamate, and glutamine by the kidney to the perfusate appear in the ordinate. It is evident that ammonia is formed from each amino acid. In addition, the kidney releases moderate amounts of glutamate and small amounts of glutamine from aspartate, slight amounts of both amino acids from alanine, and none from glycine and leucine.

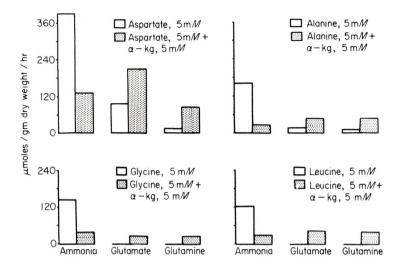

FIG. 20. Effects of α-ketoglutarate on synthesis of ammonia, glutamate, and glutamine by the isolated kidney of the chronically acidotic rat perfused with diverse amino acids. Rates shown represent addition of ammonia, glutamate, and glutamine to the perfusate from the kidney perfused with 5 mM solution of each amino acid alone (open bars) and combined with 5 mM solution of α-ketoglutarate (filled bars). Modified from Pitts (1970).

It is also evident that addition of α-ketoglutarate in equimolar amounts to the perfusing fluid containing each amino acid results, in all cases, in marked decrease of renal release of ammonia associated with substantial increase of release of glutamate and glutamine. Thus, high levels of α-ketoglutarate produced a shift in ammonia metabolism: ammonia formed from each amino acid was diverted from excretion to synthesis of glutamate and glutamine. It has already been mentioned (Section V, B, page 303) that in the rat kidney there appears to be a dual system of control of ammonia release which includes changes of the speed of the reactions of hydrolysis and synthesis of glutamine.

(2) Figure 21 illustrates the effects of α-ketoglutarate on total renal ammonia production on the chronically acidotic dog (Balagura-Baruch et al., 1970). During intravenous infusion of α-ketoglutarate, increases of renal concentrations of glutamate and α-ketoglutarate occur. In addition, total renal production of ammonia decreases and renal release of glutamate increases.

In the absence of glutamine synthetase in dog kidney, a fact well documented in studies in vitro (Rector and Orloff, 1959) and in vivo (Lyon and Pitts, 1969), glutamine synthesis is not deemed possible. Even increased formation of glutamate from α-ketoglutarate and

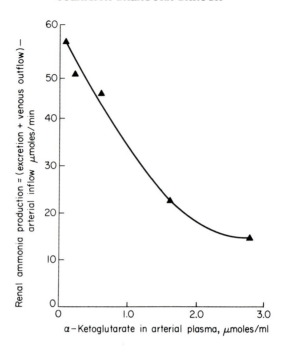

FIG. 21.   Effects of α-ketoglutarate on renal ammonia production in the chronically acidotic dog. Plasma concentration of α-ketoglutarate was increased by intravenous infusion of the substrate. From Balagura-Baruch *et al.* (1970).

ammonia, as shown in rat kidney, accounted in dog for only 25% of the total depression of ammonia release. It is doubtful whether reductive amination of α-ketoglutarate occurs to any significant extent in the acidotic dog in the absence of infusion of α-ketoglutarate. In these conditions, kidney glutamate scarcely becomes labeled during infusion of tracer amounts of $^{15}NH_4Cl$ into a renal artery (Stone and Pitts, 1967). Conceivably then, depression of ammonia production by α-ketoglutarate in dog may be due to inhibition of ammonia formation. Since kidney glutamine concentration is also elevated during infusion of α-ketoglutarate in dog, at the same time that the rates of glutamine extraction decrease, it is possible that the effects described above resulted from inhibition of ammonia formation from glutamine (Welbourne et al., 1969).

C. Regulation by End Products

α-Ketoglutarate may be converted to other organic acids in the operation of the Krebs cycle, undergoing partial or complete oxidation.

Faster removal in acidosis might, then, be due to acceleration of Krebs cycle turnover, i.e., aerobic oxidation, and/or enhancement of reactions that require cycle intermediates as substrates. Furthermore, less production of α-ketoglutarate in acidosis, if it occurs, might contribute to lowering renal concentration of this intermediate. The first two possibilities have been supported by some experimental evidence as presented below. This aspect of the control of ammonia production represents a challenging field for further investigation.

1. Utilization of α-Ketoglutarate for Gluconeogenesis

Based on findings that acidosis enhances glucose production by rat (Fuisz et al., 1965; Kamm et al., 1967) and dog (Goorno et al., 1967) cortical slices incubated with α-ketoglutarate or other glucose precursors, the following scheme of events has been proposed: In acidosis, α-ketoglutarate is consumed avidly in the formation of oxaloacetate, an immediate precursor required for reversal of glycolysis. The rate-limiting step, that of conversion of oxaloacetate to phosphoenolpyruvate, is catalyzed by phosphoenolpyruvate carboxykinase. It is thought that acidosis enhances, sequentially, the activity of this enzyme, the utilization of α-ketoglutarate in the provision of oxaloacetate for the reaction, and the supply of α-ketoglutarate from glutamate by oxidative deamination. Faster removal of glutamate results in release of inhibition of glutaminase activity. Thus, enhancement of ammonia production in acidosis is viewed as a consequence of a primary action of acidosis on a pathway in gluconeogenesis (Goodman et al., 1966; Goorno et al., 1967; Alleyne, 1968; Alleyne and Scullard, 1969).

Although this postulated scheme has attracted much attention, its reality in vivo remains to be established. In patients with hypercapnia due to chronic bronchitis and airway obstruction, Aber et al. (1966) report that consistent renal glucose production occurs, at a mean rate of 57 mg/minute and that it is inversely related to arterial pH and directly related to ammonia production. There are only two studies on dogs, described below, that are germane to the problem, since they indicate that gluconeogenesis occurs in vivo, and suggest that it may be stimulated by acidosis. First, Steiner et al. (1968) have noted that glucose concentration in renal venous blood exceeds that in arterial blood by 0.34 mg % in dogs in chronic metabolic acidosis, and that, in contrast, no differences exist in the normal state. Second, Roxe et al. (1968) have observed that the rates of incorporation of ¹⁴C label into renal venous glucose during renal intraarterial infusion of ¹⁴C-labeled precursors are faster in acidosis than in alkalosis. These studies provide some evidence for increased renal gluconeogenesis in acidosis.

Whether it indeed occurs, and whether it is the cause of adaptation of ammonia excretion, are still unanswered questions.

In all probability other factors besides reactions of gluconeogenesis participate in controlling ammonia production. Work by Preuss *et al.* (1967) exemplifies a particular situation in which acidosis increases ammonia synthesis in the absence of gluconeogenesis. Isolated cortical tubules of dog kidney incubated with glutamate produce, as expected, more glucose and ammonia at external pH of 7.1 than of 7.7. When gluconeogenesis is abolished by addition of certain ions, lowering of the external pH to 7.1 is as effective in increasing ammonia production as it is when gluconeogenesis is intact. It is becoming increasingly evident that acidosis leads to a state of "hypermetabolism" in kidney by stimulating several metabolic pathways, including those involved in gluconeogenesis, protein synthesis, amino acid degradations, lipogenesis, and oxidative reactions (Bignall *et al.*, 1968).

2. Utilization of α-Ketoglutarate in Oxidative Metabolism

Oxygen consumption by kidney slices or homogenates, incubated with glutamine, from rats in chronic metabolic acidosis exceeds that from animals in the normal state (Lotspeich, 1965). This indicates stimulation of oxidative processes by acidosis and provides additional causes for the observed (Goldstein, 1967; Alleyne, 1968) decreases of α-ketoglutarate in rat kidney in this state. In further support are the findings of greater CO_2 formation from glucose by rabbit cortical slices upon acidification of the external media (Hastings and Fanestil, 1963); of linear correlation between renal ammonia production and oxygen consumption in dog (Poppell *et al.*, 1956); and of decreased lactate production from glucose by various tissues when incubated in acid media (Katzman *et al.*, 1953). The latter observation indicates that the decrement of lactate synthesis in acidosis is due to faster incorporation of pyruvate in the Krebs cycle.

Although definite assertion of these actions in the intact animal awaits further investigation, one may surmise from Haldane's (1924) observations that they occur. This author concluded, from measurements of the respiratory quotient on himself, that carbohydrates are oxidized to a great extent in acidosis and very little in alkalosis. The findings of stimulated oxygen consumption in acidosis agree with similar findings on α-ketoglutarate consumption in rat and dog kidneys. Thus, lowering the pH of the incubating media stimulates uptake and utilization of α-ketoglutarate by rat cortical slices (Balagura, 1966). Similarly, acidosis enhances the Tm of reabsorption of α-ketoglutarate in the intact dog (Balagura and Pitts, 1964). Alkalosis, in contrast, depresses reabsorption of this substrate and may even induce secretion, especially when citrate is simultaneously given. These changes in transport are associated with higher renal concentration of α-ketoglutarate during administration of citrate than when it is given in normal acid–base balance. Greater synthesis of α-ketoglutarate from citrate and perhaps slower utilization of α-ketoglutarate may underlie the observed effects of alkalosis (Balagura and Stone, 1967).

Conditions of aerobiosis promote the supply of oxidized pyridine nucleotides. These are cofactors for the glutamate dehydrogenase reaction to proceed in the direction of oxidative deamination of glutamate to yield α-ketoglutarate and ammonia. Preuss (1968) proposes that the ratios of oxidized to reduced pyridine nucleotides are important in regulating ammonia production and that increased availability of the oxidized fractions in acidosis may be responsible, at least in part, for increased ammonia formation in acidosis.

In summary (Fig. 22), greater ammonia production in acidotic rats is associated with decrements of renal levels of glutamate and α-ketoglutarate, with enhanced utilization of α-ketoglutarate, and with stimulation of oxygen consumption. These changes may be related sequentially as follows: acidosis, by promoting aerobic oxidations and gluconeogenesis, lowers α-ketoglutarate and glutamate concentrations. The latter effect releases the glutaminase I reaction from inhibition by glutamate and, consequently, enhances ammonia synthesis. Further investigation is needed to confirm this scheme, to include actions of alkalosis in the opposite direction of acidosis, and to extend these considerations to other animal forms.

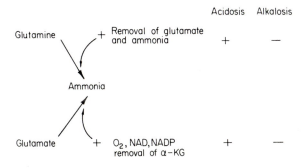

FIG. 22.   Factors influencing ammonia synthesis from glutamine (glutaminase I reaction) and from glutamate (glutamate dehydrogenase reaction). Plus sign indicates stimulation; negative sign indicates inhibition.

However it must be pointed out that our knowledge of the control of ammonia production is scant, that the scheme postulated above has not been proven, and that, even, if true, it may represent only one of many factors that influence ammonia production, such as membrane permeability of cells and mitochondria, their ionic concentrations, and the levels of activators and inhibitors whose identity is unknown at present.

3. AMMONIA LEVELS (CELL pNH₃)

No doubt that renal ammonia production is depressed by increasing pNH_3 levels in renal cortical cells, as shown in Fig. 23 from studies on acidotic dogs during infusion of ammonium chloride (Pilkington *et al.*, 1965). No doubt that oxidative reactions are inhibited by high ammonia levels (McKhann and Tower, 1961). The deleterious effects on brain tissue are attested by the high mortality rate in hepatic disease with hyperammonemia. What is not certain, though, is whether the changes of renal cell pNH_3 that occur in alterations of acid–base balance, discussed below, are of sufficient magnitude to affect metabolic reactions in the manner observed at high ammonia levels.

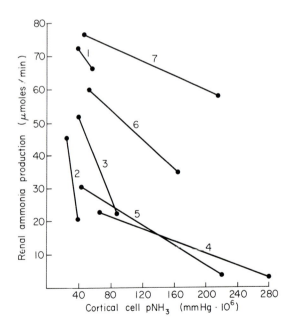

FIG. 23. Relation of renal production of ammonia to pNH_3 of cortical cells (renal venous pNH_3) in the acidotic dog. Numbers on lines correspond to experiment numbers. Left point of each pair is the control value; right point is the value during infusion of ammonium chloride. From Pilkington *et al.* (1965).

The following actions have been described *in vitro*:

(a) Ammonia inhibits the glutaminase I reaction by interacting with glutamine in a competitive manner (Sayre and Roberts, 1958). Such an effect, operating *in vivo*, would represent convenient feedback inhibition of ammonia synthesis in alkalosis, since increments of cortical cell pNH_3 have been found in this state (Denis *et al.*, 1964).

(b) Ammonia depresses oxygen consumption by cat brain slices (McKhann and Tower, 1961) and by rat liver slices and mitochondria (Recknagel and Potter, 1951; Katunuma and Okada, 1963). In explaining the latter actions as well as the toxicity produced by hyperammonemia it has been advanced that ammonia depletes the tissue of Krebs cycle intermediates by favoring reductive amination of α-ketoglutarate to form glutamate and glutamine (Recknagel and Potter, 1951; Berl *et al.*, 1962b). That this explanation may be valid for renal tissue also is indicated by formation of glutamate and glutamine by the isolated rat kidney perfused with ammonium bicarbonate and α-ketoglutarate (Pitts and Krebs, 1968, personal communication). Ammonia fixation as a means of control of its renal release has been presented above in discussing the effects of α-ketoglutarate.

(c) Additional effects of high levels of ammonia include inhibition of oxidation of pyridine nucleotides (Wedding and Vines, 1959; Katunuma and Okada, 1965), and interference with oxidative decarboxylation of pyruvate and α-ketoglutarate (McKhann and Tower, 1961). These actions, operating *in vivo*, would result in feedback inhibition of ammonia synthesis as follows: Depression of oxidative deamination of glutamate and perhaps enhancement of reductive amination of α-ketoglutarate, would result in accumulation of glutamate leading to inhibition of glutamine hydrolysis.

In man (Owen *et al.*, 1961) and dog (Denis *et al.*, 1964) hyperammonemia induced by intravenous infusion of ammonium salts depresses renal ammonia production. Under normal conditions, the kidney is the only tissue which contributes ammonia to systemic blood. Ammonia in portal blood exceeding arterial levels originates from microorganisms in the intestinal mucosa, by enzymatic action on ingested proteins, not from intestinal epithelium itself (McDermott, 1957; Summerskill, 1966). No arteriovenous differences of ammonia concentration are detected across brain and peripheral tissues in man (Bessman and Bessman, 1955) and dog (Addae and Lotspeich, 1968a). The extremely low concentration of ammonia in arterial blood, of about 0.04 μmoles/ml, reflects the major role of the liver in removing ammonia from the circulation in the phase of continuous addition to blood by kidneys and intestine.

Elevation of blood ammonia results in net ammonia uptake by brain, peripheral tissues, gastrointestinal tract, and surprisingly, by kidney (Bessman and Bessman, 1955; Owen *et al.*, 1961; Denis *et al.*, 1964; Summerskill, 1966; Addae and Lotspeich, 1968a). The renal response to hyperammonemia includes reversal of diffusion gradients between cells and peritubular blood from net addition to net uptake, depression of ammonia production, and increased urinary ammonia excretion (Owen *et al.*, 1961; Denis *et al.*, 1964). These findings led Owen *et al.* (1961) to assign to the kidney a role in lowering blood ammonia during hyperammonemia in hepatic disease. Certainly, elevation of preformed arterial ammonia results in depression of synthesis from precursor amino acids, as shown by Pilkington *et al.* (1965). These authors raised the supply of ammonia to the kidney by renal intraarterial infusion of ^{15}N-ammonium lactate. Under these conditions, the excretion of ammonia-^{14}N, the isotopic variety normally derived from precursor amino acids, decreases, whereas that of ^{15}N-ammonia increases.

The mechanisms by which renal ammonia production decreases at high blood ammonia levels could presumably involve any of the effects described *in vitro*. Whether similar mechanisms operate in increasing production in acidosis and decreasing it in alkalosis, with the small changes of cell pNH_3 occurring in these states, awaits experimental assertion. Table V illustrates the direction of the changes of cortical cell pNH_3 in various conditions. It summarizes findings in the dog by Denis *et al.* (1964), using renal venous pNH_3 as a measure of cell pNH_3. (The rationale for this measurement has been discussed on pages 267–268.)

Cell pNH_3 is determined by the balance between production rates and diffusion rates (Fig. 16). When diffusion exceeds production, cell

TABLE V

CHANGES IN CORTICAL CELL pNH_3 AND AMMONIA PRODUCTION IN VARIOUS STATES OF ACID–BASE EQUILIBRIUM[a]

Condition	Cortical cell pNH_3	Ammonia production
Acute respiratory and metabolic acidosis	↓	⇌
Acute respiratory and metabolic alkalosis	↑	↓
Chronic metabolic acidosis	↑	↑
Glutamine infusion	↑	↑
Sodium sulfate infusion	↓	⇌

[a] Increases (↑), decreases (↓), and no change (⇌), refer to comparisons between observations in altered acid–base equilibrium and in the normal state. Derived from data of Denis *et al.* (1964).

pNH_3 decreases. This situation is exemplified by the findings during acute acidosis and sodium sulfate infusion in which diffusion is favored by urine acidification (Table V). When production and diffusion increase equally, as in chronic metabolic acidosis, cell pNH_3 may not change appreciably. When production exceeds diffusion, cell pNH_3 increases. This case is illustrated by observations in acute alkalosis in which urine alkalinization depresses diffusion.

In summary, and from the evidence given, decreased ammonia production in alkalosis might conceivably be a result of elevation of cell pNH_3 levels, leading to depression of the glutaminase I reaction. This effect would be caused by a dual mechanism of competitive inhibition by ammonia and of inhibition by increased glutamate levels. The latter change would follow the depression of oxidative deamination and perhaps the enhanced reductive amination of α-ketoglutarate resulting from inhibition of aerobic oxidation by ammonia.

D. Summary

Renal cellular ammonia concentration, hence cell pNH_3, is determined by the balance between rates of ammonia production and diffusion. When both are enhanced, as in chronic metabolic acidosis, cell pNH_3 may not change appreciably. When diffusion outweighs production, as in acute acidosis, cell pNH_3 decreases. When production outweighs diffusion, as in acute alkalosis, cell pNH_3 increases.

Renal ammonia production is determined by several factors (Fig. 24), as follows: Since most of the enzyme reactions concerned with ammonia synthesis are intramitochondrial, availability of glutamine and other precursor amino acids depends not only on arterial supply to kidney, but also on the ease of transfer of precursors across membranes into renal cells and mitochondria (1, Fig. 24). Such factors as renal enzyme content and levels of activators and inhibitors determine the activities of the ammonia-forming reactions (2, Fig. 24). In all likelihood, rate limitation of ammonia production does not reside in enzyme levels and transport systems. Rather, production is probably controlled by changes of enzyme activities dependent on changes of renal levels of cofactors, ions, and end products of ammonia-forming reactions (3, Fig. 24).

Little is known on the operation of these factors *in vivo* during alterations of acid–base equilibrium of the body. The views that follow derive from studies of the effects of acidosis and alkalosis on various aspects of renal metabolism. They represent tentative, rather than proven, theo-

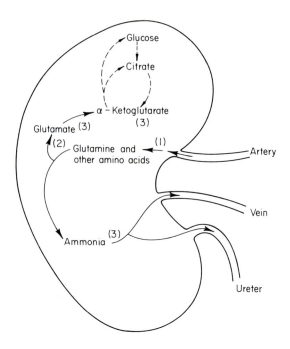

FIG. 24.   Diagram illustrating the main factors regulating renal ammonia production. (1) Precursor supply: includes arterial concentrations of glutamine and other amino acids, and permeability of renal epithelial and mitochondrial membranes to precursors. (2) Enzyme activity: includes enzyme content and levels of activators and inhibitors. (3) End-product inhibition by glutamate, α-ketoglutarate, and ammonia.

ries. Much research is still needed before a satisfactory picture of control of renal ammonia production evolves. In acidosis, the combined effects of enhanced renal oxygen consumption and gluconeogenesis lead to faster utilization of α-ketoglutarate. As a result, glutamate levels decrease by mass action effects on the glutamate dehydrogenase reaction. Oxidative deamination of glutamate is favored, in addition, by greater availability of oxidized pyridine nucleotides. As a consequence of these actions, the glutaminase I reaction is released from inhibition by glutamate. More ammonia is formed, thus, from glutamine. These effects may be strengthened by faster removal of ammonia.

Changes of pH affect multiple pathways of metabolism of carbohydrates, proteins, and lipids. Since these pathways are closely related, effects on almost any may conceivably alter others. In such a net of interrelated metabolic steps it is difficult to establish which are primarily and which are secondarily affected by alterations of pH, as is evident from the concerted effects of acidosis on renal metabolism.

ACKNOWLEDGMENTS

I am very grateful to Dr. Robert F. Pitts for his comments and criticisms of the manuscript, and for his valuable discussions of the work performed.

I also want to thank Miss Linda M. Shurland for her help in the preparation of the figures.

REFERENCES

Aber, G. M., Morris, L. O., Housley, E., and Harris, A. M. (1965). Bidirectional release of ammonium by the kidneys in patients with respiratory failure. Effect of increasing the concentration of inspired oxygen. *Nephron* **2**, 148–158.

Aber, G. M., Morris, L. O., and Housley, E. (1966). Gluconeogenesis by the human kidney. *Nature (London)* **212**, 1589–1590.

Addae, S. K., and Lotspeich, W. D. (1968a). Relation between glutamine utilization and production in metabolic acidosis. *Am. J. Physiol.* **215**, 269–277.

Addae, S. K., and Lotspeich, W. D. (1968b). Glutamine balance in metabolic acidosis as studied with the artificial kidney. *Am. J. Physiol.* **215**, 278–281.

Alleyne, G. A. (1968). Concentrations of metabolic intermediates in kidneys of rats with metabolic acidosis. *Nature (London)* **217**, 847–848.

Alleyne, G. A. O., and Scullard, G. H. (1969). Renal metabolic response to acid-base changes. I. Enzymatic control of ammoniagenesis in the rat. *J. Clin. Invest.* **48**, 364–370.

Balagura, S. (1966). Uptake and utilization of α-ketoglutarate by rat renal cortical slices. *Acta Physiol. Latinoam.* **16**, 6–12.

Balagura, S., and Pitts, R. F. (1962). Excretion of ammonia injected into renal artery. *Am. J. Physiol.* **203**, 11–14.

Balagura, S., and Pitts, R. F. (1964). Renal handling of α-ketoglutarate by the dog. *Am. J. Physiol.* **207**, 483–494.

Balagura, S., and Stone, W. J. (1967). Renal tubular secretion of alpha ketoglutarate in dog. *Am. J. Physiol.* **212**, 1319–1326.

Balagura-Baruch, S., Shurland, L. M., and Welbourne, T. C. (1970). Effects of α-ketoglutarate on renal ammonia release in the intact dog. *Am. J. Physiol.* **218**, 1070–1075.

Balinsky, J. B., and Baldwin, E. (1962). Comparative studies of waste nitrogen metabolism in Amphibia. *Biochem. J.* **82**, 187–191.

Balinsky, J. B., Cragg, M. M., and Baldwin, E. (1961). The adaptation of amphibian waste nitrogen excretion to dehydration. *Comp. Biochem. Physiol.* **3**, 236–244.

Bank, N., and Aynedjian, H. S. (1963). Measurements of tubular fluid pH in vivo in rats. *Nature (London)* **197**, 185–186.

Barker, E. S., Singer, R. B., Elkington, J. R., and Clark, J. K. (1957). The renal response in man to acute experimental respiratory alkalosis and acidosis. *J. Clin. Invest.* **36**, 515–529.

Barnett, G. D., and Addis, T. (1917). Urea as a source of blood ammonia. *J. Biol. Chem.* **30**, 41–46.

Bendall, D. S., and De Duve, C. (1960). Tissue-fractionation studies. 14. The activation of latent dehydrogenases in mitochondria from rat liver. *Biochem. J.* **74**, 444–450.

Bennett, C. M., Brenner, B. M., and Berliner, R. W. (1968). Micropuncture study of nephron function in the Rhesus Monkey. *J. Clin. Invest.* **47**, 203–216.

Berl, S., Takagaki, G., Clarke, D. D., and Waelsch, H. (1962a). Metabolic compartments in vivo. Ammonia and glutamic acid metabolism in brain and liver. *J. Biol. Chem.* **237**, 2562–2569.

Berl, S., Takagaki, G., Clarke, D. D., and Waelsch, H. (1962b). Carbon dioxide fixation in the brain. *J. Biol. Chem.* **237**, 2570-2573.

Bernstein, B. A., and Clapp, J. R. (1968). Micropuncture study of bicarbonate reabsorption by the dog nephron. *Am. J. Physiol.* **214**, 251-257.

Bessman, S. P., and Bessman, A. N. (1955). The cerebral and peripheral uptake of ammonia in liver disease with an hypothesis for the mechanism of hepatic coma. *J. Clin. Invest.* **34**, 622-628.

Bignall, M. C., Elebute, O., and Lotspeich, W. D. (1968). Renal protein and ammonia biochemistry in NH_4Cl acidosis and after nephrectomy. *Am. J. Physiol.* **215**, 289-295.

Blanchard, M., Green, D. E., Nocito, V., and Ratner, S. (1944). l-Amino acid oxidase of animal tissue. *J. Biol. Chem.* **155**, 421-440.

Bliss, S. (1941). Increased excretion of urinary ammonia in the dog following the intravenous injection of both natural and unnatural forms of certain amino acids. *J. Biol. Chem.* **137**, 217-226.

Bloomer, H. A., Rector, F. C., Jr., and Seldin, D. W. (1963). Micropuncture study of the contributions of proximal convolution, distal convolution and collecting duct to titratable acid formation. *Clin. Res.* **11**, 67.

Briggs, A. P. (1934). Excretion of ammonia and neutrality regulation. *J. Biol. Chem.* **104**, 231-238.

Bromberg, P. A., Robin, E. D., and Forkner, C. E., Jr. (1960). The existence of ammonia in blood in vivo, with observations on the significance of the NH_4^+-NH_3 system. *J. Clin. Invest.* **39**, 332-341.

Cade, R., Shalhoub, R. J., and Hierholzer, K. (1961). pCO_2 in regulating ammonia excretion by renal tubules of dogs. *Am. J. Physiol.* **200**, 881-884.

Carter, N. W., Seldin, D. W., and Teng, H. C. (1959). Tissue and renal response to chronic respiratory acidosis. *J. Clin. Invest.* **38**, 949-960.

Chinard, F. P. (1955). Comparative renal excretions of glomerular substances following instantaneous injection into a renal artery. *Am. J. Physiol.* **180**, 617-619.

Clapp, J. R., Owen, E. E., and Robinson, R. R. (1965). Contribution of the proximal tubule to urinary ammonia excretion by the dog. *Am. J. Physiol.* **209**, 269-272.

Coulson, R. A., and Hernandez, T. (1959). Source and function of urine ammonia in the Alligator. *Federation Proc.* **18**, 31.

Coulson, R. A., Hernandez, T., and Brazda, F. G. (1950). Biochemical studies on the Alligator. *Proc. Soc. Exptl. Biol. Med.* **73**, 203-206.

Cragg, M. M., Balinsky, J. B., and Baldwin, E. (1961). A comparative study of nitrogen excretion in some amphibia and reptiles. *Comp. Biochem. Physiol.* **3**, 227-235.

Damian, A. C., and Pitts, R. F. (1970). Rates of glutaminase I and glutamine synthetase reactions in rat kidney *in vivo. Am. J. Physiol.* **218**, 1249-1255.

Davies, B. M. A., and Yudkin, J. (1952). Studies in biochemical adaptation. The origin of urinary ammonia as indicated by the effect of chronic acidosis and alkalosis on some renal enzymes in the rat. *Biochem. J.* **52**, 407-412.

Denis, G., Preuss, H., and Pitts, R. F. (1964). The P_{NH3} of renal tubular cells. *J. Clin. Invest.* **43**, 571-582.

Dewan, J. G. (1938). The l(+) glutamic dehydrogenase of animal tissues. *Biochem. J.* **32**, 1378-1385.

Dickens, F., and Greville, G. D. (1933). Metabolism of normal and tumor tissue. IX. Ammonia and urea formation. *Biochem. J.* **27**, 1123-1133.

Dies, F., and Lotspeich, W. D. (1967). Hexose monophosphate shunt in the kidney during acid-base and electrolyte imbalance. *Am. J. Physiol.* **212**, 61-71.

Duda, G. D., and Handler, P. (1958). Kinetics of ammonia metabolism in vivo. *J. Biol. Chem.* **232**, 303-314.

Du Ruisseau, J. P., Greenstein, J. P., Winitz, M., and Birnbaum, S. M. (1956). Studies on the metabolism of amino acids and related compounds in vivo. IV. Blood ammonia and urea levels following intraperitoneal administration of amino acids and ammonium acetate, and the effect of arginine thereon. *Arch. Biochem. Biophys.* **64**, 355–367.

Eichel, H. J., and Bukovsky, J. (1961). Intracellular distribution pattern of rat liver glutamic-oxalacetic transaminase. *Nature (London)* **191**, 243–145.

Errera, M., and Greenstein, J. P. (1949). Phosphate-activated glutaminase in kidney and other tissues. *J. Biol. Chem.* **178**, 495–502.

Fanelli, G. M., and Goldstein, L. (1964). Ammonia excretion in the Neotenous Newt, Necturus maculosus (Rafinesque). *Comp. Biochem. Physiol.* **13**, 193–204.

Friedberg, F., and Greenberg, D. M. (1947a). Endocrine regulation of amino acid levels in blood and tissues. *J. Biol. Chem.* **168**, 405–410.

Friedberg, F., and Greenberg, D. M. (1947b). Partition of intravenously administered amino acids in blood and tissues. *J. Biol. Chem.* **168**, 411–413.

Fromm, P. O. (1963). Studies on renal and extra-renal excretion in a freshwater teleost, Salmo Gairdneri. *Comp. Biochem. Physiol.* **10**, 121–128.

Fuisz, R. E., Goodman, A. D., Kamm, D. E., Cahill, G. F., Jr., and Marble, A. (1965). Metabolic implications of renal gluconeogenesis in rate control of ammonia synthesis. *J. Clin. Invest.* **44**, 1049.

Fulgraff, G., and Pitts, R. F. (1965). Kinetics of ammonia production and excretion in the acidotic dog. *Am. J. Physiol.* **209**, 1206–1212.

Fuller, G. R., and MacLeod, M. B. (1956). Excretion of titratable acid during acute respiratory disturbances of acid-base balance. *Am. J. Physiol.* **186**, 505–510.

Gamble, J. L., Jr., Blackfan, K. D., and Hamilton, B. (1924). A study of the diuretic action of acid producing salts. *J. Clin. Invest.* **1**, 359–388.

Glabman, S., Klose, R. M., and Giebisch, G. (1963). Micropuncture study of ammonia excretion in the rat. *Am. J. Physiol.* **205**, 127–132.

Goldstein, L. (1958). Effect of NH_4Cl, ethionine and methionine on renal glutaminase I activity and urinary pH. *Federation Proc.* **17**, 372.

Goldstein, L. (1964). Relation of renal glutamine transaminase-w-amidase activity to ammonia excretion in the rat. *Nature (London)* **201**, 1229–1230.

Goldstein, L. (1965). Actinomycin D inhibition of the adaptation of renal glutamine-deaminating enzymes in the rat. *Nature (London)* **205**, 1330–1331.

Goldstein, L. (1966). Relation of glutamate to ammonia production in the rat kidney. *Am. J. Physiol.* **210**, 661–666.

Goldstein, L. (1967). Pathways of glutamine deamination and their control in the rat kidney. *Am. J. Physiol.* **213**, 983–989.

Goldstein, L., and Kensler, C. J. (1960). Factors which affect the activity of glutaminase I in the guinea pig kidney. *J. Biol. Chem.* **235**, 1086–1089.

Goldstein, L., and Schooler, J M. (1966). Regulation of ammonia production in the rat kidney. *Advan. Enzyme Regulation* **5**, 71–86.

Goldstein, L., Richterich, R., and Dearborn, E. H. (1956). Increased activity of renal glutaminases in guinea pig following prolonged administration of acid or alkali. *Proc. Soc. Exptl. Biol. Med.* **93**, 284–287.

Goldstein, L., Richterich, R., and Dearborn, E. H. (1957a). Kidney glutaminases. II: The glutamine-α-ketoacid transamination-deamidation system of the guinea pig. *Enzymologia* **18**, 261–270.

Goldstein, L., Richterich, R., and Dearborn, E. H. (1957b). Kidney glutaminases. IV. Identity of the non-phosphate-activated glutaminase with the glutamine synthesizing enzyme system. *Enzymologia* **18**, 355–365.

Goodman, A. D., Fuisz, R. E., and Cahill, G. F., Jr. (1966). Renal gluconeogenesis in acidosis, alkalosis, and potassium deficiency: its possible role in regulation of renal ammonia production. *J. Clin. Invest.* **45**, 612-619.

Goorno, W. E., Rector, F. C., Jr., and Seldin, D. W. (1967). Relation of renal gluconeogenesis to ammonia production in the dog and rat. *Am. J. Physiol.* **213**, 969-974.

Gottschalk, C. W., Lassiter, W. E., and Mylle, M. (1960). Localization of urine acidification in the mammalian kidney. *Am. J. Physiol.* **198**, 581-585.

Haldane, J. B. S. (1924). Experimental and therapeutic alterations of human tissue alkalinity. *Lancet* **i**, 537-538.

Haldane, J. B. S., and Kennaway, E. L. (1920). Experiments on the regulation of the blood's alkalinity. *J. Physiol.* (*London*) **54**, 32-45.

Hamilton, P. B. (1945). Glutamine: a major constituent of free α-amino acids in animal tissues and blood plasma. *J. Biol. Chem.* **158**, 397-409.

Handler, P., Bernheim, F., and Bernheim, M. L. C. (1949). Ammonia production by kidney slices of normal, acidotic and alkalotic rats. *Arch. Biochem.* **21**, 132-134.

Hastings, A. B., and Fanestil, D. D. (1963). Effect of CO_2 concentration on glucose-14C metabolism by rabbit kidney cortex and medulla, in vitro. *Biochem. Z.* **338**, 276-282.

Hayes, C. P., Jr., Mayson, J. S., Owen, E. E., and Robinson, R. R. (1964). A micropuncture evaluation of renal ammonia excretion in the rat. *Am. J. Physiol.* **207**, 77-83.

Henderson, L. J. (1911). A critical study of the process of acid excretion. *J. Biol. Chem.* **9**, 403-424.

Henderson, L. J., and Palmer, W. W. (1914). On the several factors of acid excretion. *J. Biol. Chem.* **17**, 305-315.

Henderson, L. J., and Palmer, W. W. (1915). On the several factors of acid excretion in nephritis. *J. Biol. Chem.* **21**, 37-55.

Hendrix, B. M., and Sanders, J. P. (1923). The effect of injections of sodium phosphates and sodium hippurate upon the excretion of acid and ammonia by the kidney. *J. Biol. Chem.* **58**, 503-513.

Holmes, B. E., and Patey, A. (1930). Production of ammonia by surviving kidney tissue. II. Studies on the possible precursors of urinary ammonia. *Biochem. J.* **24**, 1564-1571.

Holmes, B. E., and Watchorn, E. (1927). Studies in the metabolism of tissues growing in vitro. I. Ammonia and urea production by kidney. *Biochem. J.* **21**, 327-334.

Holmgård, A. (1962). Quantitative analysis of enzymes in normal and diseased kidney tissue. *Scand. J. Clin. Lab. Invest.* **14**, Suppl. 65.

Iacobellis, M., Muntwyler, E., and Griffin, G. E. (1954). Enzyme concentration changes in the kidneys of protein-and/or potassium-deficient rats. *Am. J. Physiol.* **178**, 477-482.

Iacobellis, M., Muntwyler, E., and Griffin, G. E. (1955). Kidney glutaminase and carbonic anhydrase activity and tissue electrolyte composition in potassium-deficient dogs. *Am. J. Physiol.* **183**, 395-400.

Iacobellis, M., Muntwyler, E., and Griffin, G. E. (1957). Renal glutaminase and carbonic anhydrase activities in potassium-deficient rats. *Proc. Soc. Exptl. Biol. Med.* **96**, 638-640.

Jacobs, M. H. (1940). Some aspects of cell permeability to weak electrolytes. *Cold Spring Harbor Symp. Quant. Biol.* **8**, 30-39.

Jacobs, M. H., and Stewart, D. R. (1936). The distribution of penetrating ammonium salts between cells and their surroundings. *J. Cellular Comp. Physiol.* **7**, 351-365.

Jacquez, J. A., Poppell, J. W., and Jeltsch, R. (1959). Solubility of ammonia in human plasma. *J. Appl. Physiol.* **14**, 255-258.

Kamin, H., and Handler, P. (1951a). The metabolism of parenterally administered amino acids. II. Urea synthesis. *J. Biol. Chem.* **188**, 193-205.

Kamin, H., and Handler, P. (1951b). The metabolism of parenterally administered amino acids. III. Ammonia formation. *J. Biol. Chem.* **193**, 873–880.

Kamm, D. E., Fuisz, R. E., Goodman, A. D., and Cahill, G. F., Jr. (1967). Acid-base alterations and renal gluconeogenesis: Effect of pH, bicarbonate concentration, and P_{CO_2}. *J. Clin. Invest.* **46**, 1172–1177.

Karnovsky, M. J., and Himmelhoch, S. R. (1961). Histochemical localization of glutaminase I activity in kidney. *Am. J. Physiol.* **201**, 786–790.

Katunuma, N., and Okada, M. (1963). Respiratory inhibition of TCA cycle and control of glutamic acid synthesis by ammonia in rat liver mitochondria. *Biochem. Biophys. Res. Commun.* **12**, 252–256.

Katunuma, N., and Okada, M. (1965). Effect of ammonia on decrease of pyridine nucleotide levels in the isolated rat liver mitochondria. *Biochem. Biophys. Res. Commun.* **19**, 108–113.

Katunuma, N., Huzino, A., and Tomino, I. (1966). Organ specific control of glutamine metabolism. *Advan. Enzyme Regulation* **5**, 55–69.

Katzman, R., Villee, C. A., and Beecher, H. K. (1953). Effect of increased carbon dioxide concentrations on fixed acid production in vitro. *Am. J. Physiol.* **172**, 317–323.

Klingman, J. D., and Handler, P. (1958). Partial purification and properties of renal glutaminase. *J. Biol. Chem.* **232**, 369–380.

Krebs, H. A. (1935). Metabolism of amino acids. IV. The synthesis of glutamine from glutamic acid and ammonia, and the enzymic hydrolysis of glutamine in animal tissues. *Biochem. J.* **29**, 1951–1969.

Krebs, H. A., Eggleston, L. V., and Hems, R. (1948). Synthesis of glutamic acid in animal tissues. *Biochem. J.* **43**, 406–414.

Leonard, E., and Orloff, J. (1955). Regulation of ammonia excretion in the rat. *Am. J. Physiol.* **182**, 131–138.

Levitin, H., and Epstein, F. H. (1961). Effect of potassium deficiency on renal response to respiratory acidosis. *Am. J. Physiol.* **200**, 1148–1150.

Litchfield, J. B., and Bott, P. A. (1962). Micropuncture study of renal excretion of water, K, Na, and Cl in the rat. *Am. J. Physiol.* **203**, 667–670.

Longson, D., and Mills, J. N. (1953). The failure of the kidney to respond to respiratory acidosis. *J. Physiol. (London)* **122**, 81–92.

Lotspeich, W. D. (1965). Renal hypertrophy in metabolic acidosis and its relation to ammonia excretion. *Am. J. Physiol.* **208**, 1135–1142.

Lotspeich, W. D., and Pitts, R. F. (1947). The role of amino acids in the renal tubular secretion of ammonia. *J. Biol. Chem.* **168**, 611–622.

Lyon, M. L., and Pitts, R. F. (1969). Species differences in renal glutamine synthesis *in vivo*. *Am. J. Physiol.* **216**, 117–122.

McDermott, W. V., Jr. (1957). Metabolism and toxicity of ammonia. *New Engl. J. Med.* **257**, 1076–1081.

McKhann, G. M., and Tower, D. B. (1961). Ammonia toxicity and cerebral oxidative metabolism. *Am. J. Physiol.* **200**, 420–424.

Madison, L. L., and Seldin, D. W. (1958). Ammonia excretion and renal enzymatic adaptation in human subjects, as disclosed by administration of precursor amino acids. *J. Clin. Invest.* **37**, 1615–1627.

Marriott, W. M., and Howland, J. (1918). The influence of acid phosphate on the elimination of ammonia in the urine. *Arch. Internal Med.* **22**, 477–482.

Meister, A. (1954). Studies on the mechanism and specificity of the glutamine-α-keto acid transamination-deamidation reaction. *J. Biol. Chem.* **210**, 17–35.

Meister, A. (1956). Metabolism of glutamine. *Physiol. Rev.* **36**, 103-127.

Meister, A. (1965). "Biochemistry of the Amino Acids," 2nd Ed., Vol. 2. Academic Press, New York.

Milne, M. D., Scribner, B. H., and Crawford, M. A. (1958). Non-ionic diffusion and the excretion of weak acids and bases. *Am. J. Med.* **24**, 709-729.

Milroy, T. H. (1904). The formation of uric acid in birds. *J. Physiol. (London)* **30**, 47-60.

Montgomery, H., and Pierce, J. A. (1937). The site of acidification of the urine within the renal tubule in Amphibia. *Am. J. Physiol.* **118**, 144-152.

Moyed, H. S., and Umbarger, H. E. (1962). Regulation of biosynthetic pathways. *Physiol. Rev.* **42**, 444-466.

Muntwyler, E., Iacobellis, M., and Griffin, G. E. (1956). Kidney glutaminase and carbonic anhydrase activities and renal electrolyte excretion in rats. *Am. J. Physiol.* **184**, 83-90.

Nash, T. P., and Benedict, S. R. (1921). The ammonia content of the blood, and its bearing on the mechanism of acid neutralization in the animal organism. *J. Biol. Chem.* **48**, 463-488.

O'Donovan, D. J., and Lotspeich, W. D. (1966). Activation of kidney mitochondrial glutaminase by inorganic phosphate and organic acids. *Nature (London)* **212**, 930-932.

Oelert, H., Uhlich, F., and Hills, A. G. (1968). Messungen des Ammoniakdruckes in den corticalen Tubuli der Rattenniere. *Arch. Ges. Physiol.* **300**, 35-48.

Olson, J. A., and Anfinsen, C. B. (1953). Kinetic and equilibrium studies on crystalline L-glutamic acid dehydrogenase. *J. Biol. Chem.* **202**, 841-856.

Orloff, J., and Berliner, R. W. (1956). The mechanism of the excretion of ammonia in the dog. *J. Clin. Invest.* **35**, 223-235.

Owen, E. E., and Robinson, R. R. (1963). Amino acid extraction and ammonia metabolism by the human kidney during the prolonged administration of ammonium chloride. *J. Clin. Invest.* **42**, 263-276.

Owen, E. E., and Robinson, R. R. (1965). Renal ammonia release during ammonium chloride acidosis. *Am. J. Physiol.* **208**, 58-60.

Owen, E. E., Tyor, M. P., Flanagan, J. F., and Berry, J. N. (1960). The kidney as a source of blood ammonia in patients with liver disease: the effect of acetazolamide. *J. Clin. Invest.* **39**, 288-294.

Owen, E. E., Johnson, J. H., and Tyor, M. P. (1961). The effect of induced hyperammonemia on renal ammonia metabolism. *J. Clin. Invest.* **40**, 215, 221.

Papa, S., Tager, J. M., Francavilla, A., DeHaan, E. J., and Quagliariello, E. (1967). Control of glutamate dehydrogenase activity during glutamate oxidation in isolated rat-liver mitochondria. *Biochim. Biophys. Acta* **131**, 14-28.

Patey, A., and Holmes, B. E. (1929). The production of ammonia by surviving kidney tissue. *Biochem. J.* **23**, 760-766.

Pilkington, L. A., Welch, J., and Pitts, R. F. (1965). Relationship of pNH₃ of tubular cells to renal production of ammonia. *Am. J. Physiol.* **208**, 1100-1106.

Pilkington, L. A., Young, T.-K., and Pitts, R. F. (1970). Properties of renal luminal and antiluminal transport of plasma glutamine. *Nephron* **7**, 51-60.

Pitts, R. F. (1948). Renal excretion of acid. *Federation Proc.* **7**, 418-426.

Pitts, R. F. (1966). The renal metabolism of ammonia. *Physiologist* **9**, 97-109.

Pitts, R. F. (1968a). "Physiology of the Kidney and Body Fluids," 2nd Ed., pp. 190-195. Year Book Publ., Chicago, Illinois.

Pitts, R. F. (1968b). Renal metabolism of amino acids and ammonia. *In* "Renal Transport and Diuretics," pp. 11-24. Springer, Berlin, 1969. Symposium in Feldafing in 1968.

Pitts, R. F. (1970). Metabolism of amino acids by the perfused rat kidney. *Am. J. Physiol.* (in press).

Pitts, R. F., and Alexander, R. S. (1945). The nature of the renal tubular mechanism for acidifying the urine. *Am. J. Physiol.* **144**, 239–254.

Pitts, R. F., and Pilkington, L. A. (1966). The relation between plasma concentrations of glutamine and glycine and utilization of their nitrogens as sources or urinary ammonia. *J. Clin. Invest.* **45**, 86–93.

Pitts, R. F., and Stone, W. J. (1967a). Renal metabolism and excretion of ammonia. *Proc. 3rd Intern. Congr. Nephrol., Washington, D. C.* **1**, 123–135.

Pitts, R. F., and Stone, W. J. (1967b). Renal metabolism of alanine. *J. Clin. Invest.* **46**, 530–538.

Pitts, R. F., Gurd, R. S., Kessler, R. H., and Hierholzer, K. (1958). Localization of acidification of urine, potassium, and ammonia secretion and phosphate reabsorption in the nephron of the dog. *Am. J. Physiol.* **194**, 125–134.

Pitts, R. F., DeHaas, J., and Klein, J. (1963). Relation of renal amino and amide nitrogen extraction to ammonia production. *Am. J. Physiol.* **204**, 187–191.

Pitts, R. F., Pilkington, L. A., and DeHaas, J. (1965). N^{15} tracer studies on the origin of urinary ammonia in the acidotic dog, with notes on the enzymatic synthesis of labeled glutamic acid and glutamine. *J. Clin. Invest.* **44**, 731–745.

Pollak, V. E., Mattenheimer, H., DeBruin, H., and Weinman, K. J. (1965). Experimental metabolic acidosis: The enzymatic basis of ammonia production by the dog kidney. *J. Clin. Invest.* **44**, 169–181.

Poppell, J. W., Cuajunco, F., Jr., Horsley, J. S., Randall, H. T., and Roberts, K. E. (1956). Renal arteriovenous ammonium difference and total renal ammonium production in normal, acidotic and alkalotic dogs. *Clin. Res.* **4**, 137.

Portwood, R., and Madison, L. L. (1956). The effects of glutamine loading on renal ammonia excretion and glutaminase adaptation. *Clin. Res.* **4**, 137.

Portwood, R., and Madison, L. L. (1958). The role of transaminase in the renal production of ammonia. *Clin. Res.* **6**, 288.

Preuss, H. G. (1968). Pyridine nucleotides in renal ammonia metabolism. *J. Lab. Clin. Med.* (In press).

Preuss, H. G., Ponder, D. P., and Campbell, M. S. (1967). Effects of acute pH changes on ammonia production in vitro. *Physiologist* **10**, 283.

Ratner, S., Nocito, V., and Green, D. E. (1944). Glycine oxidase. *J. Biol. Chem.* **152**, 119–133.

Recknagel, R. O., and Potter, V. R. (1951). Mechanism of the ketogenic effect of ammonium chloride. *J. Biol. Chem.* **191**, 263–275.

Rector, F. C., Jr., and Orloff, J. (1959). The effect of the administration of sodium bicarbonate and ammonium chloride on the excretion and production of ammonia. The absence of alterations in the activity of renal ammonia-producing enzymes in the dog. *J. Clin. Invest.* **38**, 366–372.

Rector, F. C., Jr., Copenhaver, J., and Seldin, D. W. (1954a). The relation of acid loads to ammonia excretion. *Clin. Res. Proc.* **2**, 93–94.

Rector, F. C., Jr., Seldin, D. W., Roberts, A. D., Jr., and Copenhaver, J. H. (1954b). Relation of ammonia excretion to urine pH. *Am. J. Physiol.* **179**, 353–358.

Rector, F. C., Jr., Seldin, D. W., and Copenhaver, J. H. (1955). The mechanism of ammonia excretion during ammonium chloride acidosis. *J. Clin. Invest.* **34**, 20–26.

Richterich, R. W., and Goldstein, L. (1957). Renal ammonia production as a model for the study of enzyme adaptation in mammals. *Experientia* **13**, 30–32.

Richterich, R. W., and Goldstein, L. (1958). Distribution of glutamine metabolizing enzymes and production of urinary ammonia in the mammalian kidney. *Am. J. Physiol.* **195**, 316–320.

Robinson, R. R., and Owen, E. E. (1965). Intrarenal distribution of ammonia during diuresis and antidiuresis. *Am. J. Physiol.* **208**, 1129–1134.

Rogulski, J., Angielski, S., Mikulski, P., and Basciak, J. (1962). Influence of maleate and N-ethylmaleimide on the synthesis of amino acids from α-ketoglutarate and ammonia in the liver and the kidney of rats. *Acta Biochim. Polon.* **9**, 27–40.

Roxe, D. M., DiSalvo, J., and Balagura, S. (1968). Renal gluconeogenesis in the intact dog. *Federation Proc.* **27**, 742.

Ruszkowski, M., Arasimowicz, C., Knapowski, J., Steffen, J., and Weiss, K. (1962). Renal reabsorption of amino acids. *Am. J. Physiol.* **203**, 891–896.

Ryber, C. (1948). On the formation of ammonia in the kidneys during acidosis. *Acta Physiol. Scand.* **15**, 114–122.

Sanslone, W. R., and Muntwyler, E. (1966). Muscle cell pH in relation to chronicity of potassium depletion. *Proc. Soc. Exptl. Biol. Med.* **122**, 900–903.

Sanslone, W. R., and Muntwyler, E. (1967). Effect of altered plasma pCO_2 on intracellular pH during potassium deficiency. *Proc. Soc. Exptl. Biol. Med.* **126**, 750–754.

Sartorius, O. W., Roemmelt, J. C., and Pitts, R. F. (1949). The renal regulation of acid-base balance in man. IV. The nature of the renal compensations in ammonium chloride acidosis. *J. Clin. Invest.* **28**, 423–439.

Sayre, F. W., and Roberts, E. (1958). Preparation and some properties of a phosphate-activated glutaminase from kidneys. *J. Biol. Chem.* **233**, 1128–1134.

Schwartz, W. B., Jenson, R. L., and Relman, A. S. (1955). Acidification of the urine and increased ammonium excretion without change in acid-base equilibrium: Sodium reabsorption as a stimulus to the acidifying process. *J. Clin. Invest.* **34**, 673–680.

Schwartz, W. B., Brackett, N. C., Jr., and Cohen, J. J. (1965). The response of extracellular hydrogen ion concentration to graded degrees of chronic hypercapnia: the physiological limits of the defense of pH. *J. Clin. Invest.* **44**, 291–301.

Seldin, D. W., Rector, F. C., Jr., Carter, N. W., and Copenhaver, J. (1954). The relation of hypokalemic alkalosis induced by adrenal steroids to renal acid secretion. *J. Clin. Invest.* **33**, 965–966.

Seldin, D. W., Teng, H. C., and Rector, F. C., Jr. (1957). Ammonia excretion and renal glutaminase activity during administration of strong acid and buffer acid. *Proc. Soc. Exptl. Biol. Med.* **94**, 366–368.

Shalhoub, R., Webber, W., Glabman, S., Canessa-Fischer, M., Klein, J., DeHaas, J., and Pitts, R. F. (1963). Extraction of amino acids from and their addition to renal blood plasma. *Am. J. Physiol.* **204**, 181–186.

Stanbury, S. W., and Thomson, A. E. (1952). The renal response to respiratory acidosis. *Clin. Sci.* **11**, 357–374.

Steiner, A. L., Goodman, A. D., and Treble, D. H. (1968). Effect of metabolic acidosis on renal gluconeogenesis in vivo. *Am. J. Physiol.* **215**, 211–217.

Stone, W. J., and Pitts, R. F. (1967). Pathways of ammonia metabolism in the intact functioning kidney of the dog. *J. Clin. Invest.* **46**, 1141–1150.

Stone, W. J., Balagura, S., and Pitts, R. F. (1967). Diffusion equilibrium for ammonia in the kidney of the acidotic dog. *J. Clin. Invest.* **46**, 1603–1608.

Sullivan, L. P. (1965). Ammonium excretion during stopped flow: a hypothetical ammonium countercurrent system. *Am. J. Physiol.* **209**, 273–282.

Sullivan, L. P., and McVaugh, M. (1963). Effect of rapid and transitory changes in blood and urine pH on NH_4 excretion. *Am. J. Physiol.* **204**, 1077–1085.

Sullivan, L. P., Wilde, W. S., and Malvin, R. L. (1960). Renal transport sites for K, H and NH_3. Effect of impermeant anions on their transport. *Am. J. Physiol.* **198**, 244–254.

Summerskill, W. H. J. (1966). On the origin and transfer of ammonia in the human gastrointestinal tract. *Medicine* **45**, 491–496.

Ullrich, K. J., and Eigler, F. W. (1958). Sekretion von Wasserstoffionen in den Sammlrohren der Saugetierniere. *Arch. Ges. Physiol.* **267**, 491–496.

Ullrich, K. J., Hilger, H. H., and Klümper, J. D. (1958). Sekretion von Ammoniumionen in den Sammelrohren der Saugetierniere. *Arch. Ges. Physiol.* **267**, 244–250.

Van Slyke, D. D., Linder, G. C., Hiller, A., Leiter, L., and McIntosh, J. F. (1926). The excretion of ammonia and titratable acid in nephritis. *J. Clin. Invest.* **2**, 255–288.

Van Slyke, D. D., Phillips, R. A., Hamilton, P. B., Archibald, R. M., Futcher, P. H., and Hiller, A. (1943). Glutamine as source material of urinary ammonia. *J. Biol. Chem.* **150**, 481.

Walker, A. M. (1940). Ammonia formation in the Amphibian kidney. *Am. J. Physiol.* **131**, 187–194.

Wallace, W. M., and Hastings, A. B. (1942). The distribution of the bicarbonate ion in mammalian muscle. *J. Biol. Chem.* **144**, 637–649.

Wallace, W. M., and Lowry, O. H. (1942). An in vitro study of carbon dioxide equilibria in mammalian muscle. *J. Biol. Chem.* **144**, 651–655.

Walter, F. (1877). Untersuchungen über die Wirkung der Saüren auf den thierischen organismus. *Arch. Exptl. Pathol. Pharmakol.* **7**, 148–178.

Watts, J. H., Bradley, L., and Mann, A. N. (1965). Total N, urea and ammonia excretions of human male subjects fed several nonessential amino acids singly as the chief source of nonspecific N. *Metab. Clin. Exptl.* **14**, 504–515.

Wedding, R. T., and Vines, H. M. (1959). Inhibition of reduced diphosphopyridine nucleotide oxidation by ammonia. *Nature (London)* **184**, 1226–1227.

Weiss, M. B., and Longley, J. B. (1960). Renal glutaminase I distribution and ammonia excretion in the rat. *Am. J. Physiol.* **198**, 223–226.

Welbourne, T. C., Shurland, L. M., and Balagura-Baruch, S. (1969). Influence of α-ketoglutarate on renal handling of glutamine in the intact dog. *Am. Soc. Nephrol.* 3rd meeting, Washington, D.C., pp. 74.

Wergedal, J. E., and Harper, A. E. (1964). Metabolic adaptations in higher animals. IX. Effect of high protein intake on amino nitrogen catabolism in vivo. *J. Biol. Chem.* **239**, 1156–1163.

White, H. L., and Rolf, D. (1952). Renal glutaminase and ammonia excretion. *Am. J. Physiol.* **169**, 174–179.

Wolbach, R. A. (1955). Renal regulation of acid-base balance in the chicken. *Am. J. Physiol.* **181**, 149–156.

Wu, H., and Sendroy, J., Jr. (1959). Pattern of N^{15} excretion in man following administration of N^{15}-labeled L-phenylalanine. *J. Appl. Physiol.* **14**, 6–10.

Yoshimura, H., Yata, M., Yuasa, M., and Wolbach, R. A. (1961a). Renal regulation of acid-base balance in the bullfrog. *Am. J. Physiol.* **201**, 980–986.

Yoshimura, H., Fujimoto, M., Okumura, O., Sugimoto, J., and Kuwada, T. (1961b). Three-step regulation of acid-base balance in body fluid after acid load. *Japan. J. Physiol.* **11**, 109–125.

6

RENAL POTASSIUM EXCRETION*

Gerhard Giebisch

I. Introduction

Among the normal constituents of extracellular fluid, potassium holds a unique position with respect to its mode of renal excretion. Unlike other ionic species, the narrow range of concentration in plasma and interstitial fluid is maintained by a complex interaction of both tubular reabsorption and tubular secretion at different levels of the nephron.

The fact that potassium clearances can significantly exceed glomer-

*Work carried out in the author's laboratory was supported by grants from the National Institutes of Health, the National Science Foundation, and the American Heart Association.

329

ular filtration rate in a variety of species and under a variety of conditions provides unequivocal proof that the kidney has a tubular mechanism for the secretion of potassium ions. However, since the potassium excreted by the mammalian kidney at a normal dietary intake amounts to only about 10-15% of the potassium in the glomerular filtrate, the role of the secretory process and the factors modifying individual transport processes at different nephron levels cannot easily be assessed by clearance methods. Nevertheless, it was postulated early and is now firmly established that even when the amount of potassium excreted into the urine is only a small fraction of that filtered most of the excreted potassium is derived from tubular secretion (Berliner, 1952; Berliner, 1961; Malnic et al., 1964; Giebisch and Windhager, 1964).

Additional evidence is available which indicates that some nephron parts must also be endowed with a powerful mechanism for transporting potassium against sizable electrochemical potential gradients from tubular lumen to peritubular fluid. This capacity of the renal tubular apparatus is demonstrated by the results of stop-flow studies (Aukland and Kill, 1961; Vander, 1961) and by the observation that the potassium concentration in the final urine may fall significantly below that of plasma water (Evans et al., 1954; Orsent-Keiles and Mc-Collum, 1941). This raises the possibility that the transport pattern may vary dramatically from one segment to another and that even the direction of net transfer of potassium may change as a function of the metabolic situation and of other intrarenal factors.

It should be clear that a three-component system of renal excretion such as that of potassium in which glomerular filtration, tubular reabsorption, and tubular secretion contribute to the urinary excretion pattern, is eminently suitable to the micropuncture approach. The exact contribution of various nephron segments to the potassium appearing in the final urine cannot accurately be defined by clearance methods since any given excretory rate can be the result of many different transport patterns at separate nephron segments. Accordingly, the more recent research efforts have been concerned with the study of renal potassium transport at the level of the single tubule. This approach has attracted considerable attention since it can provide information on many parameters of potassium transport which are not otherwise open to investigation. These studies on the mechanisms underlying renal potassium excretion have dealt mainly with two problems. First, they have provided considerable insight into the precise tubular sites of reabsorption and secretion during widely differing excretion patterns. Second, studies on single nephrons of both mammalian and amphibian kidneys have permitted an inquiry into the cellular mechanisms of transport and, importantly, into the factors controlling the net transfer rate of potassium ions.

II. Factors Affecting the Rate of Urinary Potassium Loss

It has long been known that a number of factors exert a profound effect upon the rate of urinary potassium excretion. Concentration changes of potassium in body cells, and it may be inferred that it is the concentration of potassium in some strategically localized tubule cells, affect potassium excretion: increased potassium excretion results from dehydration, whether produced by decreased water intake, increased water loss, or by the infusion of hypertonic salt solutions (Berliner et al., 1950; Mudge et al., 1950; Mudge, 1958). Common to these manipulations is a shift of fluid from the intracellular to the extracellular fluid compartment and a corresponding rise in intracellular potassium concentration. Since potassium is primarily an intracellular ion it is to be expected a priori that it is the cell potassium to which excretion would be strongly related (Berliner, 1961). On the other hand, urinary potassium loss is minimal during water diuresis (McCollum and Orent-Keiles, 1941; Berliner et al., 1950). Aside from reflecting changes in cell potassium concentration, the plasma potassium level has relatively little influence on potassium excretion.

It is also well established that changes in urinary sodium excretion have a profound effect upon the excretory rate of potassium ions (Davidson et al., 1958; Kruhoffer, 1960; Berliner, 1961; Malnic et al., 1966b). Thus, it has been proposed that secretory entry of potassium at distal nephron sites is coupled to reabsorptive movement of sodium (Berliner et al., 1954; Davidson et al., 1958; Berliner, 1961). It has been argued that to the extent that a low urinary excretion rate of sodium reflects a similarly low sodium supply to a distal secretory site of potassium, the amount of sodium at such a critical nephron site may become the rate-limiting factor in determining potassium secretion. It will become apparent that more complex factors underly the frequently parallel relationship between urinary sodium and potassium excretion.

A large body of experimental data supports the view that tubular factors related to the rate of hydrogen ion secretion or, more likely, to the acidity of secretory tubule cells, also exert a highly significant effect upon the rate of urinary potassium excretion (Berliner et al., 1951; Berliner et al., 1954; Kruhoffer, 1960; Berliner, 1961). In general, alkalinization of the urine enhances tubular excretion of potassium while in both metabolic and respiratory acidosis urinary potassium loss is curtailed. Accordingly, it has been postulated that not only potassium but also hydrogen ions are secreted into the distal tubular lumen in exchange for sodium (Berliner *et al.*, 1951; Berliner *et al.*, 1954; Berliner, 1961). However, a direct assessment of the relationship between hydrogen ion secretion and potassium secretion at the specific tubular sites involved has not generally supported the stoichiometric, reciprocal relationship to be expected from such a competitive, obligatory ion-exchange mechanism. Nevertheless, the well-known effects of alterations in the acid–base balance upon renal potassium transport underscore the central role played by the intracellular concentration of both hydrogen and potassium ions in the regulation of urinary potassium excretion.

In addition, a number of other well-defined factors are known to modify the normal pattern of potassium excretion. Most notable among these are endocrine factors, in particular adrenal mineralocorticoids: their presence is necessary to maintain adequate excretion rates at a normal dietary intake (Loeb *et al.*, 1933; Loeb, 1942). Also, the nature of the anion excreted with the urinary cation load can be shown to exert significant effects upon potassium excretion. Thus, a poorly reabsorbable anion such as phosphate, sulfate, or ferrocyanide replacing chloride has a powerful kaliuretic effect (Berliner *et al.*, 1950; Berliner, 1952; Schwartz *et al.*, 1955; Bank and Schwartz, 1960; Kruhoffer, 1960; Malnic *et al.*, 1964). The development of tolerance to potassium by a high dietary intake of this ion, a situation associated with both enhanced renal excretion and elevated uptake by extrarenal tissue, is a phenomenon illustrating the great adaptability of the renal control mechanism to alterations in potassium metabolism (Thatcher and Radike, 1947; Berliner *et al.*, 1950; Kruhoffer, 1960; Berliner, 1961; Alexander and Levinsky, 1968; Wright *et al.*, 1969). Finally, the administration of certain cationic amino acids leads to an enhanced urinary potassium excretion (Dickerman and Walker, 1964).

III. Localization of Potassium Transport in the Nephron

A. Mammalian Nephron

The contribution of various nephron segments to different excretion patterns of potassium has recently been investigated in considerable detail. These studies have dealt with the delineation of the site and the quantitation of tubular transport along the nephron in a number of vertebrates. Although the largest body of information has been obtained on rodent kidneys, studies on canine, monkey, and some amphibian tubules have also been carried out.

Concerning the proximal tubular epithelium there is general agreement that the concentration of potassium in fluid exposed to the activity of this nephron segment remains about the same as in plasma or is only slightly less (Wirz and Bott, 1954; Litchfield and Bott, 1962; Bloomer et al., 1963; Marsh et al., 1963; Malnic et al., 1964; Watson et al., 1964; Hierholzer et al., 1965; Malnic et al., 1966; Watson, 1966; Bennett et al., 1967; Bennett et al., 1968; Lechene et al., 1969; de-Rouffignac et al., 1969). Although the concentration gradients which are established across the proximal tubular epithelium are small or even absent, extensive fluid reabsorption accounts for the bulk of the filtered potassium being reabsorbed along this egment. It is noteworthy that this functional pattern is preserved in the presence of rather wide variations in urinary excretion rates, even when the amounts of potassium in the final urine significantly exceed those filtered. There is general agreement that with certain exceptions, modifications of the proximal tubular reabsorptive transport pattern do not contribute importantly to variations in urinary potassium output. Diminished reabsorption of potassium along the proximal tubule can be shown to occur during those diuretic states in which proximal tubular sodium and fluid reabsorption has been reduced, most notably after the administration of osmotic diuretics (Malnic et al., 1964), sodium salts of poorly reabsorbable anions (Malnic et al., 1966b), after expansion of the extracellular fluid compartment by infusion of isotonic sodium chloride (Landwehr et al., 1967; Khuri, R. N., Strieder, N., Wiederholt, M., and Giebisch, G., unpublished), and after those diuretics known to act on the proximal tubule (Dirks and Seely, 1969). Despite the fact that proximal net reabsorption of potassium is reduced under these conditions both the fraction and the absolute amount of potassium at the early distal tubular level are frequently set at a value some 5–10% of that filtered, not significantly different from the nondiuretic state. Also, by the time fluid has reached the distal tubule, the concentration of potassium has fallen and tubular fluid/plasma ratios are almost always significantly below unity (Marsh et al., 1963; Malnic et al., 1964; Hierholzer et al., 1965; Malnic et al., 1966b; Bennett et al., 1967; Bennett et al., 1968; Cortney, 1969; Lechene et al., 1969; Rouffignac et al., 1969). Accordingly, the ascending limb of Henle's loop, most prominently its thick part, is an important site of tubular potassium reabsorption. It appears that, similar to sodium ions, load increments of potassium escaping reabsorption from the proximal convolution under the above-described conditions are, to a large extent, reabsorbed during passage of tubular fluid along Henle's loop such that the fraction entering the distal tubule is again set at a value similar to that found normally. Microperfusion studies have confirmed that the loop of Henle can adjust its rate of reabsorption in proportion to load increments as flow rate increases (Schnermann, 1968). From the available data it appears that significantly diminished reabsorption of potassium along the proximal tubule *and* the loop of Henle may only occur during strong osmotic diuresis induced by mannitol (Malnic *et al.*, 1966b) and after administration of furosemide (Bennett *et al.*, 1967; Duarte *et al.*, 1969).

The concentration of potassium at the level of the distal tubular epithelium is predominantly determined by the activity of this nephron segment. Stop-flow microperfusion studies on distal tubules of rats support this view (Malnic *et al.*, 1966a). When a poorly penetrating nonelectrolyte, such as raffinose, is deposited into the lumen of a superficial distal loop between mineral oil droplets, steady-state concentration gradients are developed under conditions approaching zero net fluid and electrolyte movement. Tubular fluid (TF) / plasma (P) ratios of potassium are found to be quite similar to those observed under free-flow conditions (Malnic *et al.*, 1966a). The rapid attainment of steady-state concentration gradients stresses the point that the kinetics of the distal tubular potassium transport system are under many, but not all, conditions independent of volume flow rate. It will become apparent from the subsequent discussion that this transport feature has important implications with respect to the effects of variations in distal tubular volume flow rate *per se* upon urinary excretion rate of potassium.

Several investigators have drawn attention to the observation that the tubular fluid/plasma potassium ratio ranging between 3 and 13 at the tip of Henle's loop implies some reentry of potassium at this site from the collecting ducts (Giebisch et al., 1964; Marsch and Solomon, 1965; Jamison, 1968; deRouffignac and Morel, 1969). This is a consequence of the fact that concentration ratios of this magnitude cannot be accounted for by fluid abstraction alone. Little is known about the physiological importance of this process, but in view of the powerful reabsorptive capacity of the thick ascending limb of the loop, and in view of the establishment of very low intratubular potassium concentrations at the earliest distal tubular level, it is doubtful, whether recirculation of potassium plays a significant role in the overall excretion pattern of this ion.

It is the distal tubule and the collecting duct system which most dramatically modulate urinary potassium excretion. This is due to the fact that, as pointed out before, the fraction of filtered potassium escaping reabsorption by the time fluid has issued from Henle's loop is small and changes little, despite the fact that the urinary excretion rate may vary about one hundredfold (Malnic *et al.*, 1964; Giebisch *et al.*, 1965; Malnic *et al.*, 1966b; Giebisch *et al.*, 1967).

The view of a key role of the distal tubular system in regulating and determining urinary potassium excretion had previously been expressed by Berliner and his associates on the basis of a series of ingenious clearance experiments (Berliner *et al.*, 1950; Berliner, 1961). In these studies, evidence was presented that urinary potassium excretion could, under a variety of experimental conditions, be effectively dissociated from filtration rate and, thus, from the amount of potassium filtered. Since it was thought unlikely that potassium reabsorption was adjusted to match changes in filtration rate such as to maintain a constant excretion rate, it was postulated that the contribution of the filtered potassium to the urinary moiety was negligible and that the relatively constant excretion rate represented secretion at a far distal nephron site. Hence, reabsorptive activity at a more proximally located nephron segment had reduced the tubular potassium content to insignificant levels. Additional electrolyte excretion studies, in which a poorly reabsorbable anion, ferrocyanide, known to be cleared by glomerular filtration alone and, therefore, not secreted, was infused, permitted a balance sheet to be drawn of the amount of potassium minimally secreted (i.e., that potassium excreted in excess of that filtered) and the amounts of bicarbonate, chloride, sulfate, and phosphate present in the final urine. Since only a small fraction of the "minimally secreted" potassium could be covered by anions other than ferrocyanide, it was argued convincingly that none of the anions normally present in extracellular fluid were secreted with potassium. Potassium must therefore have been secreted in exchange for another cation. Sodium ions are the only cations of adequate amount for such exchange.

A distal tubular site of potassium secretion has also emerged from numerous stop-flow studies (Malvin et al., 1958; Pitts et al., 1958; Jaenike and Berliner, 1960; Sullivan et al., 1960; Aukland and Kill, 1961; Sullivan, 1961; Vander, 1961; Walker et al., 1961; Ramsay, 1964). Stop-flow patterns have been obtained in which peak concentrations of potassium representing the accumulation of potassium in far distal portions of the tubule were a uniform finding, and in which these distal secretory peaks were enhanced by those manipulations known to promote kaliuresis.

The extent of distal tubular secretion of potassium is variable and depends critically upon the metabolic situation. A direct evaluation of distal tubular function under different experimental conditions has become possible by micropuncture techniques, and has permitted an accurate description of the range of distal tubular variation in potassium handling. Figure 1 summarizes distal tubular data in two extreme conditions, emphasizing the great range of transport facilities residing within this epithelial structure (Malnic *et al.*, 1964). On the left, data from a rat on a low dietary intake of potassium are shown. On the right, data are shown from a rat in which, by various manipulations, urinary potassium excretion was maximally stimulated. It is apparent that early distal tubular concentrations of potassium are significantly below plasma levels under both experimental conditions, despite the fact that in the low-potassium animals only some 3% of the filtered potassium is excreted while in the state of maximal kaliuresis urinary excretion rate was equivalent to some 150% of the filtered potassium.

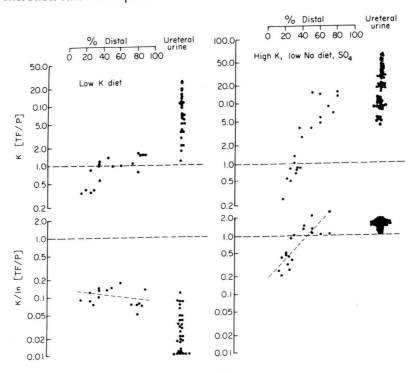

FIG. 1.   Summary of distal tubular potassium and potassium/inulin concentration ratios. *Left*: data from rats kept several weeks on a low-potassium diet. *Right*: data from rats in which potassium excretion was maximally stimulated by pretreatment with a low sodium–high potassium diet and the infusion of potassium sulfate and dichlorophenamide. From Malnic *et al.* (1964).

Distal transtubular concentration ratios rise only moderately in the former but very steeply in the latter situation, in which distal tubular peak concentrations in excess of 100 mEq/liter are not uncommon.

To evaluate these micropuncture data in terms of transtubular net movement, potassium concentration ratios are divided by the corresponding inulin ratios. The lower graphs provide information on net potassium transfer in the two situations. Continuous, albeit moderate, net reabsorption occurs in animals subjected to dietary potassium deprivation, while massive distal tubular secretion is evident in those animals in which maximal potassium excretion was induced. In these animals, some 90% of the urinary potassium has entered the lumen by way of tubular secretion. Influx of potassium from the peritubular into the luminal fluid across distal tubular epithelium determines the excretory capacity of the kidney. It is of considerable interest to note that the state of maximal urinary potassium secretion is associated with only small modifications of the reabsorptive transport pattern across the proximal tubule and Henle's loop. Despite the fact that considerably more potassium is excreted than filtered, some 80% of the filtered potassium has been reabsorbed by the time fluid enters the distal tubular system.

Comparing the amount of potassium present at the beginning of the distal tubule with that appearing in the final urine gives a rough estimate of the contribution of distal secretion to the moiety of potassium appearing in the final urine. Table I contains data obtained in the rat under a wide variety of experimental conditions. It is apparent that some three-fourths of the urinary potassium can be accounted for by distal tubular secretion under nondiuretic conditions, and the fraction is higher whenever potassium excretion has been stimulated. Notable exceptions, in which no significant addition of potassium can be demonstrated along the distal tubule, are pretreatment with a diet deficient in potassium (Malnic et al., 1964), administration of the potassium-sparing diuretic Amiloride (Merck 870) (Duarte et al., 1969), or induction of metabolic acidosis (Malnic et al., 1968; Malnic et al., in preparation). Potassium secretion along the distal convolution is also notably compromised in adrenalectomized rats (Hierholzer et al., 1965, Wiederholt and Hierholzer, 1967; Cortney, 1969).

Compared to nondiuretic conditions, potassium secretion is enhanced in the mammalian distal tubule under the following conditions: intravenous loading with hypertonic (Malnic et al., 1966b) or isotonic sodium chloride (Landwehr et al., unpublished), loading with hypertonic sodium sulfate (Malnic et al., 1966b), iso- or hypertonic potassium chloride (Malnic et al., 1966b; Malnic et al., in preparation), sodium bi-

TABLE I

Summary of Tubular Sequential Contribution to Urinary Potassium Excretion in the Rat

Experimental condition	Diet	% Filtered K Early distal tubule	% Filtered K Final urine
Antidiuresis	Control	5	17
Antidiuresis	Low K	10	3
Antidiuresis	Low Na	6	4
Antidiuresis, DOCA	Low Na	7	4
10% Mannitol i.v.	Low Na	15	30
4%NaCl i.v.	Control	8	48
Hypertonic Na_2SO_4 i.v.	Control	7	60
Dichlorphenamide i.v.	Control	10	60
10% Mannitol, isotonic KCl	Low Na	9	91
Hypertonic Na_2SO_4, KCl, dichlorphenamide	High K, Low Na	20	151
5% Mannitol in isotonic NaCl	Control	10	36
Respiratory acidosis (15% CO_2)	Control	7	29
Metabolic acidosis (HCl i.v.)	Control	10	9
Hyperventilation	Control	10	53
Acute KCl load	Control	10	68
Acute bicarbonate load	Control	12	49
Acute bicarbonate load + 15% CO_2	Control	12	38
Acute bicarbonate + KCl load	Control	15	72
Acute bicarbonate load + hyperventilation	Control	17	83
Amiloride	Control	5	5
Acute KCl load	High K	10	87
Acute K$_2$SO$_4$ load	High K	30	148

carbonate (Malnic *et al.*, 1968; Malnic *et al.*, in preparation), administration of carbonic anhydrase inhibitors (Malnic *et al.*, 1964), and induction of respiratory alkalosis (Malnic *et al.*, 1968; Malnic *et al.*, in preparation). A high dietary potassium intake enhances the distal secretory response to a standard intravenous potassium load (Wright *et al.*, 1969).

Estimates of distal tubular secretion derived from a comparison of early distal tubular with final urinary potassium moieties, and similar inferences concerning the transport properties of the collecting duct system by comparing late distal with final urinary excretion rates deserve closer scrutiny. Two important limitations of such an approach should be kept in mind. A first limitation is the inability to obtain fluid samples from the very beginning of the distal tubule. Consequently, fractions of filtered potassium present at the very beginning of the distal tubule may be significantly less than that calculated on the basis of potassium and inulin concentration ratios at the earliest distal tubular sites available for puncture. Extrapolation to zero length of the regression lines relating potassium TF/P ratios or potassium/inulin TF/P ratios to distal tubular length is open to question. As a consequence of the inability to obtain accurate estimates of the amount of potassium present either at the level of the ascending limb of Henle's loop or at the very beginning of the distal tubule, the fraction calculated to derive from distal tubular secretion represents a minimum value. Nevertheless, the view of Berliner (Berliner, 1961) of a predominantly secretory origin of urinary potassium can be considered firmly supported by direct experimental evidence under all those conditions in which significant distal tubular potassium secretion takes place. On the other hand, it should be clearly recognized that it is presently not possible to decide whether the small fraction of potassium present at the beginning of the distal tubule under conditions in which distal tubular secretion is either drastically reduced or absent, such as in the potassium-depleted animal (Malnic et al., 1964), in metabolic or respiratory acidosis (Malnic et al., 1968; Malnic et al., in preparation), or after Amiloride (Duarte et al., 1969), is of secretory origin or whether it represents potassium which has escaped reabsorption along more proximally located nephron segments. It is more likely that the latter alternative is the correct one. If secretory in origin, it would be necessary to postulate significant secretory activity at the level of either the ascending limb of Henle's loop or the first fifth of the distal tubule at a time when potassium secretion is absent along that part of the distal tubule which is available to micropuncture. Since the ascending limb of Henle's loop can be shown to be a nephron site of avid potassium reabsorption even under conditions of maximal distal tubular secretion of potassium, it appears extremely remote that a condition of complete lack of distal tubular secretory activity could be associated with secretory activity at more proximally located nephron sites.

A second limitation in the analysis of segmental contributions to urinary potassium excretion concerns uncertainties with regard to the relative contributions of superficial nephron activity to total excretory kidney function. This problem has recently received considerable attention. Evidence has been obtained indicating that in the rodent at least, there may be very significant differences in the rate of filtrate formation between superficial and deep, juxtamedullary nephron populations (Horster and Thurau, 1968). At present, virtually nothing is known about the potassium transport properties of deep nephrons and, conceivably, the potassium transport properties of juxtamedullary nephrons may be different from those of superficial nephrons. Accordingly, uncertainties arise when inferences are made concerning the contribution of either the collecting ducts or the distal tubular system to a given excretory pattern in the final urine. Caution is indicated for evaluating either distal tubular or collecting duct contributions to a given excretory pattern, particularly in species with a heterogenous nephron population (Lechene *et al.*, 1966; de Rouffignac and Morel, 1967). Even in species with homogeneous nephron populations such an approach may not be without hazard since only deep cortical nephrons extend to the very tip of the renal papilla, while superficial cortical nephrons do not. Different functional properties of various nephron groups may thus still exist.

In contrast to the distal tubule's role in the overall renal transport of potassium, which is fairly well understood, the precise contribution of the collecting ducts to urinary potassium excretion is not well defined. Although the relative importance of reabsorptive and secretory activity of the collecting ducts can be studied most directly either by microcatheterization or transmural puncture, few such studies are available. Most reports have been based on comparisons of distal fluid with final urine. On the other hand, distal tubular data are completely lacking in those herbivorous species in which a rather extensive evaluation of the tubular transport function of isolated collecting ducts *in vitro* has recently become available.*

Experimental evidence in rodents, dogs, and monkeys indicates that a significant contribution of the collecting ducts to potassium secretion occurs only rarely (Bennett *et al.*, 1967; Bennett *et al.*, 1968; Malnic *et al.*, 1964; Malnic *et al.*, 1966 b), although such evaluations are based only on a comparison of late distal with final urine excretion rates. Similarly, direct microcatheterization of single collecting ducts in the golden hamster has failed to uncover significant secretion under conditions characterized by normal excretion rates (Hilger *et al.*, 1958). Even under conditions of net renal potassium secretion (urinary potassium clearances in excess of simultaneously measured inulin clearances) at best only a moderate degree of potassium secretion could be demonstrated along the terminal collecting duct segment (Hierholzer, 1961). Although some suggestive evidence for potassium secretion along the collecting ducts is available it is doubtful whether it could, from a quan-

---

*Diezi *et al.* have very recently investigated the role of the terminal collecting ducts in determining urinary potassium excretion (Diezi *et al.*, 1969). In essence, they confirmed the conclusions arrived at by the comparison of late distal and urinary fractional excretion rates. The terminal collecting ducts abstract potassium ions from the tubular fluid in the state of dietary potassium and sodium deprivation, and a variable secretory component could be observed in strongly kaluretic states. No significant net transfer of potassium could be observed in animals on a normal potassium intake.

titative point of view, play a very significant role. Berliner had already previously argued against the notion that a large fraction of urinary potassium could be derived from secretory activity of papillary collecting duct segments (Jaenike and Berliner, 1960; Berliner, 1961). This view is based on the well-established fact that the renal medulla receives only a small fraction of the renal blood flow whereas the urinary excretion rates of potassium can continue at levels significantly exceeding that of glomerular filtration. Accordingly, it can easily be calculated that the blood supply of the papillary collecting ducts is inadequate to supply but a small fraction of the excreted potassium.

In contrast to the relatively small functional role the collecting duct system appears to play in the process of tubular potassium secretion, it can be shown that significant net reabsorption occurs under those conditions in which the fraction of potassium in the final urine is only a few percent of that filtered. The collecting duct epithelium contributes significantly to the reduction of urinary potassium excretion under conditions of dietary potassium and sodium depletion (Malnic et al., 1964; Malnic et al., 1966b) and under those conditions in which urinary sodium excretion has been drastically curtailed by the acute reduction of the glomerular filtration rate (Landwehr et al., unpublished). However, in passing it may be noted that a survey of available micropuncture data indicates that even under some of those conditions in which significant distal tubular secretion is present (for instance, after bicarbonate infusion (Malnic et al., in preparation) or during chronic potassium adaptation (Wright et al., 1969), the fraction of potassium in the final urine may be significantly less than that at the very end of the distal tubule of superficial cortical nephrons. The functional importance of this phenomenon is presently not clear. Nevertheless, the possibility has to be considered that tubular net movement of potassium occurs in three sequential steps: net reabsorption in the proximal tubule and the loop of Henle, secretion along the distal tubule, and a final step effecting again net reabsorption in the collecting duct system.

Supportive evidence for a cortical secretory origin of urinary potassium has also been derived from studies utilizing radioactive potassium in which the relative specific activities of arterial blood, renal venous blood, and of urine were compared after intravenous injection of this isotope. Morel et al. (Morel, 1955; Morel and Guinnebault, 1956; Morel, 1961; Morel et al., 1963), Black et al. (Black et al., 1956; Black and Emery, 1957), and Goldman et al. (Goldman et al., 1963) have been able to demonstrate convincingly that the specific activity of urinary potassium is quite similar to that of renal venous and tissue potassium but, prior to complete isotope equilibration, significantly different from that of arterial plasma from which filtered potassium is derived. The underlying assumption seems justified that in view of the known rapid exchange of ^{42}K with tissue potassium (Wilde, 1962), renal venous potassium contains only a negligible fraction of that potassium which has entered the kidney via the arterial blood supply but is almost completely derived from the potassium present in renal cortical tissue. Evidently, the specific activity of urinary potassium would then have to resemble closely that of the intracellular potassium pool. Rouffignac and Guinnebault have, more recently, extended their previous microinjection studies. In an investigation aimed at estimating the permeability properties of various cortical nephron segments they injected both ^{42}K and inulin-^{14}C into proximal and distal tubules as well as into cortical peritubular capillaries (de Rouffignac and Guinnebault, 1966). They confirmed the rapid exchange of peritubularly injected potassium with the cellular pool and provided evidence that radiopotassium exchanges with a cell pool of this cation before gaining access to the tubular lumen.

B. Amphibian Nephron

An evaluation of the relative contribution of the proximal tubular system to urinary potassium excretion in some aquatic amphibia has indicated that this nephron segment plays only a minor role in the modification of the filtered potassium. With one exception (Bott, 1962), several investigators have observed the concentration of potassium to increase slightly but significantly along the proximal tubule of *Necturus* (Khuri *et al.*, 1963; Oken and Solomon, 1963; Watson *et al.*, 1964). As the increase in TF/P potassium ratios was quite similar to that of inulin, no significant net reabsorption of potassium appears to occur at this site. It is therefore not surprising that the amount of potassium entering the distal tubule in aquatic amphibians relative to that filtered should be unchanged. Indeed, the recent experiments by Wiederholt *et al.* (Wiederholt *et al.*, 1969) in *Amphiuma*, an aquatic amphibian, have provided supportive evidence in that early distal potassium/inulin TF/P ratios of unity were found in the presence of widely varying distal tubular transport patterns.

These studies by Wiederholt *et al.* have also made it possible to compare distal tubular potassium transport in an amphibian nephron with that occurring in mammals (Wiederholt *et al.*, 1969). Figure 2 schematically depicts the progression of potassium concentration ratios and of net transport patterns along the distal nephron. In contrast to the mammalian distal tubule, it is apparent that tubular fluid/plasma con-

dog was studied at different levels of sodium excretion. A comparison of sodium and potassium excretion rates, expressed as the ratio of the rate of excretion of the experimental kidney to that of the control kidney, stresses several important facts. If absolute excretion rates of sodium are maintained at a relatively high level with diuretics or infusion of sodium salts, depression of filtration rate by some 35% has no significant effect upon urinary potassium excretion. In sharp contrast are results obtained when no effort is made to maintain such a high rate of sodium excretion. Sodium excretion then drops precipitously to very low levels and is consistently associated with a very marked reduction of potassium excretion as well.

Figure 5 summarizes results from a similar experimental study in the rat, showing the interrelationship between distal tubular sodium and potassium transport when glomerular filtration rate is acutely reduced by partial renal arterial clamping. Data on distal tubular sodium and potassium concentrations are compared before and after the experimental maneuver. Plotted on the abscissa are the sodium and potassium concentrations before clamping. The concentrations in re-collected samples from the same distal tubular site after clamping are plotted on the ordinate. It is apparent that the majority of points fall above the line of equality despite the observation that both the concentration and excretion rates of sodium and potassium in the final urine fell to low levels. The fact that distal sodium and potassium concentra-

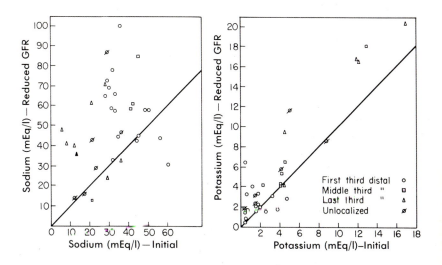

Fig. 5.　Effect of reduced filtration rate on distal tubular sodium and potassium concentration. Landwehr *et al.* (1968) and unpublished observations by the same authors.

steady-state concentration gradients of sodium are allowed to develop in the presence of a poorly reabsorbable nonelectrolyte, the sodium concentration at the early distal tubular level never drops below that of potassium (Giebisch, and Windhager, 1964; Malnic *et al.*, 1966a). Also, estimates indicate that under all tested experimental conditions, most notably those in which a sharply limited urinary sodium excretion rate is associated with a significant drop in potassium excretion, the quantity of sodium reabsorbed along the distal tubule exceeds the amount of potassium simultaneously excreted along the same nephron segment by an order of magnitude (Malnic *et al.*, 1966b). If the behavior of potassium is considered (Fig. 3, lower part) it becomes apparent that it is not dramatically diminished distal secretion but greatly enhanced tubular reabsorption at a site beyond the distal tubule, that is, along the collecting ducts, which is responsible for the very low excretion rates of potassium.

Results from studies in which distal tubular fluid samples are obtained from identical distal locations prior to and after an acute reduction in glomerular filtration rate also permit an evaluation of the main sites along the nephron where sodium and potassium transport are modified. The phenomenon has previously been incisively explored by the clearance approach by Davidson *et al.* and their key findings are depicted in Fig. 4 (Davidson *et al.*, 1958). The effect of acutely reducing filtration rate on the excretion of potassium and sodium in the

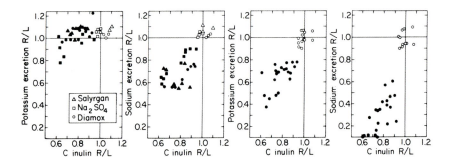

FIG. 4.   Data from experiments during acute reduction of glomerular filtration rate in the dog. *Left*: mass plot of sodium and potassium data from experiments in which a high rate of sodium excretion was maintained. *Right*: mass plot of sodium and potassium data from experiments in which sodium excretion was not maintained at high rates. Open symbols represent control clearance periods, solid symbols periods in which filtration rate in the right kidney was lowered. Data are expressed as the ratio of excretion, or as the ratio of inulin clearances, right to left kidney (R/L). From Davidson *et al.* (1958).

that of arterial plasma from which filtered potassium is derived. The underlying assumption seems justified that in view of the known rapid exchange of ^{42}K with tissue potassium (Wilde, 1962), renal venous potassium contains only a negligible fraction of that potassium which has entered the kidney via the arterial blood supply but is almost completely derived from the potassium present in renal cortical tissue. Evidently, the specific activity of urinary potassium would then have to resemble closely that of the intracellular potassium pool. Rouffignac and Guinnebault have, more recently, extended their previous microinjection studies. In an investigation aimed at estimating the permeability properties of various cortical nephron segments they injected both ^{42}K and inulin-^{14}C into proximal and distal tubules as well as into cortical peritubular capillaries (de Rouffignac and Guinnebault, 1966). They confirmed the rapid exchange of peritubularly injected potassium with the cellular pool and provided evidence that radiopotassium exchanges with a cell pool of this cation before gaining access to the tubular lumen.

B. Amphibian Nephron

An evaluation of the relative contribution of the proximal tubular system to urinary potassium excretion in some aquatic amphibia has indicated that this nephron segment plays only a minor role in the modification of the filtered potassium. With one exception (Bott, 1962), several investigators have observed the concentration of potassium to increase slightly but significantly along the proximal tubule of *Necturus* (Khuri *et al.*, 1963; Oken and Solomon, 1963; Watson *et al.*, 1964). As the increase in TF/P potassium ratios was quite similar to that of inulin, no significant net reabsorption of potassium appears to occur at this site. It is therefore not surprising that the amount of potassium entering the distal tubule in aquatic amphibians relative to that filtered should be unchanged. Indeed, the recent experiments by Wiederholt *et al.* (Wiederholt *et al.*, 1969) in *Amphiuma*, an aquatic amphibian, have provided supportive evidence in that early distal potassium/inulin TF/P ratios of unity were found in the presence of widely varying distal tubular transport patterns.

These studies by Wiederholt *et al.* have also made it possible to compare distal tubular potassium transport in an amphibian nephron with that occurring in mammals (Wiederholt *et al.*, 1969). Figure 2 schematically depicts the progression of potassium concentration ratios and of net transport patterns along the distal nephron. In contrast to the mammalian distal tubule, it is apparent that tubular fluid/plasma con-

titative point of view, play a very significant role. Berliner had already previously argued against the notion that a large fraction of urinary potassium could be derived from secretory activity of papillary collecting duct segments (Jaenike and Berliner, 1960; Berliner, 1961). This view is based on the well-established fact that the renal medulla receives only a small fraction of the renal blood flow whereas the urinary excretion rates of potassium can continue at levels significantly exceeding that of glomerular filtration. Accordingly, it can easily be calculated that the blood supply of the papillary collecting ducts is inadequate to supply but a small fraction of the excreted potassium.

In contrast to the relatively small functional role the collecting duct system appears to play in the process of tubular potassium secretion, it can be shown that significant net reabsorption occurs under those conditions in which the fraction of potassium in the final urine is only a few percent of that filtered. The collecting duct epithelium contributes significantly to the reduction of urinary potassium excretion under conditions of dietary potassium and sodium depletion (Malnic *et al.,* 1964; Malnic *et al.,* 1966b) and under those conditions in which urinary sodium excretion has been drastically curtailed by the acute reduction of the glomerular filtration rate (Landwehr *et al.,* unpublished). However, in passing it may be noted that a survey of available micropuncture data indicates that even under some of those conditions in which significant distal tubular secretion is present (for instance, after bicarbonate infusion (Malnic *et al.,* in preparation) or during chronic potassium adaptation (Wright *et al.,* 1969), the fraction of potassium in the final urine may be significantly less than that at the very end of the distal tubule of superficial cortical nephrons. The functional importance of this phenomenon is presently not clear. Nevertheless, the possibility has to be considered that tubular net movement of potassium occurs in three sequential steps: net reabsorption in the proximal tubule and the loop of Henle, secretion along the distal tubule, and a final step effecting again net reabsorption in the collecting duct system.

Supportive evidence for a cortical secretory origin of urinary potassium has also been derived from studies utilizing radioactive potassium in which the relative specific activities of arterial blood, renal venous blood, and of urine were compared after intravenous injection of this isotope. Morel *et al.* (Morel, 1955; Morel and Guinnebault, 1956; Morel, 1961; Morel et al., 1963), Black *et al.* (Black et al., 1956; Black and Emery, 1957), and Goldman *et al.* (Goldman et al., 1963) have been able to demonstrate convincingly that the specific activity of urinary potassium is quite similar to that of renal venous and tissue potassium but, prior to complete isotope equilibration, significantly different from

distal tubular function under different experimental conditions has become possible by micropuncture techniques, and has permitted an accurate description of the range of distal tubular variation in potassium handling. Figure 1 summarizes distal tubular data in two extreme conditions, emphasizing the great range of transport facilities residing within this epithelial structure (Malnic *et al.*, 1964). On the left, data from a rat on a low dietary intake of potassium are shown. On the right, data are shown from a rat in which, by various manipulations, urinary potassium excretion was maximally stimulated. It is apparent that early distal tubular concentrations of potassium are significantly below plasma levels under both experimental conditions, despite the fact that in the low-potassium animals only some 3% of the filtered potassium is excreted while in the state of maximal kaliuresis urinary excretion rate was equivalent to some 150% of the filtered potassium.

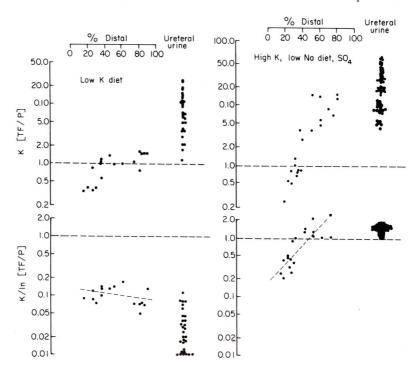

FIG. 1.   Summary of distal tubular potassium and potassium/inulin concentration ratios. *Left*: data from rats kept several weeks on a low-potassium diet. *Right*: data from rats in which potassium excretion was maximally stimulated by pretreatment with a low sodium–high potassium diet and the infusion of potassium sulfate and dichlorophenamide. From Malnic *et al.* (1964).

that, as pointed out before, the fraction of filtered potassium escaping reabsorption by the time fluid has issued from Henle's loop is small and changes little, despite the fact that the urinary excretion rate may vary about one hundredfold (Malnic *et al.*, 1964; Giebisch *et al.*, 1965; Malnic *et al.*, 1966b; Giebisch *et al.*, 1967).

The view of a key role of the distal tubular system in regulating and determining urinary potassium excretion had previously been expressed by Berliner and his associates on the basis of a series of ingenious clearance experiments (Berliner *et al.*, 1950; Berliner, 1961). In these studies, evidence was presented that urinary potassium excretion could, under a variety of experimental conditions, be effectively dissociated from filtration rate and, thus, from the amount of potassium filtered. Since it was thought unlikely that potassium reabsorption was adjusted to match changes in filtration rate such as to maintain a constant excretion rate, it was postulated that the contribution of the filtered potassium to the urinary moiety was negligible and that the relatively constant excretion rate represented secretion at a far distal nephron site. Hence, reabsorptive activity at a more proximally located nephron segment had reduced the tubular potassium content to insignificant levels. Additional electrolyte excretion studies, in which a poorly reabsorbable anion, ferrocyanide, known to be cleared by glomerular filtration alone and, therefore, not secreted, was infused, permitted a balance sheet to be drawn of the amount of potassium minimally secreted (i.e., that potassium excreted in excess of that filtered) and the amounts of bicarbonate, chloride, sulfate, and phosphate present in the final urine. Since only a small fraction of the "minimally secreted" potassium could be covered by anions other than ferrocyanide, it was argued convincingly that none of the anions normally present in extracellular fluid were secreted with potassium. Potassium must therefore have been secreted in exchange for another cation. Sodium ions are the only cations of adequate amount for such exchange.

A distal tubular site of potassium secretion has also emerged from numerous stop-flow studies (Malvin et al., 1958; Pitts et al., 1958; Jaenike and Berliner, 1960; Sullivan et al., 1960; Aukland and Kill, 1961; Sullivan, 1961; Vander, 1961; Walker et al., 1961; Ramsay, 1964). Stop-flow patterns have been obtained in which peak concentrations of potassium representing the accumulation of potassium in far distal portions of the tubule were a uniform finding, and in which these distal secretory peaks were enhanced by those manipulations known to promote kaliuresis.

The extent of distal tubular secretion of potassium is variable and depends critically upon the metabolic situation. A direct evaluation of

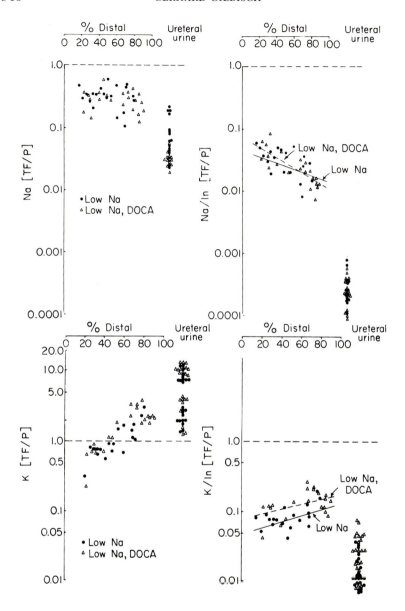

Fig. 3. Summary of distal tubular sodium and sodium/inulin concentration ratios (top) and of potassium and potassium/inulin concentration ratios (bottom). Animals were kept on a low-sodium diet for several weeks prior to the experiment. DOCA-treated animals received DOCA at a dose of 1 mg/kg for 2 weeks. From Malnic et al. (1966).

known in which pretreatment with a low-sodium diet did not appear to blunt the kaliuretic response to acute (Anderson and Laragh, 1958; Malnic *et al.*, 1966b) or chronic potassium loading (Wright *et al.*, 1969). Nevertheless, in view of some of the evidence cited the thesis has been advanced that the secretion of potassium is strongly dependent upon the availability of sodium at the distal tubular site where potassium secretion takes place (Davidson *et al.*, 1958; Berliner, 1961).

Micropuncture studies in which the concentrations of sodium, potassium, and inulin were measured in distal tubular samples under a wide variety of experimental conditions permit a direct assessment of the role of distal sodium reabsorption in the secretory process of potassium. Two experimental situations have been particularly useful to test the thesis of a limited distal tubular sodium supply. The first one is dietary sodium deprivation (Malnic *et al.*, 1966b), and the second one the acute reduction of glomerular filtration rate (Landwehr *et al.*, 1968, Landwehr *et al.*, unpublished; Davidson *et al.*, 1958). These were considered of prime importance because many examples in which a parallel change in sodium and potassium excretion has been noted fall into one of these two categories.

Figure 3 summarizes pertinent data on sodium and potassium transport along the distal tubule in rats maintained over several weeks on a low-sodium diet and excreting only some 25% of the potassium of control rats (Malnic *et al.*, 1966b). It is also well known that such pretreatment completely abolishes the urinary potassium loss normally observed after the administration of mineralocorticoids, particularly DOCA (Howell *et al.*, 1954; Seldin *et al.*, 1956; Relman, and Schwartz, 1962). On the upper left, sodium tubular fluid/plasma concentration ratios are summarized, the corresponding potassium data being shown below. Despite the fact that final urinary sodium concentrations are uniformly low and, importantly, considerably below values found in control animals, early distal tubular sodium concentrations are at least 10 times that of potassium. Thus, as shown on the upper right, the fraction of sodium entering the distal tubules amounts under these conditions to some 4–6% of that filtered. It has been a consistent observation that the most dramatic drop in sodium concentration occurs along the collecting ducts. Under those conditions in which tubular sodium conservation is maximally stimulated it is the activity of the collecting duct epithelium and not that of more proximal tubular segments which renders the final urine almost sodium-free (Malnic *et al.*, 1966b). Accordingly there is a highly significant dissociation of the main nephron site for potassium secretion and that for the establishment of maximal transtubular sodium gradients. Even under the most favorable conditions of stationary microperfusion, a situation in which

TABLE I

SUMMARY OF TUBULAR SEQUENTIAL CONTRIBUTION TO URINARY POTASSIUM
EXCRETION IN THE RAT

Experimental condition	Diet	% Filtered K	
		Early distal tubule	Final urine
Antidiuresis	Control	5	17
Antidiuresis	Low K	10	3
Antidiuresis	Low Na	6	4
Antidiuresis, DOCA	Low Na	7	4
10% Mannitol i.v.	Low Na	15	30
4%NaCl i.v.	Control	8	48
Hypertonic Na_2SO_4 i.v.	Control	7	60
Dichlorphenamide i.v.	Control	10	60
10% Mannitol, isotonic KCl	Low Na	9	91
Hypertonic Na_2SO_4, KCl, dichlorphenamide	High K, Low Na	20	151
5% Mannitol in isotonic NaCl	Control	10	36
Respiratory acidosis (15% CO_2)	Control	7	29
Metabolic acidosis (HCl i.v.)	Control	10	9
Hyperventilation	Control	10	53
Acute KCl load	Control	10	68
Acute bicarbonate load	Control	12	49
Acute bicarbonate load + 15% CO_2	Control	12	38
Acute bicarbonate + KCl load	Control	15	72
Acute bicarbonate load + hyperventilation	Control	17	83
Amiloride	Control	5	5
Acute KCl load	High K	10	87
Acute K_2SO_4 load	High K	30	148

carbonate (Malnic *et al.*, 1968; Malnic *et al.*, in preparation), administration of carbonic anhydrase inhibitors (Malnic *et al.*, 1964), and induction of respiratory alkalosis (Malnic *et al.*, 1968; Malnic *et al.*, in preparation). A high dietary potassium intake enhances the distal secretory response to a standard intravenous potassium load (Wright *et al.*, 1969).

Estimates of distal tubular secretion derived from a comparison of early distal tubular with final urinary potassium moieties, and similar inferences concerning the transport properties of the collecting duct system by comparing late distal with final urinary excretion rates deserve closer scrutiny. Two important limitations of such an approach should be kept in mind. A first limitation is the inability to obtain fluid samples from the very beginning of the distal tubule. Consequently, fractions of filtered potassium present at the very beginning of the distal tubule may be significantly less than that calculated on the basis of potassium and inulin concentration ratios at the earliest distal tu-

Distal transtubular concentration ratios rise only moderately in the former but very steeply in the latter situation, in which distal tubular peak concentrations in excess of 100 mEq/liter are not uncommon.

To evaluate these micropuncture data in terms of transtubular net movement, potassium concentration ratios are divided by the corresponding inulin ratios. The lower graphs provide information on net potassium transfer in the two situations. Continuous, albeit moderate, net reabsorption occurs in animals subjected to dietary potassium deprivation, while massive distal tubular secretion is evident in those animals in which maximal potassium excretion was induced. In these animals, some 90% of the urinary potassium has entered the lumen by way of tubular secretion. Influx of potassium from the peritubular into the luminal fluid across distal tubular epithelium determines the excretory capacity of the kidney. It is of considerable interest to note that the state of maximal urinary potassium secretion is associated with only small modifications of the reabsorptive transport pattern across the proximal tubule and Henle's loop. Despite the fact that considerably more potassium is excreted than filtered, some 80% of the filtered potassium has been reabsorbed by the time fluid enters the distal tubular system.

Comparing the amount of potassium present at the beginning of the distal tubule with that appearing in the final urine gives a rough estimate of the contribution of distal secretion to the moiety of potassium appearing in the final urine. Table I contains data obtained in the rat under a wide variety of experimental conditions. It is apparent that some three-fourths of the urinary potassium can be accounted for by distal tubular secretion under nondiuretic conditions, and the fraction is higher whenever potassium excretion has been stimulated. Notable exceptions, in which no significant addition of potassium can be demonstrated along the distal tubule, are pretreatment with a diet deficient in potassium (Malnic et al., 1964), administration of the potassium-sparing diuretic Amiloride (Merck 870) (Duarte et al., 1969), or induction of metabolic acidosis (Malnic et al., 1968; Malnic et al., in preparation). Potassium secretion along the distal convolution is also notably compromised in adrenalectomized rats (Hierholzer et al., 1965; Wiederholt and Hierholzer, 1967; Cortney, 1969).

Compared to nondiuretic conditions, potassium secretion is enhanced in the mammalian distal tubule under the following conditions: intravenous loading with hypertonic (Malnic et al., 1966b) or isotonic sodium chloride (Landwehr et al., unpublished), loading with hypertonic sodium sulfate (Malnic et al., 1966b), iso- or hypertonic potassium chloride (Malnic et al., 1966b; Malnic et al., in preparation), sodium bi-

contribution of either the collecting ducts or the distal tubular system to a given excretory pattern in the final urine. Caution is indicated for evaluating either distal tubular or collecting duct contributions to a given excretory pattern, particularly in species with a heterogenous nephron population (Lechene *et al.*, 1966; de Rouffignac and Morel, 1967). Even in species with homogeneous nephron populations such an approach may not be without hazard since only deep cortical nephrons extend to the very tip of the renal papilla, while superficial cortical nephrons do not. Different functional properties of various nephron groups may thus still exist.

In contrast to the distal tubule's role in the overall renal transport of potassium, which is fairly well understood, the precise contribution of the collecting ducts to urinary potassium excretion is not well defined. Although the relative importance of reabsorptive and secretory activity of the collecting ducts can be studied most directly either by microcatheterization or transmural puncture, few such studies are available. Most reports have been based on comparisons of distal fluid with final urine. On the other hand, distal tubular data are completely lacking in those herbivorous species in which a rather extensive evaluation of the tubular transport function of isolated collecting ducts *in vitro* has recently become available.*

Experimental evidence in rodents, dogs, and monkeys indicates that a significant contribution of the collecting ducts to potassium secretion occurs only rarely (Bennett *et al.*, 1967; Bennett *et al.*, 1968; Malnic *et al.*, 1964; Malnic *et al.*, 1966 b), although such evaluations are based only on a comparison of late distal with final urine excretion rates. Similarly, direct microcatheterization of single collecting ducts in the golden hamster has failed to uncover significant secretion under conditions characterized by normal excretion rates (Hilger *et al.*, 1958). Even under conditions of net renal potassium secretion (urinary potassium clearances in excess of simultaneously measured inulin clearances) at best only a moderate degree of potassium secretion could be demonstrated along the terminal collecting duct segment (Hierholzer, 1961). Although some suggestive evidence for potassium secretion along the collecting ducts is available it is doubtful whether it could, from a quan-

---

*Diezi *et al.* have very recently investigated the role of the terminal collecting ducts in determining urinary potassium excretion (Diezi *et al.*, 1969). In essence, they confirmed the conclusions arrived at by the comparison of late distal and urinary fractional excretion rates. The terminal collecting ducts abstract potassium ions from the tubular fluid in the state of dietary potassium and sodium deprivation, and a variable secretory component could be observed in strongly kaluretic states. No significant net transfer of potassium could be observed in animals on a normal potassium intake.

bular sites available for puncture. Extrapolation to zero length of the regression lines relating potassium TF/P ratios or potassium/inulin TF/P ratios to distal tubular length is open to question. As a consequence of the inability to obtain accurate estimates of the amount of potassium present either at the level of the ascending limb of Henle's loop or at the very beginning of the distal tubule, the fraction calculated to derive from distal tubular secretion represents a minimum value. Nevertheless, the view of Berliner (Berliner, 1961) of a predominantly secretory origin of urinary potassium can be considered firmly supported by direct experimental evidence under all those conditions in which significant distal tubular potassium secretion takes place. On the other hand, it should be clearly recognized that it is presently not possible to decide whether the small fraction of potassium present at the beginning of the distal tubule under conditions in which distal tubular secretion is either drastically reduced or absent, such as in the potassium-depleted animal (Malnic *et al.*, 1964), in metabolic or respiratory acidosis (Malnic *et al.*, 1968; Malnic *et al.*, in preparation), or after Amiloride (Duarte *et al.*, 1969), is of secretory origin or whether it represents potassium which has escaped reabsorption along more proximally located nephron segments. It is more likely that the latter alternative is the correct one. If secretory in origin, it would be necessary to postulate significant secretory activity at the level of either the ascending limb of Henle's loop or the first fifth of the distal tubule at a time when potassium secretion is absent along that part of the distal tubule which is available to micropuncture. Since the ascending limb of Henle's loop can be shown to be a nephron site of avid potassium reabsorption even under conditions of maximal distal tubular secretion of potassium, it appears extremely remote that a condition of complete lack of distal tubular secretory activity could be associated with secretory activity at more proximally located nephron sites.

A second limitation in the analysis of segmental contributions to urinary potassium excretion concerns uncertainties with regard to the relative contributions of superficial nephron activity to total excretory kidney function. This problem has recently received considerable attention. Evidence has been obtained indicating that in the rodent at least, there may be very significant differences in the rate of filtrate formation between superficial and deep, juxtamedullary nephron populations (Horster and Thurau, 1968). At present, virtually nothing is known about the potassium transport properties of deep nephrons and, conceivably, the potassium transport properties of juxtamedullary nephrons may be different from those of superficial nephrons. Accordingly, uncertainties arise when inferences are made concerning the

tions increase after reduction of filtration rate is most probably related to the prolonged passage time through the loop of Henle and more complete water equilibration, as evidenced by the increased inulin concentration ratios observed in distal tubular samples after renal arterial clamping. Additional calculations indicate, again, that the fraction of sodium reabsorbed greatly exceeds that of potassium secreted. Again, a reduced distal tubular supply of sodium is clearly not responsible for the significant suppression of potassium excretion. Rather it appears that a low sodium concentration in the final urine, achieved by more complete tubular reabsorption along the collecting ducts, leads to the enhanced reabsorption of potassium at the very same nephron level. It is the collecting duct epithelium and not the distal tubule which emerges as the main site where the most important reduction in urinary potassium output is achieved under these conditions.

The considerations cited argue convincingly against the notion that in those species in which the distal tubular epithelium is the main site of potassium secretion, the delivery of increased amounts of sodium into the distal tubule provides additional sodium ions for exchange, thereby stimulating potassium secretion. Clearly, experimental evidence proves that the amount of sodium reaching the site of distal tubular potassium secretion does not vary dramatically enough to become a rate-limiting factor in potassium secretion. Such a view would clearly demand that nephron sites proximal to the secretory site of potassium ions importantly modify tubular sodium concentration and, for instance, under conditions of maximal sodium conservation reduce the distal tubular sodium supply so as to restrict exchange for potassium. Such is not the case since it is the collecting duct, a site beyond the distal tubule, which exerts such a regulatory function.

If the tubular reabsorption of sodium and secretion of potassium are measured in micropuncture studies it can also be shown that these two operations are frequently not reciprocally related and that they can be markedly dissociated. The following examples are illustrative: (1) the infusion of sodium salts of poorly reabsorbable anions such·as sodium sulfate, during which sodium reabsorption along the distal tubule is greatly reduced and potassium secretion maximally stimulated (Malnic et al., 1966b); (2) the administration of cardiac glycosides both in rats pretreated with a low-potassium diet (Duarte et al., 1969) and in the doubly perfused *Amphiuma* kidney (Wiederholt et al., 1969), which leads to increased intratubular potassium concentration and diminished reabsorption of sodium; (3) the effect of actinomycin D in adrenalectomized, aldosterone-treated rats (Wiederholt, 1968) which results in blockage of the aldosterone effect upon sodium transport while potassium secretion is unaffected by the inhibitor. Absence of a fixed tubular exchange ratio between these two cationic species is also observed in the doubly perfused frog kidney, in which the effects on urinary potassium excretion of a stepwise reduction of sodium concentration in the aortic perfusion fluid were studied (Vogel and Tervooren, 1964) While changes in sodium excretion undoubtedly exert a significant effect upon the tubular transport pattern of potassium, experimental evidence does not appear to confirm the notion that sodium ions are required for a tightly coupled carrier-mediated exchange. Accordingly, it is inappropriate to consider that an increased distal tubular sodium load provides more sodium for exchange and thereby stimulates potassium secretion. Alternative modes by which sodium ions may affect potassium transport will be discussed subsequently.

While the relationship between tubular transport of sodium and potassium in the distal tubule can be assessed rather directly, such has not yet been done with respect to the collecting ducts. Most information on the functional properties of this nephron segment have been obtained by comparison of late distal concentration ratios and excretion rates with similar parameters in the final urine. It should be clearly kept in mind that at this very terminal nephron segment the concentration of sodium may reach very low levels and that experimental evidence obtained so far does not exclude a coupled cation-exchange mechanism. Alternatively, in the presence of a low anion permeability and a low sodium load, maintenance of electroneutrality demands exchange between cellular potassium and luminal sodium whenever tubular potassium secretion takes place. This situation differs from carrier-mediated exchange. However, some experimental evidence obtained in perfusion studies *in vitro* on single collecting ducts of the rabbit are consistent with coupled sodium for potassium exchange and the presence of active potassium secretion (Grantham *et al.*, 1970). The functional importance of such a process is presently not clear, but it seems probable that its quantitative role in the overall secretory process of potassium and, thus, in urinary potassium excretion is relatively small.

V. Role of Adrenal Mineralocorticoids in Renal Tubular Potassium Transport

In addition to their marked effects on cellular electrolyte transport of sodium and potassium, mineralocorticoids also modify the renal tubular transport of potassium. States of adrenal insufficiency are charac-

terized by potassium retention and low excretion rates while administration of mineralocorticoids, after a significant time delay, typically
promotes urinary loss of potassium. The stimulation of urinary potassium excretion is frequently associated with increased tubular reabsorption of sodium, and as discussed previously, an adequate dietary sodium supply coupled with a normal urinary excretion rate is necessary
to demonstrate the kaliuretic effects of mineralocorticoids. A close
survey of the available experimental evidence indicates that sodium
and potassium effects can frequently be dissociated (Hierholzer and
Ebel, 1968). In the first place, no fixed relationship exists between the
ability of a variety of mineralocorticoids to effect kaliuresis and sodium
retention. Thus, normalization of sodium balance in adrenalectomized
animals may be produced by rather small amounts of aldosterone
which do not alter urinary potassium excretion rates, while larger doses
do induce the kaliuretic effect (Swingle et al., 1954). On the other hand,
in dogs with intact adrenals a significant kaliuretic effect can be observed after injection of aldosterone into one renal artery without modifying urinary sodium excretion (Barger et al., 1958). A comparative
study of the effects of different steriods in unanesthetized rats provides
evidence that different steriods can be similarly potent in inducing sodium retention but have significantly different effects with respect to
their kaliuretic effects (Fimognari et al., 1967). In a recent study (Fimognari et al., 1967) increasing dietary potassium intake was shown to
modify markedly the effects of aldosterone. In rats on a stock diet, a
significant decrease in sodium excretion was seen after aldosterone
administration, not accompanied by significant kaliuresis. On the other
hand, a highly dramatic increase in urinary potassium excretion was
regularly observed in animals pretreated with a low-potassium diet.
Another line of evidence to support the thesis that sodium and potassium excretion are not interrelated in a direct, stoichiometric relationship and that the effects of aldosterone on potassium transport are not
intimately coupled to tubular sodium transport derives from an analysis of the mineralocorticoid "escape" phenomenon: the observation
that continuous administration of mineralocorticoids promotes a sustained urinary loss of potassium (provided that such losses are replaced
in the diet) although the kidney "escapes" from the sodium-retaining
effect of the steroid (August and Nelson, 1964). Finally, several investigators have demonstrated unequivocally that Actinomycin D, a potent
agent known to inhibit the incorporation of amino acids into RNA (Fimognari et al., 1967), significantly inhibits the antinatriuretic response
of aldosterone in adrenalectomized rats but is entirely without action

on its kaliuretic effect (Williamson, 1963; Fimognari *et al.*, 1967; Wiederholt, 1968). This dissociation of aldosterone effects occurs at the distal tubular level (Wiederholt, 1968; Hierholzer and Ebel, 1968).

Studies on single tubules provide direct evidence that the main site of action of mineralocorticoids is localized at the distal tubular level. No major effect can be demonstrated on fractional potassium reabsorption along the proximal tubule (Wiederholt and Wiederholt, 1968; Cortney, 1969), although the absolute amounts reabsorbed are frequently reduced as filtration rate is diminished in adrenal insufficiency. However, the effects of adrenalectomy are most clear-cut at the distal tubular level, particularly its second half. While potassium concentration normally increases significantly along this part of the nephron, adrenalectomy reduces this ability (Hierholzer *et al.*, 1965; Stolte *et al.*, unpublished). Stationary microperfusion studies confirm that it is the distal tubular epithelium where effects of aldosterone upon potassium transport can be shown most precisely. The concentration gradient of potassium ions across the later part of the distal tubular epithelium is sharply reduced in adrenalectomy (Hierholzer *et al.*, 1965). Figure 6 summarizes pertinent results. In addition, Cortney and others observed that net secretion of potassium along the distal tubule and the col-

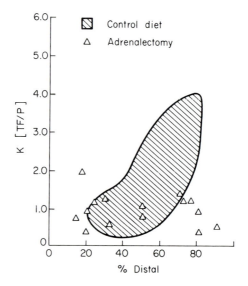

FIG. 6. Summary of transtubular potassium concentration ratios observed in stationary microperfusion experiments of distal tubules in the rat. Contour diagram indicates range of values in control animals. From Hierholzer *et al.* (1965).

lecting ducts is reduced in the adrenalectomized rat (Cortney, 1969; Stolte *et al.*, unpublished). Thus, it appears that an adequate level of circulating adrenal mineralocorticoids is necessary for maintainance of normal secretory capacity of potassium ions along the terminal nephron segment.

VI. Role of Hydrogen Ions in Renal Tubular Potassium Transport

It is a frequent observation that there exists an important reciprocal relationship between urinary acidity and potassium excretion. Thus, potassium excretion rises when the urine has been made alkaline by the administration of sodium bicarbonate (Burnett and Burrows, 1950; Kruhoffer, 1950; Franglen *et al.*, 1963; Roberts *et al.*, 1953; Toussaint and Vereerstraeten, 1962) or administration of the carbonic anhydrase inhibitor acetazolamide (Berliner *et al.*, 1951). Likewise, respiratory alkalosis accelerates potassium excretion (McCance and Widdowson, 1936; Stanbury and Thomson, 1952). Conversely, respiratory acidosis following carbon dioxide inhalation is frequently associated with a decrease in urinary potassium excretion (Denton *et al.*, 1952; Barker *et al.*, 1957) and infusions of acid into the portal circulation of the avian kidney are followed by a rapid and significant fall in potassium excretion (Orloff and Davidson, 1959). It has also long been known that administration of potassium salts raises urine pH (Loeb *et al.*, 1932; Winkler and Smith, 1942; Wolf, 1947; Berliner *et al.*, 1950; Fuller *et al.*, 1955; Orloff and Davidson, 1959; Rector *et al.*, 1962), while depletion of the body stores of potassium enhances the reabsorption of bicarbonate and the excretion of ammonia and titrable acid (Roberts *et al.*, 1953; Fuller *et al.*, 1955; Giebisch *et al.*, 1955b). A reciprocal relationship has also been observed between potassium and hydrogen ion excretion in the diurnal excretory rhythm (Mills and Stanbury, 1954). These studies have been taken to suggest the possibility of competition of these two ion species for a common secretory mechanism (Berliner, 1952; Berliner, 1961).

The role of potassium in determining hydrogen ion secretion is discussed in considerable detail in Chapter 4 of this volume (Rector). It suffices to mention at this point that there exists clear-cut evidence that hypokalemia stimulates hydrogen ion secretion in the proximal convoluted tubule (Rector *et al.*, 1964a), a site of extensive potassium reabsorption. Apparently, the renal effects of changes in potassium metabolism are not limited to those distal portions of the nephrons where potassium ions are secreted. Rector has convincingly argued that the

observation of accelerated hydrogen ion secretion in the proximal tubule of potassium-depleted animals is strong evidence that potassium
ions also influence hydrogen secretion by some mechanism other than
competition for a secretory pathway. It is most likely that potassium
depletion lowers intracellular pH and thereby stimulates increased
proximal hydrogen excretion (Rector *et al.*, 1964a; Rector, Chapter 4 of
this volume).

Since the distal tubular epithelium is the main site of potassium secretion, recent interest has focused on this as the most likely site to
demonstrate the profound effects of primary acid–base disturbances on
tubular potassium transport. To gain insight into the relationship between intratubular pH, rate of tubular bicarbonate reabsorption and
potassium transfer at the distal tubular level, Malnic *et al.* have carried
out a series of micropunctures in rats in which these parameters were
measured simultaneously (Malnic *et al.*, 1968; Malnic *et al.*, in preparation). Figure 7 summarizes estimates of the extent of distal tubular po-

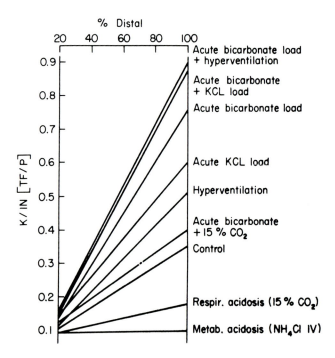

Fig. 7. Summary of distal tubular potassium secretion, plotted as a function of
tubular length during control conditions and during various acid–base disturbances.
From Malnic *et al.* (unpublished observations), and Giebisch and Malnic (1970).

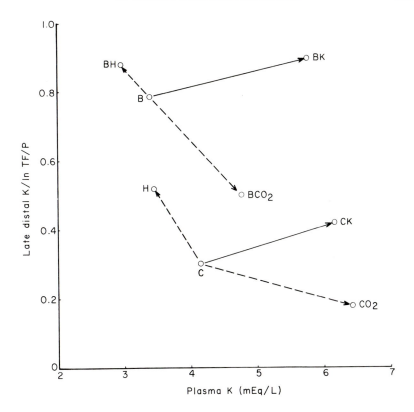

F IG. 8. Summary of distal tubular potassium secretion, plotted as a function of plasma potassium level, during control and during various acid–base disturbances. C denotes control conditions (5% mannitol in 0.8% NaCl); CO_2, 15% CO_2; H, mechanical hyperventilation, CK, acute i.v. KCl loading; B, bicarbonate loading; BCO_2, bicarbonate loading + 15% CO_2; BH, bicarbonate loading plus mechanical hyperventilation; BK, bicarbonate loading + i.v. KCl loading. From Giebisch and Malnic (1969).

tassium secretion in a variety of experimental conditions. It is quite apparent that tubular activity prior to the distal tubule does not significantly modify urinary excretion rate since there is relatively little variation in the fraction of potassium entering the distal tubule under the different conditions. Furthermore, it is clear that, again, the distal tubular epithelium emerges as the main site where changes in the urinary excretion rate for potassium are effected by modulation of distal tubular secretion rate. Figure 8 relates distal tubular transport patterns of potassium to plasma potassium levels. Since the fraction of potassium entering the distal tubule varies little, late tubular potassium/inulin concentration ratios are a fairly accurate reflection of relative secretion.

Three experimental conditions were superimposed upon the control state, characterized by a mean late distal tubular potassium/inulin TF/P ratio of 0.35 at a plasma potassium level of 4.0 mEq/liter. Both respiratory and metabolic acidosis depress distal secretory activity despite the fact that they induce a sharp rise in plasma potassium. The latter is an extrarenal response due to the shift of potassium from tissue upon acidification of the body fluids (Giebisch et al., 1955a; Swan et al., 1955). It is also apparent that acute hyperventilation resulting in respiratory alkalosis increases distal tubular secretion of potassium associated with a slight but significant fall in plasma potassium. Intravenous loading with sodium bicarbonate also induces a powerfully enhanced distal secretion in the presence of a drop in plasma potassium. Changes in pCO_2, superimposed on a bicarbonate load, have effects qualitatively similar to those in animals with normal bicarbonate levels. Breathing 15% CO_2 drops distal secretion while further alkalinization by mechanical hyperventilation pushes the secretory activity of the distal tubules to an even higher level than that achieved by bicarbonate infusion alone.

It is also of interest to compare the effect of an acute intravenous potassium load in normal and alkalotic animals. Although this maneuver leads to a rise in plasma potassium level and an increase in distal secretion in both conditions, the increment in absolute secretion rate achieved in alkalotic animals is significantly larger than that in the normal animals (Fig. 8). Some evidence indicates that extracellular alkalinization leads to intracellular alkalosis and an increase in intracellular potassium (Giebisch et al., 1955; Swan et al., 1955; Brown and Goott, 1963; Cohen et al., 1967; Struyvenberg et al., 1968). The latter fact is also supported by the finding of a decrease in plasma potassium levels subsequent to extracellular alkalinization. If these results can be extended to the distal tubule, the bicarbonate effect, i.e., stimulation of distal tubular potassium secretion, could be mediated by an increase in intracellular potassium levels. If it is assumed that the intracellular potassium content is elevated in bicarbonate-loaded animals the enhanced secretory response subsequent to potassium administration in bicarbonate-loaded rats may mean that the elevation of extracellular potassium levels is now even more effective in further increasing intracellular potassium stores. As a consequence, it would be also more effective in stimulating distal tubular potassium secretion.

Recently it has become possible to evaluate the extent of distal tubular potassium secretion as a function of tubular *in situ* pH (Malnic *et al.*, 1968; Malnic *et al.*, in preparation). Utilizing an antimony electrode system (Vieira and Malnic, 1968) pH is measured *in situ* and *in vitro* at the same tubular site from which tubular fluid has been withdrawn for the analysis of potassium and inulin. It has been found that an increase in intratubular pH is generally associated with increasing potassium secretion rates. A second interesting observation is made that, at almost identical intratubular pH values, elevation of pCO_2 depresses distal potassium secretion (Malnic et al., 1968; Malnic et al., in preparation). Similarity of intratubular in situ pH at different pCO_2 levels can be achieved by the balance of increased bicarbonate load and elevated tubular reabsorption rate of bicarbonate. In respiratory acidosis, filtered bicarbonate is known to be increased. Increased bicarbonate reabsorption is also a well known renal response to elevation of arterial pCO_2 (Dorman et al., 1954). It is reasonable to infer that intracellular pH of distal tubule cells was more acid when animals were breathing high levels of CO_2. The point of particular importance is that this situation, i.e., depression of tubular potassium secretion at identical intratubular pH but differing intracellular pH, permits a rather direct assessment of the role of intracellular pH changes in regulating potassium transport. Intracellular acidosis, independently of intratubular pH, diminishes distal tubular potassium secretion.

Difficulties arise when the thesis of a reciprocal relationship between potassium and hydrogen ion secretion is evaluated by a direct comparison of distal tubular bicarbonate reabsorption and potassium secretion (Giebisch and Malnic, 1970; Malnic et al., in preparation). By comparing the absolute rates of potassium and hydrogen ion secretion (the latter estimated from the calculated rate of bicarbonate reabsorption), these two transport processes can be evaluated in a number of acid-base disturbances and compared to those of animals in a normal acid-base status. Such an analysis indicates that a consistent reciprocal relationship between rates of potassium and hydrogen ion secretion does not hold. Most notably, subsequent to the infusion of sodium bicarbonate, distal tubular potassium secretion is markedly elevated at a time of increased bicarbonate reabsorption. On the other hand, potassium and hydrogen ion secretion are reduced in chronic metabolic acidosis. Limitations of this approach should be clearly kept in mind. First, it is assumed that tubular bicarbonate reabsorption truly reflects distal tubular hydrogen ion secretion. Although most available evidence favors this view (Rector, Chapter 4 of this volume), it is not unequivocally proven at the high distal tubular bicarbonate levels which obtain in situations like bicarbonate infusion, hyperventilation, or the superposition of bicarbonate loading on respiratory alkalosis. Under such conditions, a favorable gradient for diffusion of bicarbonate ions from lumen to peritubular fluid exists (high tubular bicarbonate levels, significant intratubular electronegativity). In view of the demonstrated finite permeability of proximal tubules to bicarbonate (Bank and Aynedjian, 1967) an uncertainty is introduced when hydrogen ion secretion rate is calculated from bicarbonate reabsorption. An overestimate of actual hydrogen ion secretion would obtain. Nevertheless, it is almost certain that distal tubular hydrogen ion secretion is enhanced, and not reduced during bicarbonate loading and the excretion of an alkaline urine. This is a consequence of continued hydrogen secretion as evidenced by a significant disequilibrium pH (Rector, Chapter 4 of this volume; Rector *et al.*, 1965; Vieira and Malnic, 1968) and the presence of much larger quantities of proton acceptors (bicarbonate buffer) in the lumen. Second, the rate of hydrogen ion secretion could be underestimated when based on the rate of distal tubular bicarbonate reabsorption alone when the bicarbonate concentration is low and other intratubular buffers such as phosphate or ammonia may act as proton receptors. Both processes must be small: net secretion of ammonia along the distal tubule is small at best even in acidotic rats (Glabman *et al.*, 1963; Hayes *et al.*, 1964) and the absence of significant intratubular pH changes along the distal tubule excludes sizable titration of nonbicarbonate buffers (Vieira and Malnic, 1968; Rector *et al.*, 1965). It seems that the magnitude of ionic bicarbonate reabsorption and non-bicarbonate-related hydrogen ion secretion is probably too small to seriously invalidate the conclusions based on bicarbonate reabsorption, namely, relative independence of distal H^+ and K^+ transport. It seems more attractive to assume that alkalinization increases, and acidification lowers intracellular potassium concentration, or the size of a distal intracellular potassium transport pool, and directly affects the electrochemical potential gradient, and thus, the driving force of potassium ions across the luminal cell boundary. There is presently no direct evidence in support of a consistent, tight, reciprocal coupling between distal tubular hydrogen ion and potassium transport, such as would be expected if these ion species were to compete for a common carrier of limited supply at the luminal cell membrane.

VII. The Development of Potassium Tolerance

Animals challenged with a large dose of potassium are protected against the lethal effects of hyperkalemia by extrarenal and renal mechanisms. There develops tolerance with the repeated administration of potassium salts. In 1947 Thatcher *et al.* (Thatcher and Radike, 1947) found that rats could be made resistant to lethal doses of potassium by prior repeated potassium administration. The development of tolerance was associated with both a more rapid excretion of the exogenous potassium load as well as a smaller increase in the plasma concentration of potassium. In the dog, the phenomenon was studied by Berliner *et al.*, who confirmed the basic finding of enhanced renal excretion, demonstrated the occurrence of net potassium secretion by clearance methods in this situation, and suggested that the renal response was not mediated by increased mineralocorticoid activity (Berliner *et al.*, 1950).

More recently, Alexander and Levinsky have focused their attention on the extrarenal aspects of the phenomenon (Alexander and Levinsky, 1968). Despite prior nephrectomy, rats fed a high-potassium diet maintained lower plasma potassium levels for at least 2 hours after an acute potassium challenge. From their studies it appears that, at least in the development of the short-term extrarenal potassium tolerance, the adrenal cortex plays an important role. Not only did prior adrenalectomy abolish adaptation, but both rats fed a low-sodium diet as a stimulus to aldosterone secretion as well as adrenalectomized rats given large amounts of desoxycorticosterone, developed adaptation to potassium loading. Additional experiments were highly suggestive that this adaptation depends on a chronic increase in aldosterone secretion.

Wright *et al.* have recently undertaken a micropuncture study of the renal aspects of potassium adaptation (Wright *et al.*, 1969). In a distal tubular re-collection study in which the response to a standard intravenous potassium load was compared in animals with normal and elevated dietary potassium intake, clear evidence was obtained that the distal tubular epithelium is the nephron site responding with a significantly enhanced secretory response. (Figure 9 gives a representative example.) Confirmatory evidence was also obtained that the plasma levels of potassium remain markedly lower in the adapted animals. Renal adaption is small within the first week of potassium feeding but increases progressively. It is of interest that a high dietary potassium intake promotes urinary sodium loss, as evidenced by the significantly lower sodium excretion which develops compensatorily in animals kept on a high potassium intake for several weeks. This markedly accentuates the kaliuretic response in such animals when the potassium load is given as the sulfate salt, presumably by increasing distal intratubular electronegativity. Potassium-adapted animals receiving an intravenous potassium sulfate load develop the steepest known distal transtubular concentration gradients of potassium, reaching values in excess of 100 meq/liter. It was not possible to mimic the distal tubular response to potassium loading by dietary sodium deprivation, an observation which tends to minimize the role of adrenal stimulation in the development of the chronic renal phase of adaptation.

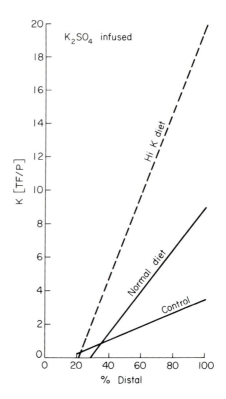

FIG. 9.   Response of distal tubular epithelium of rat kidneys to an intravenous potassium sulfate load (0.1 mM/min · kg). Data from a re-collection study in which fluid was collected from the same distal tubular site prior to and after an acute potassium load. Control TF/P potassium ratios were similar in animals kept on a normal or high potassium diet. It is apparent that animals kept on a high dietary potassium intake (20 mEq/day) respond with a larger increase of distal TF/P potassium ratios subsequent to a potassium sulfate challenge. From Wright *et al.* (1969).

VIII. The Effects of Some Drugs on Renal Tubular Potassium Transport

Many but not all diuretics increase the urinary excretion of potassium. It appears that most of the kaliuretic agents fall into one of three classes: (1) those which are effective in promoting urinary water and sodium loss; (2) those which inhibit carbonic anhydrase and, thus, alkalinize the urine; and (3) those which exhibit pH-independent effects upon the distal tubular epithelium promoting specifically the establishment of steeper potassium concentration gradients, resulting in the excretion of urine rich in potassium. The action of drugs upon potassium transport of the first type appears to be nonspecific, since it has been observed that there is no difference in urinary potassium loss when, at similar excretion rates of sodium, the effects of these diuretics are compared with those achieved by sodium chloride infusions alone (Suki *et al.*, 1965).

Some diuretics suppress urinary potassium loss. For instance, mercurial diuretics can be shown to be specific inhibitors of potassium secretion, particularly when the latter has been stimulated (Berliner *et al.*, 1950; Mudge *et al.*, 1950; Berliner *et al.*, 1951). These effects can be dissociated from the diuretic effects of these drugs since, in the dog, amounts too small to promote diuresis and sodium loss effectively depress potassium excretion (McBride *et al.*, 1958). Another group of drugs, represented by agents such as triampterene (Baba *et al.*, 1964) and amiloride (Merck 870) (Baer *et al.*, 1967; Bull and Laragh, 1968) specifically depress potassium excretion at a time when sodium excretion is moderately stimulated. Finally, spironolactones affect renal tubular potassium secretion by their anti-aldosterone effect (Liddle, 1966).

The kaliuretic effect of many natriuretic drugs, most notably mercurials, furosemide, ethacrinic acid, chlorothiazide, and hydrochlorothiazide has frequently been interpreted to be due to depression of sodium reabsorption proximal to the site of potassium secretion, thereby accelerating sodium–potassium exchange in the distal tubule by providing a more adequate supply for greater utilization of secretory capacity. However, in view of the fact that the normal supply of sodium ions to the main site of potassium secretion, i.e., the distal tubule, is never rate-limiting to begin with, this restricted supply hypothesis is clearly untenable. An alternative explanation for at least part of the kaliuretic effect of such drugs is the following: There is good evidence that the distal tubular secretory system for potassium ions frequently, but not always, behaves as a flow-limited system. Stated differently, a given transtubular concentration gradient will be maintained irrespective of distal volume flow rate. An inescapable consequence of this fact is that distal secretion rate varies directly with flow rate. Supportive evidence for this thesis can be found along three lines of argument. First, an extensive study indicates the absence of significant differences between free-flow and steady-state concentration gradients across the distal tubular epithelium under a wide variety of experimental conditions, underscoring the point that variations in flow rate have a minimal effect upon the generation of transtubular concentration gradients (Malnic *et al.*, 1966a; Giebisch *et al.*, 1967). Secondly, a direct comparison of distal transepithelial concentration gradients of potassium at different volume flow rates achieved by either graded furosemide administration (Duarte *et al.*, 1969) or by graded urea or saline diureses

(Khuri et al., unpublished) indicates that these gradients were unaffected by changes in fluid delivery into the distal tubular system. Hence, the absolute and relative urinary excretion rate of potassium varied inversely with the extent of fluid reabsorption along the terminal nephron. For instance, after furosemide net secretion of potassium obtains at the most brisk diuresis, net reabsorption occurs when the administration of smaller amounts of furosemide promotes only a moderate urinary fluid loss (Duarte *et al.*, 1969). Confirming the results of Suki *et al.* (Suki *et al.*, 1965), there was, at comparable excretion rates of sodium, no significant difference in potassium excretion between furosemide-treated and saline-infused animals.* As a final point in support of the thesis that flow rate per se is an important factor determining potassium secretion in the distal tubule is the recent observation by Morgan and Berliner (Morgan and Berliner, 1969). In a series of distal tubular perfusion experiments *in vivo* evidence was obtained that, at a given tubular site, the concentration of potassium was independent of changes in flow rates. Again, distal secretion rate of potassium varied directly with flow rate.

The capacity of a number of drugs, most notably azetazolamide and, to a smaller extent, chlorothiazide to enhance potassium secretion is probably related to increased delivery of fluid into the distal tubules due to decrease in fluid reabsorption at more proximal nephron sites (Dirks and Seely, 1969) and to its alkalinizing effect on distal tubular fluid (Vieira and Malnic, 1968). Both effects are important since derivatives of chlorothiazide which retain their diuretic activity but have lost their carboanhydrase-inhibiting activity are significantly less effective in promoting urinary potassium loss (Farley and Orloff, 1964).

Another group of drugs affecting the renal transport of potassium are the cardiac glycosides. Although these agents are very powerful inhibitors of sodium extrusion and potassium uptake in many cell systems, as well as effective inhibitors of oriented transport in several *in vitro* systems (Ussing, 1960), their renal effects upon potassium transfer are variable and depend, to a considerable extent, upon the experimental situation and the species investigated. The rat is relatively insensitive to various digitalis glycosides and even small effects on potassium excretion necessitate either intraarterial injection into the renal artery (Ramsay and Sachs, 1967) or sensitization by pretreatment with a potas-

---

*However, early distal potassium TF/P and potassium/inulin TF/P ratios have been found to be elevated after furosemide administration (Duarte *et al.* 1969; Morgan *et al.* 1970). This indicates that this diuretic agent inhibits fluid and potassium reabsorption along the ascending limb of Henle's loop. This effect adds to the kaluresis achieved solely by increased distal tubular volume flow.

sium-deficient diet (Duarte *et al.*, 1969). Excretion rates of potassium are either unaffected by strophantidin or depressed in animals receiving an exogenous potassium load (Orloff and Burg, 1960; Cade *et al.*, 1961). In the dog, and the chicken, potassium loading also protects the kidney against the glycoside effect on sodium transport (Orloff and Burg, 1960; Cade *et al.*, 1961). In the perfused kidney, on the other hand, such a protective effect could not be observed consistently (Rosenfeld et al., 1969). In the perfused amphibian kidney, the addition of relatively large amounts of ouabain depresses potassium reabsorption which normally occurs along the distal tubule (Vogel and Suchheim, 1962; Vogel *et al.*, 1963; Vogel and Tervooren, 1965; Wiederholt *et al.*, 1969). The conclusion appears justified that cardiac glycosides are most effective in modifying tubular potassium transfer when potassium reabsorption is stimulated along the distal tubular epithelium. The inhibition of strophantidin-diuresis and strophantidin-induced effects on renal potassium transfer by exogenous potassium loading is quite consistent with similar antagonistic effects in many membrane transport systems (Ussing, 1960). It should be noted that the effects of cardiac glycosides upon renal tubular potassium transport are associated with widely varying excretion patterns of sodium: on the one hand, significant sodium loss may occur with or without kaliuresis (Orloff and Burg, 1960), and, on the other hand, enhanced urinary potassium loss may be accompanied by sodium diuresis or may occur in the absence of a change in sodium excretion (Ramsay and Sachs, 1967). Increase in distal tubular potassium concentration subsequent to the administration of ouabain can be shown to occur at a time when the sodium concentration along this nephron segment is elevated and net reabsorption either unchanged or decreased (Duarte *et al.*, 1969; Wiederholt *et al.*, 1969). Thus, evidence for distal tubular reciprocal coupling between sodium and potassium transport cannot be obtained in glycoside-treated animals.

Recently a number of potassium-sparing natriuretic agents have become available and their ability to promote potassium retention makes them useful adjuncts in the treatment of various edematous states. These agents, being only mild diuretics, depress urinary potassium and hydrogen ion secretion and promote sodium bicarbonate loss. Hyperkalemia is a frequent occurrence (Bull and Laragh, 1968). Interpretations derived both from stop-flow (Baer *et al.*, 1967) and clearance experiments (Baba et al., 1964) have implied a direct distal tubular effect. Direct micropuncture experiments have fully confirmed this notion (Duarte *et al.*, 1969). Even in the presence of only mild natriuresis, amiloride completely suppresses distal secretion of potassium at a time when the transepithelial electrical potential difference across this nephron segment is significantly reduced (Duarte *et al.*, 1969).

IX. Mechanism of Tubular Potassium Transport

A. Potassium Reabsorption

The operation of a reabsorptive mechanism acting on potassium ions along the renal tubule is well documented. Potassium/inulin clearance ratios in the great majority of observations are less than unity, but even the concentration of potassium ions in the final urine may be less than that in plasma (Black and Milne, 1952; Fourman, 1952; Blahd and Bassett, 1953; Lowe, 1953). In addition, micropuncture studies on mammalian nephrons indicate that the proximal convolution, the loop of Henle, the distal tubule, and the collecting duct all possess the intrinsic capacity of net transfer of potassium from lumen to peritubular fluid. Active transport is usually defined as net movement of an ion species against an electrochemical potential gradient (Ussing, 1960). Accordingly, for an assessment of whether active transport is present or not, knowledge of the direction and magnitude of the electrical potential difference across well-defined nephron segments is necessary. While there is general agreement that the distal tubular lumen of the rat is significantly electronegative with respect to the peritubular fluid (Giebisch and Windhager, 1964), there is some controversy as to whether the same is true with respect to the proximal tubule. While several investigators had previously reported the lumen of the proximal tubule of the rat to be electrically negative by some 20 mV (Giebisch and Windhager, 1965), Frömter and Hegel have more recently cast serious doubt on the existence of a significant transtubular potential difference across proximal tubules of rat kidney (Frömter and Hegel, 1966). Although the conclusion of these authors that no significant electrical potential difference exists is accepted by the majority of investigators, the most recent experimental work by Grantham, Burg, and Orloff (1970), by Seely and Boulpaep (1970), and by de Mello and Malnic (unpublished observations) has made a reevaluation of the whole problem desirable. These authors observed a small but significant potential difference (lumen −2 to −4 mV negative with respect to the peritubular fluid). Burg *et al.* (1970) observed, even in completely isolated and perfused proximal tubules of the rabbit, a small but significant potential difference. Recordings were made by the use of axial recording electrodes, a method devoid of some of the potential shortcomings associated with tubular microelectrode penetrations.

A consideration of the electrochemical potential gradient of potassium ions across the proximal tubular epithelium has led many investigators to conclude that an active transport step is involved in some or all of the reabsorptive movement of potassium. This conclusion is based on the observation that in several experimental conditions the transtubular concentration ratio of potassium may fall below unity (Bloomer *et al.*, 1963; Marsh *et al.*, 1963; Malnic *et al.*, 1964; Rector *et al.*, 1964b; Malnic *et al.*, 1966b). Similarly, microperfusion of single proximal tubules with isotonic raffinose regularly yields small but significant concentration gradients of potassium ions (Marsh *et al.*, 1963; Malnic *et al.*, 1966a; Wiederholt, 1968). These observations alone would suggest that some active potassium reabsorption takes place along the proximal convoluted tubule. Obviously, this conclusion would be reinforced if, indeed, a significant electrical difference (lumen negative) could be shown to exist across the mammalian proximal tubule. It should be noted that on the basis of free-flow micropuncture studies in which no significant proximal transtubular concentration gradient of potassium ions was found, and accepting Frömter and Hegel's observation of zero electrical potential difference, Bennet *et al.* have concluded that potassium reabsorption in the proximal convoluted tubule is passive (Bennett *et al.*, 1968). This conclusion may need some reevaluation in the light of the recent findings of Burg *et al.* and others that a small but significant transepithelial potential difference (lumen negative) exists across mammalian proximal tubules.

Some observations on proximal tubular potassium transport indicate that, in general, the absolute rate of reabsorption is related to the rate of proximal tubular fluid transport and, thus, to the rate at which sodium ions are pumped from lumen to peritubular fluid space (Giebisch and Windhager, 1964). The nature of this interrelation is unresolved at present but it would appear that some of the mechanisms for maintaining glomerulotubular balance involve also the proximal tubular reabsorption of potassium ions. Thus, the acute reduction of glomerular filtration rate does not significantly change the concentration of potassium ions in proximal tubular fluid at a time when the absolute rate of fluid reabsorption is drastically reduced (Watson, 1966). This indicates that the absolute rate of reabsorptive net transfer has decreased to a similar extent. Thus, even in the presence of some evidence in favor of active proximal potassium reabsorption, some coupling to sodium or fluid movement appears to be operative and to participate in the overall regulation of proximal potassium transport. Since, in principle, coupling or interaction between transepithelial solute movement has been demonstrated (Ussing, 1966; Biber and Curran, 1968), and since, furthermore, many different transport processes occur at the proximal tubular level, the interrelationship between net potassium movement and that of other ion species deserves close scrutiny. It is of some interest, within this context, that in the dog nephron, the reduction of fractional tubular sodium transport in the proximal tubule subsequent to extracellular fluid volume expansion does not materially change fractional potassium transport (Watson, 1966). Also, increased hydrogen ion secretion in potassium-depleted rats, as evidenced by an enhanced capacity of the proximal convoluted tubule to reabsorb bicarbonate ions, does not materially change the fractional rate of proximal tubular potassium reabsorption (Rector *et al.*, 1962; Malnic *et al.*, 1964). Similarly, proximal tubular potassium transfer is also rather insensitive to carbonic anhydrase inhibition (Malnic *et al.*, 1964; Watson, 1966). These observations clearly indicate that the proximal transport pattern of potassium ions has some independence from both the sodium and the hydrogen ion transfer systems.

Concerning the possible site of an active potassium transport mechanism in proximal tubule cells, it is most reasonable to assume the luminal cell membrane to be the site of an active potassium pump (Blommer *et al.*, 1963; Marsh *et al.*, 1963; Giebisch and Windhager, 1964; Malnic *et al.*, 1964; Malnic *et al.*, 1966a; Giebisch *et al.*, 1967). If either a small transtubular electrical potential difference or a small potassium concentration gradient is present ($P_{tub} < P_{pl}$) the concentration gradient of potassium ions across the luminal cell membrane exceeds that to be expected from the electrical potential difference. It can be calculated that an exclusively passive distribution of potassium ions across the luminal cell boundary without the presence of an active reabsorptive potassium pump would result in intratubular potassium concentrations in excess of those commonly observed.

Clear-cut evidence is available that distal tubular potassium reabsorption is an active process. This is based on the observation that free-flow and steady-state concentration gradients of less than unity have been observed at a time when a significant electrical potential difference (lumen negative) exists (Giebisch and Windhager, 1964; Malnic *et al.*, 1964; Malnic *et al.*, 1966a; Malnic *et al.*, 1966b; Giebisch *et al.*, 1967). Also, direct evidence is available that net reabsorption occurs against a significant electrical potential difference. It will be pointed out subsequently that the overall transepithelial potential difference across single distal tubule cells is the consequence of two finite potential steps, a larger one (some 70–90 mV) across the peritubular cell boundary (cell negative with respect to peritubular fluid) and a smaller one (20–40 mV) across the luminal cell membrane (cell negative with respect to lumen). Were it not for an active reabsorptive mechanism for potassium ions at the luminal cell membrane, the smaller electrical potential difference across this boundary would be insufficient to prevent leakage of potassium ions into the tubular lumen, and a rise in distal tubular potassium concentration above that experimentally observed.

B. Potassium Secretion

The problem of the nature of net secretory potassium transfer and the factors modifying this process at the distal tubular level have recently been investigated in some detail. One line of approach has been to compare the electrical driving force acting on potassium ions with the free-flow concentration differences actually achieved across this nephron segment (Malnic et al., 1964; Malnic et al., 1966a; Malnic et al., 1966b; Giebisch et al., 1967). Utilizing the Nernst equation, and comparing the experimentally observed concentration differences with those theoretically possible by passive transtubular distribution according to the electrical driving force, allows one to decide whether active transport participates in potassium secretion. Under a wide variety of experimental conditions, including those in which maximal distal tubular potassium concentrations were achieved, it was consistently observed that the concentration ratios were considerably lower than would be expected if potassium ions were to distribute passively according to the electrical driving force. Accordingly, potassium movement under free-flow conditions always proceeds down an electrochemical potential gradient. From such studies it may be concluded that under all conditions tested no evidence for active potassium secretion was obtained and that the electrical driving force, i.e., the distal transepithelial potential difference (lumen negative) could be adequate to account for the observed magnitude of distal transtubular potassium concentration differences. Figure 10 summarizes pertinent data.

A second line of approach is aimed toward throwing some light upon the cause of the apparent disequilibrium of potassium ions across the distal tubular epithelium ($K_{tub} < K_{expect}$). Under conditions in which net fluid movement was almost completely abolished (Malnic et al., 1966a), distal transepithelial potassium concentration gradients have been compared with the electrical potential difference. Figure 11 schematically depicts the method and some results. Essentially, a small luminal segment is filled with a nonreabsorbable nonelectrolyte solution (Gertz, 1962). Ions move into the lumen until a limiting concentration difference is reached. At that point active movement and passive leak balance each other such that a state of zero net flux of fluid and solute is

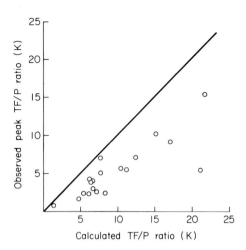

Fɪɢ. 10.   Summary of transtubular concentration ratios, calculated by the Nernst equation for the distal tubule, compared to the observed maximal tubular fluid/plasma concentration ratios. Data from free-flow and stationary microperfusion experiments. From
Giebisch *et al.* (1967) and from Malnic *et al.* (unpublished observations).

achieved. As discussed in some detail (Kashgarian *et al.*, 1963; Marsh *et al.*, 1963; Malnic *et al.*, 1966a), the imposed reduction of net fluid movement reduces solute flux asymmetry and minimizes solvent drag effects. The fact that steady-state conditions obtain after a finite time period also minimizes the role of variations in tubular volume flow rate upon the development of potassium concentration gradients. Accordingly, a comparison of concentration gradients with the electrical potential difference is much simplified under these conditions. Figure 11 summarizes the experimental approach and gives some results.

    Three aspects of the results obtained by such stationary microperfusion experiments are of significance. First, a comparison of steady-state concentrations achieved across early and late distal tubular segments indicates that it is the late distal tubule which varies the magnitude of potassium concentration gradients. Second, the magnitude of this late distal concentration gradient is always below that expected from passive distribution according to the electrical potential difference measured under these conditions (Malnic *et al.*, 1966a). Finally, by microperfusion methods one can also study the effects of changes in the electrical driving force upon the transtubular distribution of potassium ions across the distal tubular epithelium. Such information can be obtained by changing the transepithelial potential difference by the deposition, into a distal tubule, of different solutions known to alter the electrical potential difference, and observing the effects upon the tubular potassium concentration (Malnic *et al.*, 1966a). Such experiments have clearly shown that the transepithelial potential difference is a powerful factor in determining the magnitude of the distal potassium concentration gradient. Reduction of intratubular electrical negativity reduced intratubular potassium concentrations. On the other hand, an augmentation of the transepithelial driving force, by a variety of maneuvers, making the tubular lumen more negative with respect to the peritubular fluid, increases intratubular potassium concentration. A consistent observation in such perfusion studies was the finding that, again, the achieved concentrations of potassium were considerably less than those expected from a purely passive distribution according to the electrical potential difference. This fact is of considerable importance because it clearly indicates that factors other than the electrical driving

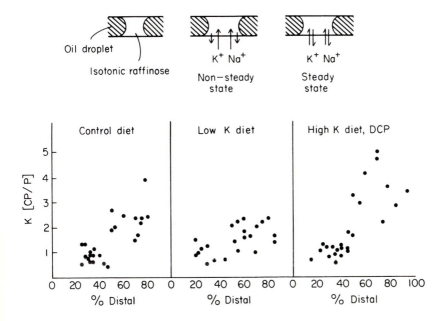

FIG. 11. Schematic presentation of stationary microperfusion method using a poorly permeant nonelectrolyte solution as perfusion fluid (top) and summary of distal transtubular potassium steady-state concentration ratios during isotonic raffinose perfusion. From Giebisch *et al.* (1967).

force are able to modify the extent to which potassium ions accumulate within the distal tubular lumen.

Figure 12 shows the model of a single distal tubule cell which incorporates those functional elements thought to be of primary importance in distal tubular potassium transport (Giebisch *et al.*, 1967). It includes the following features: (1) A high intracellular potassium concentration is maintained by a peritubular ion pump, effecting sodium extrusion and potassium accumulation. It should be noted that direct evidence for either active potassium uptake across the peritubular cell boundary or for tight coupling between transmembrane movement of sodium and potassium at the distal tubular cell level is presently lacking. (2) Electrical asymmetry is maintained such that the potential difference across the peritubular cell membrane significantly exceeds that across the luminal cell border. This inequality of electrical potential differences results in the overall transepithelial potential difference and renders the lumen electronegative with respect to the peritubular fluid pool. Accordingly, an inwardly directed driving force for potassium ions exists such as to effect net transfer into the lumen. Magnitude and direction of potassium transfer across the luminal cell border would be controlled by two important parameters: (1) the electrochemical potential gradient across the luminal cell boundary determining the magnitude of passive diffusion from cell into lumen, and (2) the strength of a reabsorptive pumping mechanism located also at the luminal cell membrane and effecting the active movement from tubular lumen into the distal tubule cell.

Since this cell model differs in important aspects from the frequently cited distal potassium–hydrogen–sodium exchange model, the supporting evidence should be considered. It rests on a consideration of

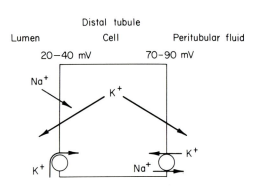

FIG. 12.   Schematic presentation of some properties of distal tubule cells. From Giebisch *et al.* (1967).

the respective electrochemical potential differences across individual cell membranes and the demonstrated absence of direct stoichiometric relationships between distal tubular potassium and sodium transport on the one hand, and between potassium and bicarbonate (hydrogen) ion transport on the other.

A comparison of the magnitude of the electrical driving force with the observed transepithelial concentration gradient under all tested conditions, both free-flow and steady-state, indicates that it is unnecessary to invoke active potassium secretion at the distal tubular level. Calculations indicate that the electrical potential difference is an adequate driving force to account for the magnitude of transepithelial concentration differences achieved (Fig. 10). Accordingly, it is not necessary to postulate an active secretory potassium pump. Also, direct estimates of the transtubular potassium conductance (i.e., the current flowing from lumen to peritubular fluid for a given electrical driving force when potassium is the main current-carrying ion species) are possible. Such measurements indicate that the distal tubular potassium conductance is of such magnitude as to permit passive influx of potassium into the electronegative lumen at a rate comparable to that actually observed (Giebisch and Malnic, 1969). However, active secretion is not excluded by such experiments (see below with respect to peritubular potassium transport).

From a number of considerations it also appears certain that electrochemical equilibrium for potassium ions across the distal tubular epithelium is prevented by active reabsorptive transport out of the lumen (Malnic et al., 1966a). Operation of a mechanism opposing the passive inward movement of potassium along the electrochemical potential gradient results in observed free-flow and steady-state intraluminal concentrations of potassium below those expected from electrochemical equilibrium. Active reabsorptive net movement of potassium can occur, under certain conditions, across the distal tubular epithelium in mammalian kidneys and is normally taking place in distal tubules of amphibian kidneys. In the mammal, under the majority of experimental conditions, reabsorptive flux across the luminal cell membrane is masked by more extensive and passive movement of potassium from cell into lumen. A shift in the balance between luminally directed passive potassium leak and the strength of the reabsorptive pump activity is the key mechanism by which potassium transport is regulated at the distal tubular level. Morel has also concluded, on the basis of stop-flow analyses, that active potassium reabsorption must be present at the distal tubular level and that movement of potassium into the lumen may be passive (Morel and Guinnebault, 1956).

Three factors are of particular importance in determining the electrochemical potential difference effecting inwardly directed potassium movement, and thus, setting the driving force for passive potassium movement into the lumen: (1) the electrical potential difference, (2) the intracellular potassium concentration, and (3) the potassium conductance of the luminal cell membrane. There follows a discussion of these factors in some detail.

The electrical properties of distal tubules have been studied extensively in both mammalian and amphibian kidneys (Kashgarian *et al.*, 1963; Giebisch *et al.*, 1966; Giebisch, 1968; Sullivan, 1968). Since it is not only possible to measure transepithelial potential differences but also to impale single distal tubule cells and record stable transmembrane potential differences, a fairly accurate assessment of the behavior of both the peritubular and the luminal cell membranes is possible. A comparison of the relative ionic conductances of the peritubular and luminal cell membrane has indicated important differences, thus furthering an understanding of the genesis of the distal transepithelial potential difference. Based on the effectiveness of specific ionic substitutions in altering the electrical potential difference across the two cell membranes, some inferences may be made with respect to the contribution of a given ion species to the overall ionic conductance.

The results of such experiments have shown that the peritubular cell membrane of single distal tubule cells both in the rat and in *Amphiuma*, an aquatic amphibian, is highly potassium-selective (Giebisch *et al.*, 1966; Sullivan, 1968), and thus, similar to many other excitable and nonexcitable cells. In sharp contrast the luminal cell membrane is less selective with respect to its ionic conductance properties. A number of ions, most notably potassium *and* sodium, contribute to the ionic currents, and thus, to the diffusion potential across this cell membrane (Giebisch *et al.*, 1966; Sullivan, 1968; Malnic and Giebisch, unpublished). Given finite conductances to both potassium and sodium (and, to a much lesser degree, also to chloride), it would be expected that replacement of both cationic species by a less permeant cation (such as choline) would increase the potential difference across the luminal cell membrane and, accordingly, reduce the overall transepithelial potential difference by reducing the extent of asymmetrical cell polarization. This is a consequence of the direction of the concentration differences between cell interior (high K, low Na) and the tubular lumen (low K, variably low Na). Another factor of importance in the reduction of the electrical potential difference across the luminal cell boundary and, hence, in the generation of the overall transepithelial potential difference, is the low chloride conductance of the distal tubular epithelium

(Malnic and Giebisch, unpublished). It limits the chloride current and thus, reduces polarization of the luminal cell boundary. The combination of the described conductance properties, i.e., a relatively high potassium and sodium conductance and a low chloride conductance, tends to make the tubular lumen continuous with the cell interior (-70 to -90 mV). This is of obvious importance for potassium movement into the lumen: it effectively reduces the electrical force which opposes loss of potassium from the cell interior into the tubular lumen. It is obvious from these considerations that the relative depolarization of the luminal cell membrane is of great functional importance. It is responsible for unequal electrical cell polarization, for the generation of the transepithelial potential difference and, hence, for one of the main driving forces of potassium movement into the tubular lumen.

A number of factors modifying urinary potassium secretion may operate by initiating an alteration in distal transepithelial potential difference. Such an effect of the electrical driving force upon transtubular potassium distribution has been suggested. It would explain the observation that potassium is excreted at a higher rate when multivalent anions such as sulfate or ferrocyanide replace chloride ions (Sullivan *et al.*, 1960; Berliner, 1961; Morel, 1961; Sullivan, 1961; Clapp *et al.*, 1962; Malnic *et al.*, 1964; Malnic *et al.*, 1966a) or when poorly reabsorbable univalent anions such as phosphate constitute a larger than normal fraction of the urinary anion load (Lemieux et al., 1964). Distal tubular potential differences are augmented in this situation. Amiloride reduces the distal tubular potential difference (Duarte *et al.*, 1969). It appears from transepithelial conductance studies that acute changes in luminal pH do not affect transepithelial distal potassium conductance (Giebisch and Malnic, 1969; Malnic and Giebisch, unpublished).

It has been pointed out that the normal transepithelial potential difference across the distal tubules is significantly affected by the concentration of sodium ions within the distal tubular lumen. The fact that the magnitude of the electrical potential difference is sensitive to luminal sodium concentration may be of importance in the coupling between sodium reabsorption and potassium secretion in the final urine. If the electrical potential difference across the collecting ducts, as across the distal tubular epithelium, is dependent upon the concentration of sodium ions, diminished intratubular negativity and reabsorptive loss from the collecting ducts might be expected whenever the sodium concentration and electrical negativity are reduced. Potassium reabsorption is most extensive along the collecting duct under these very conditions when sodium reabsorption is almost complete. Some coupling effects between sodium concentration and potassium secretion along both distal tubules and collecting ducts may thus be mediated electrically.*

The effective intracellular potassium concentration is probably another major determinant of distal tubular secretory rate of potassium ions. A number of factors that modify potassium transport may do so by changing the effective intracellular potassium concentration. Cell potassium concentration may be altered osmotically by changes in body hydration (Mudge et al., 1950; Berliner, 1961). Alterations may also be caused by changes in the potassium uptake across the peritubular cell boundary. This may, in part, be an active process. If a fraction of this potassium uptake were active, changes in the transport rate at this site would affect intracellular potassium concentration and thus, indirectly, also the electrochemical potential gradient acting on potassium movement across the luminal cell membrane. Suppression of cellular potassium uptake may be the mechanism by which cardiac glycosides (Orloff and Burg, 1960), mercurial diuretics (Bowman and Landon, 1967), and lack of adrenal mineralocorticoids (Woodbury and Koch, 1957; Kruhoffer, 1960; Hierholzer and Ebel, 1968) all reduce distal tubular potassium secretion. It is also likely that alterations in the acid–base status affect intracellular potassium concentration. The kaliuretic effect of alkalinizing extracellular body fluids is likely to be mediated, at least partially, by an increase in intracellular potassium ions of distal tubule cells, similar to extrarenal effects of such acid–base disturbances (Giebisch et al., 1955b; Swan et al., 1955). On the other hand, the suppression of distal tubular potassium secretion observed both during acute respiratory or metabolic acidosis may be mediated by a reduction in cellular potassium content subsequent to intracellular acidosis (Giebisch et al., 1955; Swan et al., 1955; Cohen et al.,

---

*Recent studies by Grantham et al., (1970) in perfused, isolated collecting ducts of rabbits have shown that at very low perfusion rates intratubular potassium concentrations may be higher than those expected from passive distribution. Under these conditions it is possible that sodium ions become limiting for potassium secretion. The functional importance, in particular, the quantitative role of this process, is presently not clear. In rodents (Malnic et al., 1964; Malnic et al., 1966b), the dog (Bennett et al., 1967), and the monkey (Bennett et al., 1968) the collecting ducts play only a minor role in potassium secretion. Sodium depletion in the rat, although effective in rendering final urine almost sodium-free, does not limit the ability of the kidney to secrete potassium ions copiously when challenged by an exogenous potassium load (Anderson and Laragh, 1958; Malnic et al., 1966b). However, it is possible that in herbivorous animals like the rabbit, adaptation to high potassium intake includes active secretory movement across the collecting duct epithelium. A comparison of late distal with final urinary potassium excretion rates in rats kept on a high potassium intake for several months has not shown significant net addition of potassium at tubular sites beyond the distal tubule (Wright et al., 1969).

1967; Struyvenberg *et al.*, 1968). Finally, it is most reasonable to expect that the development of potassium tolerance in the distal tubule of potassium-adapted animals is also related to an increase in the intracellular potassium pool, thereby effectively augmenting the driving force for potassium accumulation in the distal tubule.

The problem of the role of intracellular potassium in distal tubule cells with respect to the functional state of the potassium transport system has recently been investigated in *Amphiuma* by Wiederholt *et al.* (Wiederholt et al., unpublished). As pointed out before, extensive distal tubular net reabsorption occurs normally in this amphibian kidney, but may be replaced by strong secretion when the animal is exposed to a high potassium intake or after the administration of a carboanhydrase inhibitor (Wiederholt *et al.*, 1969). It has recently become possible to assess individual unidirectional flux components and the transport pool of potassium ions under these different conditions. One of the most significant findings was the observation that coincident with the reversal of net transport from reabsorption to secretion there occurred a very dramatic increase in the intracellular transport pool of potassium, i.e., in that fraction of cell potassium which exchanges readily with the transported tracer. This increase was due to enhanced peritubular active uptake of potassium ions into distal tubule cells. This underscores the importance of a critical fraction of intracellular potassium in regulating the rate of potassium secretion. Evidence from studies on mammalian kidney cortex slices also indicates that cell potassium may be distributed between more than one compartment. The distribution of potassium between various compartments is affected by several factors, such as changes of pH in the medium as well as *in vivo*, and suggests that such potassium compartmentation may be of physiological significance (Foulkes, 1962).

It is also likely that the mechanism underlying the increase in potassium concentration along the distal tubule which is observed in a wide variety of experimental conditions could be, in part, related to a gradual increase in the magnitude of the intracellular potassium pool and thus, presumably, to an increase of intracellular potassium concentration along the distal tubule (Giebisch and Windhager, 1964). Although this problem has not yet been studied directly by comparing the transport pool size at different points along the distal tubule, it may be inferred from the following considerations. Figure 13 summarizes data obtained in rat kidneys, based on the simultaneous measurements of sodium and potassium concentrations and the extent of fluid reabsorption as a function of tubular length. It is obvious that the rate of sodium reabsorption per unit length of the distal tubule falls as fluid passes along this part of the tubule. The decline in reabsorptive rate

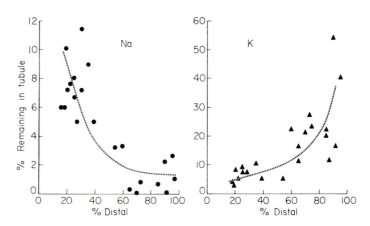

FIG. 13. Fraction of filtered sodium and potassium remaining or appearing in tubular fluid as a function of distal tubular length. Data from Malnic *et al.* (1964); figure from Giebisch and Windhager (1964).

coincides with a fall in tubular sodium concentration and makes it highly likely that commensurate with this fall in intratubular sodium concentration the intracellular transport pool and the concentration of sodium within distal tubule cells may also decline. This decrease in sodium concentration suggests a rise in intracellular potassium concentration if isoosmotic conditions are to be maintained. Such an increase in the intracellular transport pool, and presumably of the potassium concentration in a critical cell compartment could then be the cause of the enhanced secretion rate of potassium along the second half of the distal tubular epithelium.

Another factor which undoubtedly contributes to the observed increase in intratubular potassium concentration is the increase in the transepithelial potential difference along the distal tubule. A careful reinvestigation utilizing improved methods of electrode localization has indicated that, contrary to previous findings, the potential difference increases along the distal tubule (Wright, 1970). Although the mechanism underlying this change in transepithelial potential difference is not clear, the observed potential profile along the distal tubule would aid sodium reabsorption along the early part of the distal tubule and potassium secretion along the terminal part of this nephron segment.

At present it is difficult to assess the role of changes in the potassium permeability of the luminal cell boundary and of the role of changes in the strength of the reabsorptive potassium pump in modifying potassium transport across the distal tubule. Conceivably, both could modify distal potassium transport. With the exception of studies using ouabain which, under appropriate conditions, blocks reabsorptive potassium transport little is known of how these transport parameters change as a function of distal tubular length and what role they play in the many situations in which the rate of potassium transport is altered.

Recent evidence has demonstrated unequivocally that distal tubular volume flow rate is an essential factor which deserves consideration in any analysis of the factors regulating distal tubular potassium transport. Figure 14 shows the relationship to be expected between transepithelial concentration gradients, excretion rate, and tubular and urine flow rate in diffusion and flow-limited systems. When the concentration profile along the distal tubule is compared over a wide range of flow rates of tubular fluid, it appears that the distal potassium transport system is flow-limited (Khuri et al., unpublished). This is demonstrated by the important observation that similar concentration gradients are maintained across the distal tubular epithelium at increasingly higher flow rates. This situation obtains in various types of graded diureses such as those brought on by urea or saline infusions, or after furosemide administration. The excretion rate of potassium varies directly

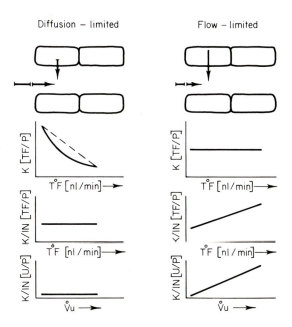

Fig. 14. Schematic presentation of expected behavior of distal transepithelial potassium concentration ratios and of fractional distal tubular and urinary potassium excretion in a diffusion-limited and flow-limited system. From Khuri et al. (unpublished).

with urine flow rate, and its relationship to distal tubular sodium reabsorption has yet to be assessed. A recent microperfusion study of single distal tubules in which flow rate was varied over a wide range also supports the view that the kinetics of inwardly directed diffusion of potassium ions into the distal tubular lumen is such that flow rate is the limiting factor in determining the rate of excretion (Morgan and Berliner, 1969). A notable exception is found in the state of potassium depletion and in other conditions such as water diuresis in which potassium excretion is initially low (Kruhoffer, 1960; Rector, personal communication). If distal tubular flow rate is gradually increased in rats having a minimal potassium excretion rate subsequent to dietary potassium deprivation, transtubular concentration gradients of potassium fall progressively and both distal tubular and urinary excretion rate remain constant. Apparently, under conditions of maximal tubular potassium conservation the kinetics of the potassium transport system are those of a diffusion-limited system in which, independent of flow rate, a fixed amount of potassium is entering the distal tubule per unit time (Khuri *et al.*, unpublished). It is presently not clear which functional parameters are responsible for the transformation from flow-limited into diffusion-limited transport system. However, it is clear that changes in distal tubular and urine flow rate per se are one of the important factors deserving close scrutiny in the analysis of those variables determining urinary excretion rate of potassium.

ACKNOWLEDGMENTS

I wish to express my gratitude to Dr. R. W. Berliner and to Dr. F. Wright for constructive comments and to Mrs. M. B. MacLeod for most valuable editorial assistance.

REFERENCES

Alexander, E. A., and Levinsky, N. G. (1968). *J. Clin. Invest.* **47**, 4.
Anderson, Helen M., and Laragh, John H. (1958). *J. Clin. Invest.* **37**, 323–331.
August, J. T., and Nelson, D. H. (1964). *J. Clin. Invest.* **38**, 30.
Aukland, K., and Kiil. (1961). *Scand. J. Clin. Lab. Invest.* **13**, 87–99.
Baba, W. I., Tudhope, G. R., and Wilson, G. H. (1964). *Clin. Sci.* **27**, 181–193.
Baer, J. E., Jones, C. B., Spitzer, A. S., and Russo, H. F. (1967). *J. Pharmacol. Exptl. Theor.* **157**, 472–485.
Bank, N., and Aynedjian, H. S. (1967). *J. Clin. Invest.* **46**, 95–102.
Bank, N., and Schwartz, W. B. (1960). *J. Clin. Invest.* **39**, 1516–1525.
Barger, A. C., Berlin, R. D., and Tulenko, J. F. (1958). *Endocrinology* **62**, 804.
Barker, E. S., Singer, R. B., Elkinton, J. R., and Clark, J. K. (1957). *J. Clin. Invest.* **36**, 515–529.
Bennett, C. M., Brenner, B. M., and Berliner, R. W. (1968). *J. Clin. Invest.* **47**, 1.
Bennett, C. M., Clapp, J. R., and Berliner, R. W. (1967). *Am. J. Physiol.* **213**, 1254–1264.
Berliner, R. W. (1952). *Federation Proc.* 11, 3.

Berliner, R. W. (1961). *Harvey lectures* **55**, 141-171.
Berliner, R. W., Kennedy, T. J., and Hilton, J. G. (1950). *Am. J. Physiol.* **162**, 348-367.
Berliner, R. W., Kennedy, T. J., and Orloff, J. (1951). *Am. J. Med.* **11**, 274-282.
Berliner, R. W., Kennedy, T. J., and Orloff, J. (1954). *Arch. Int. Pharmacodyn.* **47**,3-4.
Biber, T. U. L., and Curran, P. F. (1968). *J. Gen. Physiol.* **51**, 606-619.
Black, D. A. K., Davies, H. E. F., and Emery, E. W. (1956). *Clin. Sci.* **15**, 277-283.
Black, D. A. K., and Emery, E. W., (1957). *Brit. Med. Bull.* **13**, 7-10.
Black, D. A. K., and Milne, M. D. (1952). *Clin. Sci.* **11**, 397-415.
Blahd, W. H., and Bassett, S. H. (1953). *Metabolism* **2**, 218-224.
Bloomer, H. A., Rector, F. C., and Seldin, D. W. (1963). *J. Clin. Invest.* **42**, 277-285.
Bott, A. Phyllis. (1962). *Am. J. Physiol.* **203**, 662-666.
Bowman, F. J., and Landon, E. J. (1967). *Am. J. Physiol.* **213**, 1209-1217.
Brown, E. B., and Goott, G. (1963). *Am. J. Physiol.* **204**, 765-770.
Bull, M. B., and Laragh, J. H. (1968). *Circulation* **37**, 45-53.
Burnett, C. H., Burrows, B. A., Commons, R. R., and Towery, B. T. (1950). *J. Clin. Invest.* **29**, 175-186.
Cade, J. R., Shalhoub, R. J., Canessa-Fischer, M., and Pitts, R. F. (1961). *Am. J. Physiol.* **200**, 373-379.
Clapp, J. R., Rector, F. C., and Seldin, D. W. (1962). *Am. J. Physiol.* **202**, 781-786.
Cohen, R. D., Simpson, B. R., Goodwin, F. J., and Strumin, L. (1967). *Clin. Sci.* **33**, 233-247.
Cortney, M. A., (1969). *Am. J. Physiol.* **216**, 589-598.
Davidson, D. G., Levinsky, and Berliner, R. W. (1958). *J. Clin. Invest.* **37**, 548-555.
Denton, D. A., Maxwell, M., McDonald, I. R., Munro, J., and Williams, W. (1952). *Australian J. Exp. Biol. Med. Sci.* **30**, 489-510.
Dickerman, H. W., and Walker, W. Gordon. (1964). *Am. J. Physiol.* **206**, 403-408.
Diezi, J., Michaud, P., Aceves, G., and Giebisch, G. (1969). *Fed. Proc.* **29**, 271.
Dirks, J. H., and Seely, J. F. (1969). *Annual Rev. Pharmacol.* **9**, 73-101.
Dorman, P. J., Sullivan, W. Jr., and Pitts, R. F. (1954). *J. Clin. Invest.* **33**, 82-89.
Duarte, C., Chomety, F., and Giebisch, G. (1969). *Clin. Res.* 17, 428.
Earley, L. E., and Orloff, J. (1964). *Annual Rev. Med.* **15**, 149-166.
Evans, B. M., Hughes Jones, N. C., Milne, M. D., and Steiner, S. (1954). *Clin. Sci.* **13**, 305-316.
Foulkes, E. C. (1962). *Am J. Physiol.* 203, 655-661.
Fourman, P. (1952). *Lancet* **262**, 1042-1044.
Franglen, G. T., McGarry, E., and Spencer, A. G. (1963). *J. Physiology* **121**, 35-45.
Fimognari, G. M., Fanestil, D. D., and Edelman, I. S. (1967). *Am. J. Physiol.* **213**, 954.
Frömter, E., and Hegel, U. (1966). *Arch. Ges. Physiol.* 291, 107-120.
Fuller, G. R., Macleod, M. D., and Pitts, R. F. (1955). *Am. J. Physiol.* **182**, 111-118.
Gertz, K. G. (1962). *Proc. 32 Intern. Congr. Physiol. Sci. Leiden* 370-371.
Giebisch, G. (1968). *J. Gen. Physiol* **51**, 315s-325s.
Giebisch, G. (1969) *Nephron.* **6**, 260-281.
Giebisch, G., Berger, L., and Pitts, R. F. (1955a). *J. Clin. Invest.* **34**, 231.
Giebisch, G. Macleod, M. B., and Pitts, R. F. (1955b). *Am. J. Physiol.* **183**, 377-386.
Giebisch, G., Klose, R. M., and Malnic, G. (1967). *Bull. of the Swiss Academy of Med. Sciences* **23**, 287-312.
Giebisch, G., and Malnic, G. (1969). *In* "Symposium of Renal Transport and Metabolism." Springer, Berlin, Vienna, New York, 123-138.
Giebisch, G., and Malnic, G., 1970. *Proc. IV. Internat. Congr. Nephrol. Stockholm*, Vol. 1, 181-194.
Giebisch, G., Malnic, G., Klose, R. M., and Windhager, E. E. (1966). *Am. J. Physiol.* **211**, 560-568.

Giebisch, G., and Windhager, Erich. (1964). *Am. J. Med.* **36**, 643-660.

Giebisch, G., Windhager, E. E., and Malnic, G. (1965). *Proc. 23 Intern. Congr. Physiol. Sci.,* Tokyo, 167-175.

Glabman, S., Klose, R. M., and Giebisch, G. (1963). *Am. J. Physiol.* **205**, 127-132.

Goldman, A. G., Yalow, A. A., and Grossman, J. (1963). *Clin. Sci.* **24**, 287-299.

Grantham, J. J., Burg, M., and Orloff, J. (1970). *J. Clin. Invest.* **49**, 1815-1826.

Hayes, C. P., Jr., Mayson, J. S., Owen, E. E., and Robinson, R. R. (1964). *Am. J. Physiol.* **207**, 77-83.

Hierholzer, K. (1961). *Am. J. Physiol.* **201**, 318-324.

Hierholzer, K., and Ebel, H. (1968). *Proceedings, VI. Symposium der Gesellschaft für Nephrologie, Wien*, 223-241.

Hierholzer, K., Wiederholt, H., Holzgrene, H., Giebisch, G., Klose, R. M., and Windhager, E. E. (1965). *Pflugers Arch. Ges. Physiol* **285**, 193-210.

Hilger, H. H., Klumper, J. D., and Ullrich, K. J. (1958). *Pflugers Arch. Ges. Physiol.* **267**, 213-237.

Horster, M., and Thurau, K. (1968). *Arch. Ges. Physiol.* **301**, 162-181.

Howell, S. David, and Davis, James O. (1954). *Am. J. Physiol.* **179**, 359-363.

Jaenike, J. R., and Berliner, R. W. (1960). *J. Clin. Invest.* **39**, 481-490.

Jamison, R. L., (1968). *Am. J. Physiol.* **215**, 236-242.

Kashgarian, M., Stockle, H., Gottschalk, C. W., and Ullrich, K. J. (1963). *Arch. Ges. Physiol.* **277**, 89-106.

Kennedy, Jr., T. J., Winkler, J. H., and Dunning, M. F. (1949). *Am. J. Med.* **6**, 790-794.

Khuri, R. N., Goldstein, D. A., Maude, D., Edmonds, C., and Solomon, A. K. (1963). *Am. J. Physiol.* **204**, 743-748.

Khuri, R. N., Wiederholt, M., Argulian, S., and Giebisch, G. (unpublished).

Kruhoffer, P. (1950). "Studies on water-electrolyte excretion and glomerular activity in the mammalian kidney." Rosenkilde and Bagger, Copenhagen.

Kruhoffer, P. (1960). "Handbuch der experimentellen Pharmakologie" (O. Eichler and A. Farah, eds.), p. 293. Springer, Berlin, Gottingen, Heidelberg.

Landwehr, D. M., Klose, R. M., and Giebisch, G. (1967). *Am. J. Physiol.* **212**, 1327-1333.

Landwehr, D. M., Klose, R. M., and Giebisch, G. (unpublished).

Landwehr, D. M., Schnermann, J., Klose, R. M., and Giebisch, G. (1968). *Am. J. Physiol.* **215**, 687-695.

Landwehr, D. M., Schnermann, J., Klose, R. M., and Giebisch, G. (unpublished).

Lechene, C., Corby, C., and Morel, F. (1966). *Compt. Rend. Acad. Sci.* **262**, 1126.

Lechene, C., Morel, F., Guinnebault, M., and de Rouffignac, C., 1969. *Nephron* **6**, 457-477.

Lemieux, G., Warren, Y., Gervais, M. (1964). *Am. J. Physiol.* **206**, 743-749.

Liddle, G. W. (1966). *Ann. N. Y. Acad. Sci.* **139**, 466-470.

Litchfield, J. B., and Bott, P. A. (1962). *Am. J. Physiol.* **203**, 667-670.

Loeb, R. F. (1941-1942). *Harvey lectures* **37**, 100-128.

Loeb, R. F., Atchley, D. W., Benedict, E. M., and Leland, J. (1933). *J. Exptl. Med.* **57**, 775-792.

Loeb, R. F., Atchley, D. W., Richards, D. W., Benedict, E. M., and Driscoll, M. E. (1932). *J. Clin. Invest.* **11**, 621-639.

Lowe, K. G. (1953). *Clin. Sci.* **12**, 57-62.

Malnic, G., and Giebisch, G. (unpublished).

Malnic, G., Klose, R. M., and Giebisch, G. (1964). *Am. J. Physiol.* **206**, 674-686.

Malnic, G., Klose, R. M., and Giebisch, G. (1966 a). *Am. J. Physiol.* **211**, 548-559.

Malnic, G., Klose, R. M., and Giebisch, G. (1966 b). *Am. J. Physiol.* **211**, 529-547.

Malnic, G., Mello-Aires, M., and Giebisch, G. (1968). *Federation Proc.* **27**, 695.

Malnic, G., Mello-Aires, M., and Giebisch, G. (in preparation).

Malvin, R. L., Wilde, W. S., and Sullivan, L. P. (1958). *Am. J. Physiol.* **194**, 135–142.

Marsh, D., and Solomon, S. (1965). *Am. J. Physiol.* **208**, 1119–1128.

Marsh, D. J., Ullrich, K. J., and Rumrich, G. (1963). *Pflugers Arch. Ges. Physiol.* **277**, 107–119.

McBride, W. O., Weiner, I. M., and Mudge, G. H. (1958). *Federation Proc.* **17**, 107.

McCance, R. A., and Widdowson, E. M. (1936). *Proc. Roy. Soc. London, Ser. B* **120**, 228–239.

Mills, J. N., and Stanbury, S. W. (1954). *Clin. Sci.* **13**, 1.

Morel, F. (1955). *Helv. Physiol. Pharm. Acta.* **13**, 276–294.

Morel, Fransois. (1961). *In* "Proceedings of the First International Congress on Nephrology", pp. 16–39. S. Karger, Basel, New York.

Morel, F., and Guinnebault, M. (1956). *Helv. Physiol. Acta* **14**, 255–263.

Morel, F., McLean, R., Lechene, C., and Guinnebault, M. (1964). *In* "Proceedings of the Second International Congress on Nephrology", Series 78, pp. 552–554. Excerpta Medica, Amsterdam, New York.

Morgan, T., and Berliner, R. W. (1969). *Am. J. Physiol.* **217**, 992–997.

Morgan, T., Tadokoro, M., Martin D., and Berliner, R. W. (1970). *Am. J. Physiol.* **218**, 992–997.

Mudge, G. H. (1958). *Bull. N. Y. Acad. Med.* **34**, 152–162.

Mudge, G. H., Ames III, A., Foulks, J., and Gilman, A. (1950). *Am. J. Physiol.* **161**, 151–158.

Mudge, G. H., Foulks, J., and Gilman, A. (1950). *Am. J. Physiol.* **161**, 159–166.

Oken, D., and Solomon, A. K. (1963). *Am. J. Physiol.* **204**, 377–380.

Orent-Keiles, E., and McCollum, E. V. (1941). *J. Biol. Chem.* **140**, 337–352.

Orloff, J., and Burg, M. (1960). *Am. J. Physiol.* **199**, 49–54.

Orloff, J., and Davidson, D. G. (1959). *J. Clin. Invest.* **38**, 21–30.

Pitts, R. F., Gurd, R. S., Kessler, R. H., and Hierholzer, K. (1958). *Am. J. Physiol.* **194**, 125–134.

Ramsay, A. G. (1964). *Am. J. Physiol.* **206**, 1355–1360.

Ramsay, A. G., and Sachs, G. (1967). *Proc. Soc. Exptl. Biol. Med.* **126**, 294–298.

Rector, Jr., F. C. (in preparation). *In* "The Kidney" (Rouiller and Muller, eds.), Vol. III. Academic Press, New York.

Rector, Jr., F. C., Bloomer, H. A., and Seldin, D. W. (1964a). *J. Clin. Invest.* **43**, 1976–1982.

Rector, F. C., Bloomer, H. A., and Seldin, D. W. (1964 b). *J. Lab. Clin. Med.* **63**, 100–105.

Rector, Jr., F. C., Buttram, H., and Seldin, D. W. (1962). *J. Clin. Invest.* **41**, 611–617.

Rector, Jr., F. C., Carter, N. W., and Seldin, D. W. (1965). *J. Clin. Invest.* **44**, 278–290.

Relman, A. S., and Schwartz, W. B. (1962). *Yale J. Biol. Med* **24**, 540–558.

Roberts, K. E., Magida, M. G., and Pitts, R. F. (1953). *Am. J. Physiol.* **172**, 47–54.

Rosenfeld, S., Kraus, L., McCullen, A., Low, W., and Morales, J. (1969). *Proc. Soc. Exptl Biol. Med.* **130**, 65–71.

de Rouffignac, C., and Guinnebault, M. (1966). *Nephron* **3**, 175–197.

de Rouffignac, C., Lechene, C., Guinnebault, M., and Morel, F., *Nephron*, in press.

de Rouffignac, C., and Morel, F. (1967). *Arch. Ant. Microscop. Morph. Exp.* **56**, 123.

de Rouffignac, C., and Morel, F. (1969). *J. Clin. Invest.* **48**, 474–486.

Schmermann, J. (1968). *Arch. Ges. Physiol.* **300**, 255–282.

Schwartz, W. B., Jenson, R. L., and Relman, A. S. (1955). *J. Clin. Invest.* **34**, 673–680.

Seely, J. F., and Boulpaep, E. L. (1970). *Fed. Proc., Fed. Am. Soc. Exp. Biol.* **29**, 272.

Seldin, D. W., Welt, L. G., and Cort, J. H. (1956). *Yale J. Biol. Med.* **29**, 229–247.

Stanbury, S. W., and Thomson, A. E. (1952). *Clin. Sci.* **11**, 357–374.

Stolte, H., Wiederholt, M., and Hierholzer, K. (unpublished).

Struyvenberg, A., Morrison, R. B., and Relman, A. S. (1968). *Am. J. Physiol.* **214**, 1155–1162.

Suki, W., Recotr, Jr., F. C., and Seldin, D. W. (1965). *J. Clin. Invest.* **44**, 1458–1469.

Sullivan, L. P. (1961). *Am. J. Physiol.* **201**, 774–780.

Sullivan, L. P., Wilde, W. S., and Malvin, R. L. (1960). *Am. J. Physiol.* **198**, 244–254.

Sullivan, W. J. (1968). *Am. J. Physiol.* **214**, 1096–1103.

Swan, R. C., Axelrod, D. R., Seip, M., and Pitts, R. F. (1955). *J. Clin. Invest.* **34**, 1795–1801.

Swingle, W. W., Maxwell, R., Ben, M., Baker, C., LeBrie, S. J., and Eisler, M. (1954). *Endocrinology* **55**, 813–821.

Thatcher, J. S., and Radike, A. W. (1947). *Am. J. Physiol.* **151**, 138–146.

Toussaint, C., and Vereerstraeten, P. (1962). *Am. J. Physiol.* **204**, 768–772.

Ussing, H. H. (1960). *In* "Handbuch der experimentellen Pharmacologie," p. 49. Springer Verlag, Heidelberg.

Ussing, H. H. (1966). *Ann. N.Y. Acad. Sci.* **137**, 543–555.

Vander, A. J. (1961). *Am. J. Physiol.* **201**, 505–510.

Vander, A. J., Wilde, W. S., and Malvin, R. L. (1961). *J. Theoret. Biol.* **1**, 236–243.

Vieira, F. L., and Malnic, G. (1968). *Am. J. Physiol.* **214**, 710–718.

Vogel, G., and Suchheim, S. (1962). *Pflugers Arch.* **276**, 312–316.

Vogel, G., Kroger, W., Tervooren, U., Kolzer, M., and Rott, G. (1963). *Pflugers Arch.* **277**, 502–512.

Vogel, G., and Tervooren, U. (1964). *Pflugers Arch.* **281**, 356–364.

Vogel, G., and Tervooren, U. (1965). *Pflugers Arch.* **284**, 103–107.

Walker, W. G., Cooke, C. R., Payne, J. N., Baker, C. R. F., and Andrew, D. J. (1961). *Am. J. Physiol.* **200**, 1133–1136.

Watson, J. F. (1966). *J. Clin. Invest.* **45**, 8.

Watson, J. F., Clapp, J. R., and Berliner, R. W. (1964). *J. Clin. Invest.* **43**, 595–605.

Wesson, Jr., L. G. (1965). *In* "Handbuch der Urologie" (Alken, Dix, Weyrauch and Wildbolz, eds.), pp. 1–386. Springer-Verlag, Berlin.

Wesson, Jr., L. G. (1969). "Physiology of the Human Kidney." Grune and Stratton, New York.

Wiederholt, M. (1968). *Abstr. 2nd Ann. Congr. Am. Soc. Nephrology, Washington,* 70.

Wiederholt, M., and Hierholzers, K. (1967). *Abstr. V Symposium d. ges. f. Nephrologie, Lausanne.*

Wiederholt, M., Sullivan, W. J., and Giebisch, G. (1969). *Federation Proc.* **28**, 649.

Wiederholt, M., Sullivan, W. J., Giebisch, G., Solomon, A. K., and Curran, P. F. (unpublished).

Wiederholt, M., and Wiederholt, B. (1968). *Arch. Ges. Physiol.* **302**, 57–78.

Wilde, W. S. (1962). *In* "Potassium in Urineral Metabolism" (C. L. Cowar and F. Bronner, eds.), Vol II, Part B, pp. 73–108. Academic Press, New York.

Williamson, H. E. (1963). *Biochem. Pharmacol.* **12**, 1449.

Windhager, E. E., and Giebisch, G. (1965). *Phsyiol. Rev.* **45**, 214–244.

Winkler, A. W., and Smith, P. K. (1942). *Am. J. Physiol.* **138**, 94–103.

Wirz, H., and Bott, P. A. (1954). *Proc. Soc. Exptl. Biol. Med.* **87**, 405–407.

Wolf, A. V. (1947). *Am. J. Physiol.* **148**, 54–68.

Woodbury, D. M., and Koch, A. (1957). *Proc. Soc. Exptl. Biol. Med.* **94**, 720.

Wright, F., Strieder, N., Baechtold, N., and Giebisch, G. (1969). *Abstr. IV Int. Congr. Nephrol., Stockholm.*

Wright, F. (1970). *Fed. Proc.* **29**, 272.

Author Index

Numbers in *italics* refer to the pages on which the complete references are listed.

A

Abboud, F. M., 40, *70*
Aber, G. M., 298, 311, *319*
Abramson, R. G., 142, 168, 171, *201, 203*
Aceves, G., 340, *379*
Addae, S. K., 300, 301, 315, 316, *319*
Addis, T., 279, *319*
Agmon, J., 158, *199*
Ahlquist, R. P., 40, *58*
Alexander, E., 183, *203*, 332, 359, *378*
Alexander, R. S., 211, 213, 223, *250*, 256, *325*
Alleyne, G. A. O., 308, 311, 312, *319*
Alving, A. S., 20, *69*
Ames, A., III, 331, 361, 374, *381*
Amiel, C., 84, *124*
Anastasakis, S., 171, *188*
Anderson, H. M., 345, 374, *378*
Anderson, J., 110, 118, 120, *123*, 159, *197*
Andersson, B., 175, *186*
Andrew, D. J., 335, 344, *382*
Anfinsen, C. B., 284, 289, *324*
Angielski, S., 284, 287, 289, *326*
Ankeney, J. L., 153, *198*
Anslow, W. P., Jr., 158, *186*
Ansorge, H., 35, *66*
Arasimowicz, C., 273, *326*
Archibald, R. M., 255, 271, 279, *327*
Arcila, H., 137, 138, 139, 166, *186, 196*
Ardill, B. L., 155, *186*
Argulian, S., 377, 378, *380*
Arky, R. A., 157, 185, *204*
Armstrong, G. G., Jr., 174, *197*
Arrizurieta-Muchnik, E. E., 177, *186*
Ashley, M. M., 182, *202*
Asshauer, E., 118, *121*
Åström, A., 41, *58*
Atchley, D. W., 159, *198*, 241, *249*, 332, 353, *380*
Atkins, E. L., 235, 241, *247*

August, J. T., 161, 162, *186*, 351, *378*
Aukland, K., 10, 22, 25, 43, 51, 55, 56, 58, *59*, *63*, 84, 120, *121*, 137, 156, 180, *186, 196*, 330, 335, *378*
Axelrod, D. R., 356, 374, *382*
Ayer, J. L., 211, *250*
Aynedjian, H. S., 5, 19, *63*, 141, 142, *193*, *196*, 272, *319*, 358, *378*

B

Baba, W. I., 169, 171, 172, 173, *186, 197*, 361, 363, *378*
Baechtold, N., 332, 338, 341, 345, 359, 368, 374, *382*
Baer, J. E., 173, *187*, 361, 363, *378*
Bahlmann, J. O., 150, 182, *187*
Baines, A. D., 130, 148, *187*
Baker, C., 351, *382*
Baker, C. R. F., 335, 344, *382*
Balagura, S., 256, 260, 262, 264, 265, 266, 267, 270, 271, 278, 285, 311, 312, 313, *319, 326*
Balagura-Baruch, S., 308, 309, 310, *319*, *327*
Baldamus, C. A., 85, 114, *126*, 155, 159, 161, *204*
Baldwin, D. S., 153, *187*
Baldwin, E., 281, 292, *319, 320*
Balinsky, J. B., 281, 292, *319, 320*
Bálint, P., 4, 22, 35, *59*, 137, 153, *187*
Ball, W. C., Jr., 144, *190*
Banfield, W. G., 46, *65*, 75, *124*
Bank, N., 5, 19, *63*, 141, 142, 164, 171, *187*, *193*, *196*, 230, 235, *247*, 272, *319*, 332, 358, *378*
Banks, R. O., 134, *192*
Barajas, L., 12, *59*
Barber, J. K., 158, *187*
Barclay, A. E., 44, *69*

383

Subject Index

401